The Students' Handbook for Studying Health and Social Care

This book provides students with the essential context, knowledge and practice skills required to succeed in your health and social care degree.

Students doing a health and social care degree make a real difference to people's lives every day in incredible and inspiring ways. Choosing to study health and social care gives you the opportunity to acquire a wide range of essential context, knowledge and practice skills that positively transform both your life and the lives of many others. This book uniquely presents these essential context, knowledge and practice skills in one essential place, to provide students with a comprehensive understanding of the requirements of doing a health and social care degree.

Topics covered in the book include health and social care legislation, demographic change, children's rights, disability, mental health, anatomy and physiology, health and social care regulation, communication skills, teamwork and leadership and reflective practice. It is an indispensable learning resource for health and social care students wishing to succeed in their degree and beyond in a wide range of both health and social care settings, as well as a wide variety of other settings, such as schools, community settings and welfare organisations.

Clive Sealey is a Senior Lecturer in Social Policy and Theory in the School of Health and Wellbeing, University of Worcester, UK. His interests are in social policy-related issues linked to poverty, policy and theory. He obtained his PhD in social policy from the University of Birmingham in 2009. His previous book publications are *Social Policy Simplified* (2015), *Social Policy, Service Users and Carers* (2022), *Applying Social Policy to Criminal Justice Practice* (2023) and *An Introduction to Child and Adolescent Mental Health* (2025).

The Students' Handbook for Studying Health and Social Care

Essential Context, Knowledge and Practice Skills for Doing a Successful Degree

Edited by Clive Sealey

Routledge
Taylor & Francis Group
LONDON AND NEW YORK

Designed cover image: Getty Images

First published 2026
by Routledge
4 Park Square, Milton Park, Abingdon, Oxon OX14 4RN

and by Routledge
605 Third Avenue, New York, NY 10158

Routledge is an imprint of the Taylor & Francis Group, an informa business

British Library Cataloguing-in-Publication Data
A catalogue record for this book is available from the British Library

ISBN: 978-1-032-61929-3 (hbk)
ISBN: 978-1-032-60852-5 (pbk)
ISBN: 978-1-032-61930-9 (ebk)

DOI: 10.4324/9781032619309

Typeset in Sabon
by KnowledgeWorks Global Ltd.

Contents

Figures

Tables

Learning Boxes

Contributors

Each of the following contributors to *The Students' Handbook for Studying Health and Social Care* are affiliated with the School of Health and Wellbeing, University of Worcester, Worcestershire, UK:

Naomi Blaikie
Emily Byrne
Kirsty Fraser
Dawn Goodall
Daniel Howarth
Denisse Levermore
Lisa Mauro-Bracken
Janet Osbaldiston
Lisa Porter
Clair Rees
Rebecca Weston

1 Welcome to your health and social care degree!

Clive Sealey

The aims of this chapter are to:

- **Outline what this book is about**
- **Detail who this book is for**
- **Provide a brief outline of the book's structure chapters**

Introduction

Welcome to your health and social care degree!

This book is to help you in studying for your health and social care degree. The study of health and social care at university covers a wide range of topics, ranging from anatomy and physiology to health conditions to well-being to care to legislation. Indeed, unlike some courses, it is very likely the case that no two health and social care degree courses are the same. By choosing to study health and social care, you have given yourself the opportunity to acquire knowledge and learn skills that positively transform both your life and the lives of many others. There are not many things that are certain to happen in your life, but it is certain that health and social care is something that we have all used in the past and are likely to use in the future.

This chapter outlines the key aims of the book in terms of its focus on providing students with the essential context, knowledge and skills of studying health and social care. It defines and brings together these themes to explain in detail why these are important to doing a successful health and social care degree. It also provides a brief outline of the structure of the book and subsequent chapters.

Why study health and social care?

For many students, studying health and social care is the start of a personal journey of discovery that never ends. It is likely to be the start of an exciting and rewarding part of your life that will very likely lead you onto greater things in the future. Studying health and social care is different from studying many other degrees because of its focus on trying to solve real-life issues that can literally be a matter of life and death. This is a degree where the possibility of changing your life and the lives of others occurs on a daily basis, from the time we are born to the time we die, 'from cradle to grave' (Sealey, 2015). It is also possible to literally see right in front of your eyes the difference that you are making. Having taught many health and social care students over many years, I have seen how the learning from the degree can transform how you think, act, feel and behave in

DOI: 10.4324/9781032619309-1

many positive ways that changes lives. For example, I have seen how learning has led to students making significant changes in how they live their lives. Similarly, I have seen how learning has led to people changing their perspectives on life and how they do things in their life. And I have seen how going out in practice makes people grow as individuals and take on responsibilities that they would not have dreamed of before starting the degree.

What is also often overlooked is the positive effect that studying health and social care can make to other people. We can say that health and social care has transformed our society from what it was in the past, and it is very likely that it continues to do so in the future. For example, if we consider the fact that over the last 50 years or so, people are living much longer than they did, are surviving diseases and conditions that would have killed them, such as cancer, and many more people are participating in society in ways that they would not have been able, these have all occurred due to significant developments in health and social care.

Studying health and social care enables individuals to work in a wide variety of specific health and social care settings, such as hospitals and care homes, as well as a wide range of other settings, such as schools, community settings and welfare organisations. For example, we have all been to see a GP and/or been to a hospital, and we are all likely to need help with washing, dressing or feeding at some time in the future. This means that unlike some other subjects, it is directly relevant to everyone, and its effects are felt by everyone. These effects directly occur when you apply the skills that you learn on this course. In lots of circumstances, these effects can seem small, such as helping someone with personal care. However, these small effects can make a huge difference to the lives of individuals, as it can be the difference between being able to be part of the community and not being part of the community. For example, helping someone with personal care helps them to play, work, socialise and interact, which can make a huge difference to their lives. This reinforces the point made above that studying health and social care is something that enables you to make a difference to the lives of many others, and our own, on a daily basis, right in front of your eyes.

What is health and social care?

A good place to start your degree is to define what we mean by health and social care, as this helps to begin to understand the context of what studying health and social care is about. Before doing this, a word on the terms that we use. We usually use the term 'health and social care' as a shorthand to mean 'health care and social care'. So when used from this point onwards in this book, unless specified otherwise, health and social care means health care and social care.

There is no single accepted definition of health and social care, but there are individual definitions of 'health' and 'social care' that we can use to help us understand them better.

The simplest way to define health is as the physical absence of disease, illness or injury or disability. This definition has the benefit of being simple to understand and apply. This would mean, for example, that when someone has a disease, illness, injury or disability, they are unhealthy, and when they do not, they are healthy. It also means that treatments can be easy to develop and apply specifically for when disease, illness, injury or disability occurs. However, if we define health simply as the physical absence of disease, injury, illness or disability, this would mean that how an individual feels about their health becomes irrelevant, as we are only concerned with the physical presence of disease, illness, injury or disability that we can see. For instance, consider where someone says that they have a headache, this would be hard to consider as ill health, as we cannot see the headache. We could run diagnostic tests which could show that something causing the headache, such as a tumour, but this would take time and expense. In the meantime, the individual would have to live their lives as if they are healthy, regardless of the pain that they would be in. So defining health narrowly as the absence of disease, illness or injury or disability could have some negative effects for the individual.

This is one of the reasons that health is not usually defined in this way. The most commonly used definition of health is from the World Health Organization (WHO) (1948), which states that 'Health is a state of complete physical, mental and social wellbeing and not merely the absence of disease or infirmity'. This is a wider definition of health than above, as it includes not just physical health but also mental health and social well-being. It has the benefit of helping us to see that health is about more than the physical absence of something, but also about how a person feels about their health. So, for example, while a person may appear physically well, they may not be feeling mentally well, and this would enable us to try to treat them in this state as well. For this reason and other reasons, it is this wider definition of health rather than the narrow definition above that is usually how health is defined.

In specific relation to health care, the Department of Health and Social Care (2022:20) provides a definition of health needs as:

> the treatment, control, management or prevention of a disease, illness, injury or disability, and the care or aftercare of a person with these needs (whether or not the tasks involved have to be carried out by a health professional).

Although this refers to health needs, this definition is relevant to health care as it identifies treatment control, management, prevention, care and aftercare as what should happen when health needs occur. We can use this definition of health needs to define health care as:

> a broad range of measures such as treatment, control, management, prevention, care and aftercare to meet physical, mental and social wellbeing health needs.

Having defined health care, we can now look to define social care. Sealey *et al.* (2022a: 3) provide a definition of social care as:

> Social care is an all-inclusive term for a broad range of services designed to meet the practical daily living needs of individuals both inside and outside the home. These daily living needs can be specific such as washing, feeding, dressing, mobility and toileting. Daily living needs can also be more abstract such as maintaining independence and social interaction, enabling the individual to play a fuller part in society, protecting them in vulnerable situations, helping them to manage complex relationships and (in some circumstances) accessing a care home or other supported accommodation. For this reason, social care includes working with a very broad range of individuals including children, older people, people with mental health problems, people with learning disabilities and disabled people.

This is clearly a much longer definition of health! One of the reasons for this is that social care covers such a wide range of needs and circumstances that a short definition would not be possible (Humphries, 2023). The key emphasis in the definition above is on 'daily living needs' and how the key focus of social care is on either meeting these or enabling these to be met. In contrast to physical health, it identifies that needs can be both concrete, such as dressing, and abstract, such as social interaction. The other key point of note from the definition is that social care is for everyone, not just for old people as is often thought (Humphries, 2023). People can have social care needs throughout their lives, from birth, through to childhood, adolescence, adulthood and older life.

From the definitions of health and social care, we can identify two important features of health and social care. The first is that both health and social care conditions can occur at any time and at any age in an individual's life. Just as someone can have cancer at any time in their life, so they can have mental health issues at any time in their life. This means that health and social care meets needs throughout the lifetime which can occur at any time.

The other key point to note is that often, people can have more than one health and social care condition at the same time, and these can be linked to each other. For example, a person with diabetes may also have high blood pressure that is caused by their diabetes or they may have depression that is linked to their diabetes. This is known as **co-morbidity and multi-morbidity** (Learning Box 1.1).

Both co-morbidity and multi-morbidity conditions can reflect health and social care needs, and often require both health and social care. Additionally, there are also health conditions which can be caused by both physical and mental health factors, such as myalgic encephalomyelitis (ME), also known as chronic fatigue syndrome (CFS). This means that treatment is required for both its physical and social causes. This is why health and social care should be seen as equal to each other, and not as one being more important than another. It often happens that health is seen as more important than social care, and more resources are often devoted to health care than social care (Sealey *et al.*, 2022b). However, the reality is that health and social care are just as important as each other, and should not be seen as having anything other than having **parity of esteem** (Learning Box 1.2) in relation to each other.

Learning Box 1.1: Co-morbidity and multi-morbidity

Co-morbidity and multi-morbidity are two terms that mean similar but distinct things.

Co-morbidity is when a person has two or more health conditions, where one of the conditions occurs directly from the other condition. For example, a person may have obesity as the main condition, and high blood pressure as a co-morbid condition caused by the obesity. Or they may have autism as a main condition, and epilepsy as a co-morbid condition caused by autism.

Multi-morbidity is when a person has two or more health conditions, but they are not caused by each other. For example, a person may have an infectious disease and sight loss, which are not caused by each other. Or they may have arthritis and depression, which are not caused by each other.

Learning Box 1.2: Parity of esteem

Parity of esteem here refers to viewing and treating health and social care as equal in terms of value and worth. The notion of parity of esteem has come to prominence in specific relation to mental health (Owens *et al.*, 2022), but mental health is just one aspect of health and social care. Parity of esteem would mean that health care would not be prioritised over social care in terms of funding and resources, and so would mean social care would be better able to meet the needs of individuals. The beneficial outcomes from parity of esteem between health and social care would include quicker and better access to social care, and greater choice for individuals to choose how they receive care (Owens *et al.*, 2022).

From the definitions above, we can see that at the heart of studying health and social care is understanding what health and social care needs are, and identifying appropriate care to meet these needs. The importance of studying health and social care is evident from the fact that we are all likely to need health and social care at any time during our lifetime, with each possibly causing a need in the other. This means that they should be seen as equal to each other.

Who is this book for?

This book aims to provide students with a good understanding of the essential context, knowledge and practice skills for doing a successful health and social care degree, regardless of where or how the degree is undertaken. The book is written as a course textbook for undergraduate students studying health and social care degrees. However, there is an increased emphasis on the importance of health and social care to allied health professionals, such as nursing, midwifery, physiotherapy and occupational therapy, and the book could also be of interest to these students. Also, the structure of the book means that it is possible for students of other linked degrees to use specific chapters of interest to them.

The structure of the book

This book is written as a course textbook rather than as a module textbook. Accordingly, the book is divided into three sections, focusing on the essential context, knowledge and practice skills that you require to undertake a health and social care degree course.

Part 1: The essential context of health and social care

The context section of the book focuses on outlining and analysing the current circumstance that exists in health and social care. This includes chapters on the transition into higher education (HE), legislation, demographic change, and quality assurance and regulation.

Chapter 2: The transition into university for health and social care students

This chapter explores some of the common issues facing students moving into HE to study a health and social care degree. The chapter recognises that many health and social care students may be commencing university through the 'non-traditional' routes and may be looking to juggle work, family and new study commitments. It also offers guidance on students who may be moving away from home for either study and/or accommodation, enabling both groups of students to get the best from their course experience. This aims to help you understand some of the feelings you may be experiencing as well as offer some generic advice on how to prepare.

Chapter 3: Health and social care in the context of social, demographic and technological change – Who cares?

The chapter outlines in detail how social, demographic and technological changes are not only impacting on health and social care now, but also how they have the potential to impact on health and social care in the future. The chapter focuses, in particular, on the effects on health and social care changes on the family, the increased ageing population and improvements in technologies. This includes a discussion of both the positive and negative effects of these changes, and the current and future potential impact of these changes on who provides health and social care in the future.

Chapter 4: Understanding health for health and social care practice

Health is a fundamental aspect of human life, influencing our ability to live fully and achieve our potential. However, defining health is not straightforward. This chapter aims to provide a better understanding of health as a way to improve practice. It outlines different definitions of health and considers the implications of these definitions. The chapter identifies issues that influence the definitions of health, such as historical factors, subjective and objective factors, the multidimensional nature of health, and the individual's perspective of health. The chapter concludes by outlining the beneficial effects that understanding health can provide for health and social care practice.

Chapter 5: Understanding mental health for health and social care

This chapter presents key issues for health and social care in relation to mental health. It starts by explaining the current context of mental health as a way to contextualise its significance to health and social care. It then outlines two key definitions of mental health and explores the significance of these definitions. This is followed by detailing the importance of distinguishing between mental health, mental illness and mental disorder. It then describes key mental health legislation and diagnoses that you are likely to come across in practice. This leads on to a discussion of the significance of mental health stigma. The chapter concludes with a brief outline of key mental health treatments.

Chapter 6: Legislation/Laws guiding health and social care practice

Legislation/law is comprehensive in nature, affecting all aspects of our everyday life, as well as affecting what we do in practice. This means that knowing what the legislation/law is and how this affects what we can do as practitioners is very important for health and social care practitioners. The chapter starts with a discussion of what legislation/law is, and provides a simple definition of legislation. The chapter then discusses the importance of legislation/law for health and social care, as this may not always be apparent. The chapter concludes by briefly linking ten key health and social care practice behaviours to key legislation/law. The focus is on detailing the importance of these legislation/laws to health and social care practice.

Chapter 7: Regulation in health and social care: Improving the quality of care?

When people access health and social care services, they do so with the expectation that it will be of a certain quality. One way to try to ensure that care services are of good quality is through the use of regulation. This chapter analyses the functions and purposes of regulation to clarify the importance that regulation serves within the context of health and social care. It then examines the processes of regulation for health and social care to provide an understanding of how it works. This includes key bodies involved in the process of regulation. Finally, the chapter provides a critical analysis of the process of regulation to consider whether regulation can improve the quality of care.

Part 2: Essential knowledge for studying health and social care

This part of the book outlines and analyses key knowledge that is important for studying health and social care. This includes chapters on sociological theories, anatomy and physiology, defining care, children's rights, equality and anti-oppressive practice, disability, children and young people's mental health, disability, older adults and mental health.

Chapter 8: Key sociological theories for health and social care

This chapter identifies the importance of sociological theories to health and social care practice. The chapter looks at ways in which studying sociological theories support health and social care practitioners to develop a deeper understanding of the complex interplay between individuals and society, enabling more effective and accountable practice. To do this, the chapter embarks on a sociological journey through time to see the different ways in which theorists have attempted to explain and understand the world in which we live.

Chapter 9: Core models of health

Working in health or social care can involve many different roles and working alongside many different professionals, who may bring different understandings of health with them, which affects the care provided. This chapter explores three predominant perspectives, or 'models' of health that significantly shape our understanding and approaches to care, the medical model, the social model and the biopsychosocial model (BPS). Understanding how health is defined and framed is important for health and social care students because it informs understanding of their own working practices (and that of others), and to be clear on what is and what is not relevant to care. This enables students to have a better understanding of the systems and processes within which they are working.

Chapter 10: The importance of anatomy and physiology for health and social care

This chapter outlines how and why an understanding of anatomy and physiology is important to health and social care practice. The chapter starts with brief outlines of both anatomy and physiology, in terms of what they mean individually. It then outlines the importance of linking anatomy and physiology together. Finally, it explains three specific beneficial outcomes of understanding of anatomy and physiology for health and social care.

Chapter 11: Safeguarding in health and social care: Progressive, proactive and preventative actions for practice

This chapter focuses on outlining the meaning of safeguarding and keys factors that can reduce safeguarding issues and concerns. It outlines the difference between a narrow and a wide definition of safeguarding, the significance of this difference and how this is reflected in legislation. It outlines nine factors which lead to progressive, proactive and preventative action on safeguarding. This provides students with a clear understanding of what safeguarding is, and also a clear outline of action you can take in practice to progressively, proactively and preventatively deal with safeguarding issues and concerns.

Chapter 12: Children and young people's mental health

This chapter focuses on the importance of good mental health and the impact of poor mental health in relation to children and young people's development and lifelong health and well-being. The chapter explores and identifies key factors that can negatively affect the mental health of children/young people. These include the cost-of-living crisis, negative experiences using social media, the global COVID-19 pandemic, abuse and neglect, the impact of racism and poor parental mental health. The chapter then outlines factors that can help to enable good mental health for children and young people, such as supportive relationships, resilience and development milestones.

Chapter 13: The rights of children and young people within health and social care settings

This chapter provides an overview of children's and young people's rights within health and social care settings. It emphasises the importance of understanding and upholding these rights to ensure the well-being and protection of children and young people. The chapter details how the existence of rights can positively affect the everyday lives of children and young people, while at the same time acknowledging that attitudes towards children's rights can vary by society and culture. The chapter is particularly relevant for professionals who will be working with children and young people. It also holds significance for those working with adults, as the principles of rights and protections are universally applicable.

Chapter 14: Disability: Perspectives, experiences and implications for health and social care practice

This chapter aims to help you consider academic and cultural ideas around disability and explore, or begin to explore, your own ideas, values and beliefs around disability. The chapter explores some factors and possible examples of discriminatory issues ideas which while working as a health and care professional are likely cause oppression for people with a disability. The chapter uses Thompson's (2021) PCS model as a framework to raise your awareness of issues that affect your service users, such as your own thoughts and beliefs, their thoughts and beliefs, legislation and societal attitudes.

Chapter 15: Anti-discriminatory and anti-oppressive ACTion for health and social care

This chapter details the importance of anti-discriminatory and anti-oppressive practice for health and social care. The chapter firstly defines what anti-discriminatory and anti-oppressive practice are, and links them to relevant legislation. The chapter then briefly details relevant anti-discrimination and anti-oppressive practice legislation. It then explains why and how anti-discriminatory and anti-oppressive practice can impact on the quality of health and social care that you provide. The chapter concludes by proposing Awareness, Challenging and Transformation as an ACTion strategy that you can use to provide and promote anti-discriminatory and anti-oppressive practice.

Chapter 16: Healthy ageing: The future of health and social care?

This chapter considers how continued 'growth' throughout the life-course, especially in older age, can have a beneficial impact on the future of health and social care. It challenges the traditional notion of inevitable decline into old age, and the increased demands this in turn places on the economy as our population ages. It argues that embracing the concept of 'growing in age' as the norm and recognising older adults as a diverse group with varying health and social care needs are key elements to altering the perception of ageing. As the ageing population grows, older adults are increasingly recognised for their potential contributions to societal development, and ensuring their abilities are incorporated into policies and programmes is essential for fostering inclusive growth.

Part 3: Essential practice skills for health and social care

This section of the book outlines and analyses essential practice skills for studying and practice in health and social care. This includes chapters on reflective practice, communication skills, placement skills and leadership and teamworking.

Chapter 17: Being a reflective practitioner within health and social care settings

Reflection is a vital part of health and social care practice. This chapter provides a broad overview of reflective practice to help you understand the basics of the reflective process and guide you towards the skills and resources needed to reflect effectively. This chapter helps you to understand the importance of reflection, be able to structure your reflective practice by using recognised models, understand how to write reflectively for university assignments, identify barriers to being able to reflect effectively, and engage in exercises to enable you to start reflecting.

Chapter 18: Communication skills for practice

This chapter explores a range of communication skills that are used in health and social care. It introduces some of the underpinning theories of and about communication. This is designed to help both emerging and experienced practitioners develop their communication skills for use in their practice, as well as develop their own understanding of what makes good communication.

Chapter 19: Placements skills for health and social care students

As a student studying health and social care at the university, it is almost certain your course has some form of placement. The chapter uses Patricia Benner's (1984) five-stage 'novice to expert' theory as a way to explain what to expect when on placement. This provides a good understanding of what is likely to be your experience while on placement. The chapter offers suggestions and guidance for you regardless of what stage of learning you are at, with the aim of helping you progress through the stages as your placement develops and your knowledge and skills increase.

Chapter 20: Leadership and teamworking – The foundations of organisational culture in health and social care practice

This chapter explores leadership styles and teamworking. Research shows that effective leadership and teamwork are vital for delivering high-quality health and social care, directly influencing organisational culture which improves care. The chapter examines their practical application in health and social care settings and highlights their role in enabling a positive organisational culture that supports enhanced patient and service user outcomes.

Chapter 21: Ten essential context, knowledge and skills for doing a successful health and social care degree

This chapter is a summary of the book. It identifies ten key themes that run through the book, as a way to highlight essential context, knowledge and skills for studying health and social care.

Learning boxes

The book uses learning boxes to make key issues and concepts clearer, as above. Where an issue or concept has a learning box, it is highlighted with bold text. In some instances, learning boxes appear in another chapter. Please refer to the list of key learning boxes on page xi.

References

Benner, P.E. (1984) *From Novice to Expert: Excellence and Power in Clinical Nursing Practice*. Menlo Park, CA: Addison-Wesley Pub. Co., Nursing Division.

Department of Health and Social Care (2022) *National Framework for NHS Continuing Healthcare and NHS- funded Nursing Care*. Available at https://assets.publishing.service.gov.uk/government/uploads/system/uploads/attachment_data/file/1170290/National-Framework-for-NHS-Continuing-Healthcare-and-NHS-funded-Nursing-Care_July-2022-revised_corrected-July-2023.pdf (Accessed 31 March 2025).

Humphries, R. (2023) *Ending the Social Care Crisis: A New Road to Reform*. Bristol: Policy Press. Available at https://doi.org/10.46692/9781447364474

Owens, J. *et al.* (2022) 'Parity of esteem and systems thinking: A theory informed qualitative inductive thematic analysis', *BMC Psychiatry*, 22(1), p. 650. Available at https://doi.org/10.1186/s12888-022-04299-y

Sealey, C. (2015) *Social policy simplified: connecting theory with people's lives*. London ; New York, NY: Palgrave Macmillan.

Sealey, C., Fillingham, J. and Unwin, P. (2022a) 'Social policy, service users and carers: Proposals for improving policy and practice', in C. Sealey, J. Fillingham, and P. Unwin (eds.) *Social Policy, Service Users and Carers*. Cham: Springer International Publishing, pp. 211–222. Available at https://doi.org/10.1007/978-3-030-69876-8_13
Sealey, C., Unwin, P. and Fillingham, J. (2022b) 'Introduction', in C. Sealey, J. Fillingham, and P. Unwin (eds.) *Social Policy, Service Users and Carers*. Cham: Springer International Publishing, pp. 1–14. Available at https://doi.org/10.1007/978-3-030-69876-8_1
Thompson, N. (2021) *Anti-Discriminatory Practice: Equality, Diversity and Social Justice*. 7th edn. London: Macmillan Education UK (Practical Social Work Ser).
World Health Organization (1948) *Constitution of the World Health Organization*. Available at https://www.who.int/about/governance/constitution (Accessed 31 March 2025).

Part 1

The essential context of health and social care

2 The transition into university for health and social care students

Rebecca Weston

The aims of this chapter are to:

- **Describe the difference experiences that health and social care students can have before they start university**
- **Identify issues for students to navigate in their first few weeks of university**
- **Detail a range of support services available to helps at university**

Introduction

Coming to university is a big decision. Whether you are just completing your college course at the end of your mandatory education, or you are choosing to return to study after a break from education, there will be something that has motivated your decision to complete your UCAS form and apply for your chosen course, coupled with the commitment you have made to complete that course.

This chapter explores some of the common issues faced by students moving into Higher Education (HE) to study a health and social care degree. Students on health and social care courses tend to fall into two categories. The first of these are 'traditional' students, meaning students who go to school, then to college or sixth form, and then to university. The second of these are 'non-traditional' or 'mature student', who go to school, have some life experiences such as work or family and then go to university. The chapter recognises that many health and social care students may be commencing university through the 'non-traditional' routes and may be looking to juggle work, family and new study commitments. For example, UCAS reports that in 2019, 40% of students recruited onto Social Work courses are aged over 30, compared to 29% of students recruited onto nursing courses (UCAS, 2020). Furthermore, the Office for Students (OfS) (2020) recognise that the 'non-traditional' routes into HE can include Access to HE courses, professional experience and distance learning. The case studies of Stacy Ann and Swani below highlight these different routes and explore the expectations each student may have for university.

It also offers guidance on students who may be moving away from home either for study and/or for accommodation, enabling both groups of students to get the best from their course experience. To do this effectively, this chapter adopts the use of two vignettes of students arriving at universities having come from both traditional and non-traditional backgrounds and experiences. This aims to help you understand some of the feelings you may be experiencing, as well as offer some generic advice on how to prepare for university.

DOI: 10.4324/9781032619309-3

Case study: Stacey-Ann

Stacey-Ann is 36 years old, and works in a residential care setting, a job she has done for 13 years. She left school at 16 with three GCSEs and started a BTEC at her local college. Unfortunately, due to her Dad becoming ill and requiring care from her and her Mum, she left college to support her Mum and Dad whilst working a range of part-time jobs. When she was 22, her son was born and once he started attending nursery and then school, Stacey-Ann was able to find more regular work in her first care role.

During the COVID-19 pandemic, Stacey-Ann was encouraged to take on more responsibility in her current job, and now her son and younger daughters are older and all at school, Stacey-Ann has been exploring her options to continue her education. At a *Careers and Options* evening at her son's school, she spoke with an admissions tutor from the local university who dispelled her belief that 'she was too old to study now' and encouraged her to go along to an open day specifically for applicants who had been away from education for a while. Stacey-Ann attended and has applied for a place on a health and social care degree course. Because she did not complete her BTEC, she had to write an essay to support her application onto the course (which she found terrifying) and then have an informal interview where she could discuss her extensive experience in care settings. Stacey-Ann holds an unconditional offer for her course, which is at a university close to where she lives and works.

Case study: Swani

Swani is 18 and in his last year at sixth form college. He did quite well in his GCSEs, but unfortunately not well enough for him to take up his place at the local FE college which did impact his choices for sixth form. Swani is studying the Level 3 BTEC in health and social care and finding to his surprise that not only is he enjoying it, but he is getting really good grades and predicted a DDD (triple distinction). He has particularly enjoyed the module on Biology, despite hating the subject at GCSE, as the focus on the human body and systems has fascinated him. He enjoyed the work experience aspect of the course, although felt that he was really out of his depth when working with older people, however, he got a good report and passed the assessment.

Swani lives at home with his parents, two younger brothers and a much younger sister. His Gran also lives with them, which sometimes makes studying a little difficult, as the house is quite small and there always seems to be someone wanting something from the kitchen, which is where, once the evening meal is over, Swani sets out to study. Away from study, Swani is a keen footballer who has played in his local club throughout most of his teens. They do have an 18–21 age team that he believes he could be good enough for, but is worried that moving away to university would discount him from trying out.

At his recent Careers Tutorial, his tutor expressed frustration that Swani was yet to make a decision about university and even course options. Swani agreed to look at some courses that might interest him and initially applied for a course in Paramedic Science. However, competition was tough and his only offer was from a university over 150 miles away. Swani realised at that point that he wanted to remain close to his family, where he could visit regularly, but also have his own space in university accommodation. He also reassessed his course choice, but this was after the UCAS deadline, so applied for a degree in health and social care at a university local to him. Swani received a conditional offer based upon his predicted grades for his Level 3 BTEC.

Comparing Stacy-Ann's non-traditional and Swani's traditional circumstances

In terms of their experiences, Swani's route to university could be described as a traditional route, whilst Stacy-Ann's route could be described as non-traditional. There are some similarities and differences which may be typical of both traditional and non-traditional health and social care students. In terms of similarities, their application to study the health and social care occurred either not as a first choice or following a long time out of education. This means that they may be some uncertainty about their choice of degree. Also, they may both need to work to fund their degree, as the loans and grants that they receive may not be enough.

In terms of differences, younger students like Swani tend to live away from home, whilst mature students with caring responsibilities tend to live at home and commute to university. This means that their experience of 'university life' is different. For those living at home, this can make it harder to integrate into the course and the university. According to the OfS (2020), mature students also tend to be less confident about their academic skills, as a consequence of being out of education for so long. Mature students can lack in confidence when comparing themselves to younger students who have come to university via traditional routes. Furthermore, mature students may be more likely to have family or work commitments, making attending a traditional university timetable difficult. Their caring responsibilities also mean that they are not able to devote as much of their available time to their studies. As a traditional student, Swani may have financial difficulties due to living away from home, which can also mean that he is not able to devote as much of his available time to his studies.

Getting started – Induction

Regardless of a student's route into university, once an offer is 'firmly accepted' (this is a term from UCAS which indicates that a student has committed to choosing one course at one university), as the university start date draws closer, information is sent out about course registration and an induction programme. In Stacy-Ann's case, because her offer is 'unconditional' (meaning she has already met all of the entry requirements for the course), this will come through automatically. For Swani, a 'conditional' offer means that the university is waiting for confirmation that the entry requirements have been met, in this case, that Swani's BTEC qualifications match or exceed the offer made. Once this happens, the same information will be sent to all students in that position too.

Induction at most universities is an organised event, taking place over the week before lectures formally start. Many universities co-ordinate academic activities with their Student Union, so that new students get a mixture of course information and social activities. These are all designed to help students make connections both with people on their course and the wider university (Hamlin *et al.*, 2024).

Induction weeks at university are an essential part of a student's journey through HE (Morgan, 2012; Yorke and Longden, 2008). Whether you are moving away from home into halls of residence or other student accommodation for the first time, the start of your university course represents major changes to your home life, regular routine and potentially financial situation, and heading onto campus for that first day is probably one you will remember for a long time (Burroughs, 2019).

The type of activities you can expect will vary. If you are moving onto campus, there will be a set time frame given for this, which is usually just before the actual induction timetable starts. If you are a commuting student, it may be that your first experience of being on campus as a student is when you arrive to start your first induction session.

On the actual first day of your course, there are many more things that might happen on that first day. Some administrative tasks that may occur are:

- Course or module registration
- Obtaining the University Wi-Fi log-in and password
- Accessing your teaching timetable
- Course-specific tasks, especially if there is a placement element involved. This might include completing placement paperwork, checking on the status of DBS applications and health questionnaires.
- Talks from academic librarians
- Introduction to student services
- Welcome from the Student Union

When starting your scheduled induction, it can feel overwhelming, in terms of how much information you are given, how easy finding the campus or rooms are and the number of different people you might meet. Sometimes, new students are also grappling with new technologies – a new laptop, phone, new software. Students can have very different experiences of induction, both negative and positive, as exemplified by Swani's and Stacy-Ann's case studies.

Swani's experience: Imposter syndrome

Understandably, the physical act of coming onto campus can bring with it a high degree of stress and/or anxiety (Chapman, 2015). One of the reasons for this can be due to 'imposter syndrome' (Clance and Imes, 1978). This is where new students start to feel that once they meet the other students on their course, and the lecturers, they will be quickly 'found out' and asked to leave the university. This can also be exacerbated by interactions with other students, either on the same course or are your new house mates. Consider the following quote from Swani talking about his experience of his first few nights in halls before the course started:

> 'I'm sharing a university flat with four other guys. They seemed quite nice, although I think they've already bonded because three of them are doing sports courses and the last guy is doing Physio, but he's like this awesome sports guy. I didn't like to mention that I wanted to try out for my local team, it seemed so lame in comparison to what they all do ....'

The above quote shows that Swani has already 'ranked' himself against his house mates and rather than embracing the common factors between them has decided to hide that part of himself from them. Whilst this example is not going to result in Swani being asked to leave university, it does illustrate how imposter syndrome can take our thoughts and self-beliefs and project them onto how we feel others think of us (Wilkinson, 2020).

Stacy-Ann's experience – Extended induction

Meanwhile, Stacy-Ann is having quite a different experience of induction. Because her offer had been unconditional, she has been in constant contact with her tutor over the summer. Living quite close to the university has meant that she was able to visit on an open day and also again, to have a campus tour and meet some of the course-teaching team. This 'extended induction' (Morgan, 2012) has built her confidence prior to the course start date, and means that she is familiar with the campus layout, knows who her Personal Tutor is and where their office is situated. In addition, Stacy-Ann has been able to engage with student services prior to the commencement of her course, meaning she has received an assessment for dyslexia and now has a package in place to support her additional needs.

This notion of an extended induction has been proven to result in better outcomes for students who engage with it (Morgan, 2023). Whilst it may not be possible to extend it too far before the start of the course, many universities do offer opportunities to visit, meet the team and engage with student services once they make an offer (Morgan, 2012).

Making a success of induction

Whatever the model or type of induction you will experience, there are things that you can do to make it successful for you and your needs. Quite often, induction can pass in a bit of a blur. Students are often focussed on getting started on their course properly, so the induction can sometimes feel a little bit irrelevant, but universities and student unions will encourage new students to make the most of this week. Morgan (2012) recommends that universities start their induction process before the timetabled week of induction. Lizzio's (2006) 'Five Senses' Framework (2006) suggests that making connections to develop an own sense of identity as being key to student success at university, and the induction process is probably the best place to start this as it will be the time when students are not fully engaged in lectures, assessments or (especially for health and social care students) placements.

If, like in Swani's case, you are starting university and living on campus, there may be many activities available to you during this week, and quite possibly, the problem may be that there is too much choice. Alternatively, a commuter and/or mature student such as Staccy-Ann may feel that the physical distance from university can lead to feelings of disconnect and missing out on part of the student experience.

Burroughs (2019) recommends planning your induction days as carefully as you can, based upon information provided by your institution or course. This can include

- If driving into university, check out local car parks and car park prices. How far do you need to walk from your car to campus?
- If using public transport, how reliable is it? Can you get an earlier bus/train and spend the time having a relaxing coffee or familiarising yourself with your surroundings?
- If you have moved into halls of residence or other university accommodation and have made friends with your house mates, can you arrange a time to catch up during the day to share stories?
- If you are taking a laptop or other device, make sure it is fully charged. You might decide to take a charger, but many teaching rooms have limited power supplies, so go in charged up and ready!
- If you have been given any course materials for the day, be environmentally friendly (and friendly to your wallet!) and avoid printing off reams. Chances are you will be provided with print-outs and however you might feel about reading online, digital citizenship is a necessary skill to develop at HE as part of your 'graduate attributes' (JISC, 2024).

- Pack a lunch and take a drink. Eating on campus may feel exciting and a great way to meet people, but until you know the prices, it can get very costly very quickly.
- Get a notebook and something to write with. Using devices is great; however, there can be something spontaneous about jotting something down on paper, especially if you have been given a stack of information (you will be!).
- Try not to panic if you do not remember it all! Try to remember one important (to you) thing from the day. It could be the number of the teaching room your first lecture is in, the name of the student who you did the paired activity with, or how to log onto your student homepage.

Universities try to address many challenges (as identified above and more) during their induction week. Some activities begin before this formal week, especially if, like Swani, you are staying in university accommodation, or a brief 'bridging' course to support students returning to learning like Stacey-Ann.

Experiencing the first few weeks

In the first full week of your lectures, you can expect to learn about each of the modules you will be studying in the first semester. You should also expect to receive information on assessments, deadlines and how to access academic support both within the course and wider university. It is recommended that you do take this support, whatever your route into university or previous academic experience. Universities and individual courses have their own expectations of how students' complete assignments, how they reference sources, and what referencing style is used, and it is very important that you are aware of this in your initial weeks.

Increasingly, universities are responding to supporting students making an academic transition into HE by setting **a formative academic task** (Learning Box 2.1) in the early weeks of study (Matheson, 2018). The reasons for this can be to help students better understand some of the university's processes and systems, to help students obtain feedback on their work in a supportive manner, and to use both the process of submitting work electronically and responding to feedback as robust preparation for early summative assessments.

Learning Box 2.1: Key academic terms

Formative academic task: formative simply means that it is helping you 'form' or develop your writing style. Feedback is usually provided but it will not contribute to your final module or course grade.

Summative academic task: this is an assessment that 'sums up' or is you demonstrating how you have understood a topic in relation to the module, learning outcomes and assessment brief. It is marked (graded) and will count towards the final module and/or course grade.

Assignment brief: the instructions for successfully completing an assignment in relation to the structure, what to include and how to meet the learning outcomes (see below).

Learning outcomes: what you have to demonstrate you have achieved through completion of the assignment/module.

Swani's experience – Adapting to living independently away from home

Alongside the academic aspect of university, students are adapting to many changes. For Swani, a big change for him is having to plan meals and shop for food, as well as all that comes from living in shared, student accommodation. Swani is used to a busy household, with lots of distractions at different times of the evening and weekends. However, all of Swani's extended family were aware of his goals to study well and gain a place at university, and this gave him a certain degree of power within the household. His Mum supported his goal by excusing him from household chores and rewarding good grades with unexpected gifts. In his university flat, Swani does have his own study space, but the constant sound of flat doors opening and closing, fragmented pieces of conversation and cooking smells coming from the kitchen gives rise to a different distraction. Similarly, there is no one around to place a plate of food, cup of tea or keep the canned drinks stocked up for those study breaks – Swani must do that himself now!

Stacy-Ann's experience – Striving to be student and a mother

In a similar vein, Stacy-Ann returns from her lectures often tired, exhilarated and desperate to sit down and reflect on her day before planning that evening's study session. However, her three children all returning from their own experiences of education often have to be helped with completing their own homework, passing on any requirements for the following day at school, organising plans for the weekend, and all before their dinner. As Stacy-Ann manages all of this on her own, it is usually quite late before she can get that time of reflection on the day, and then the study she hoped to do whilst things were still fresh gets pushed back to two or three hours across the next week. There is a course 'WhatsApp' group that someone set up, Stacy-Ann finds it useful, but many of the messages arrive at the peak time she is tending to her children's needs, and she is feeling as though she is rapidly falling behind.

These first few weeks at university are challenging for both the reasons experienced by the two case studies, and many others as well – there is no universal experience of beginning university. However, there are some common factors that can present themselves as challenges with some ideas on how to mitigate their impact.

Managing own study time

When students start university, no matter what their educational experience has been like, there is great emphasis placed on independent learning, development of own study skills and fitting this in around the rest of your week. If you are reading this having just received your university timetable, with potentially a maximum of 12 hours teaching on it each week, you would be forgiven for wondering what all the fuss is about. Whether like Swani, you have recently completed sixth form college where your 25 hours each week are carefully timetabled, or you are returning to study after a gap like Stacy-Ann who also works 12-hour shifts in a care setting, the prospect of 'only' 12 hours of lectures each week can lure students into a sense of freedom and good intentions.

For example, you might consider your timetable alongside your work and perhaps family commitments and think that 'yes, the additional reading will be easy', 'I can join that study group to meet online each week', and 'I will write up all my lecture notes each week, keep my files organised and prepare for my assignments fully'. However, for all of this to happen, it takes organisation from the part of the student. A recent

Learning Box 2.2: Procrastination

Procrastination refers to the avoidance of completing a task or activity that you perceive as being difficult or unpleasant, often by prioritising other tasks or activities instead. For example, you have an essay to plan (difficult) for your tutorial. You are worried that your tutor will be critical of your essay plan, so you avoid doing it. Instead, you decide to write up a Christmas present list for your family. By doing this, you are avoiding the actual thing that requires organisation and planning by replacing it with a different activity that also requires organisation and planning. This can actually convince you that you are still doing something useful, even though you will not be sharing your Christmas present list with your tutor as a way to demonstrate your organisational skills.

cohort of students reflecting upon their previous study experiences described **procrastination** (Learning Box 2.2) as the major barrier to them developing good study habits. The same cohort of students also listed 'asking for help' as being difficult because they felt it showed them as 'not good enough'.

Asking for help

Earlier, we looked at how 'imposter syndrome' can be a barrier to asking for help. You might have noticed that from the example given above around procrastination, there are similarities – you avoid the essay planning activity because you feel that when you go and see your tutor, they will 'see through you' and suggest that you leave the course. So rather than show them something that indicates that you would like some help, you draw up a Christmas present list instead, as this can reinforce to you that you are actually very good at organising and planning some things.

Who can help me, and how?

Whilst all of this may feel daunting, there are many people and services situated within the university who can help. Quite often, these additional services get overlooked by students, particularly at the start of the first academic year, when students are busy navigating timetables, finding their way around campus, making new friends and trying to understand their university's IT system, Virtual Learning Environment (VLE), and develop effective study skills.

This section highlights some of the additional services offered by your university that are available to all students and not generally situated within your specific course team. The last source of help, your Personal Academic Tutor, will be situated within your course or subject team, but is also an important point of contact and support so is included here.

Academic support

The additional academic services will vary depending upon the university you are studying at, but outside of your immediate course team, there should be a central 'hub', either physical or virtual, that can inform you of what is available. For example, you should be able to access an academic liaison librarian, or library skills service. Part of your university induction will have introduced you to specific services and the contact information should be centrally available via either a course handbook, VLE, or information around campus.

Some universities may have specialist study skills portals or departments that you can utilise. Often, the fact that these are centrally located instead of within courses or departments can feel more supportive, as you can attend with flat mates, who may be on other courses and they may have a range of ways to seek help. This can include in person, online, via a chatbot or email service, or webpages produced by the university that are bespoke to their academic expectations and requirements.

National Union of Students

The National Union of Students (NUS) is a body independent of individual universities and is a union that represents 'university and college students across the UK' (NUS, 2024). If they are affiliated, there will be a student union building or area on your campus, and all UK students are automatically members once registered at the university. As they are independent of Higher Education Institutes (HEIs), they can give independent and objective advice on a range of matters, from complaints about your course, to volunteering opportunities, to seeking support in Academic Integrity meetings or other representations. In the first few weeks of starting university, your course will look to electing or appointing a course representative who liaises between course teams, students and the wider Student Union, both informally and through course meetings.

Student support services

If you are looking for support relating to health and wellbeing, most university campuses will have a referral process for a range of services such as counselling services. There may also be the opportunity to register with a doctor's surgery and there will be links to local sexual health clinics, health promotion opportunities on and around campus and a student welfare service that can support a wide range of health and social issues. This includes supporting students who become pregnant during their studies, housing support, mental health support or are struggling financially.

Personal Academic Tutor

Your Personal Academic Tutor is usually an academic member of your course team who is your 'named' tutor. Different institutes will use different terminology and organise this in ways relevant to their course and student requirements, but a common model is that your academic tutor supports you from the start of your university course, all the way through to graduation. It is usual to be introduced to them during either induction or at the very latest, within the first week of your lectures starting.

Academic tutoring can look different depending where you are studying, but one major difference some new students may notice is that however it looks, it is very different from 'tutors' at college or school. For example, whilst your academic tutor may introduce themselves to you initially, the onus will probably be on you to contact them if you wish to meet for a tutorial. This can be challenging for many first-year students, especially if their academic tutor is not currently teaching them. Some students avoid contacting their academic tutor for some of the following reasons:

- They are not aware of what issues or concerns they can contact their academic tutor for.
- Their academic tutor does not teach them; therefore they are not very visible and sending an email can feel scary.
- Students worry that contacting their academic tutor can be a sign of weakness, or not being able to cope on a university course.
- They are introduced to them in induction and then forget who they are, but are not told where to find that information.

Thankfully, many universities are becoming more responsive to these concerns and encourage their academic tutors to be more proactive in building positive relationships with their tutees. Some examples of good practice can include:

- Your academic tutor contacts all their tutees and offers a drop-in session or 'group meeting' to introduce themselves to you all.
- Time given within curriculum (teaching) time to facilitate academic tutoring.
- Formative activities being overseen by academic tutors, or students asked to have a tutorial with their individual academic tutor within the early weeks of the first semester.

However your course organises their academic tutoring, it is definitely within your best interest to overcome any initial nerves or concerns and either accept that invitation from your academic tutor, or take a deep breath and send an email to them yourself.

Summary

This chapter has highlighted some possible issues that you may face when starting on your health and social care degree. It has used the experiences of Swani as a traditional student and Stacey-Ann as a non-traditional student to outline different experiences of student transition into HE. Through the experiences of Swani and Stacey-Ann, relevant support systems have been identified for new students, including Personal Academic Tutoring, Student Union and student services. Also explored are key themes identified as important for new students, including imposter syndrome, living away from home for the first time and juggling caring responsibilities, full-time work and full-time study. This chapter hopefully helps you to navigate the first few weeks of your study, to enable you to flourish and develop as you progress on the degree.

References

Burroughs, C. (2019) *The Return to Study Handbook: Study Skills for Mature, Distance and Workplace Learners*. London: Kogan Page.

Chapman, A. (2015) 'Using the assessment process to overcome imposter syndrome in mature students', *Journal of Further and Higher Education*, 41(2), pp. 112–119. https://doi.org/10.1080/0309877X.2015.1062851

Clance, P.R. and Imes, S.A. (1978) 'The imposter phenomenon in high achieving women: Dynamics and therapeutic intervention', *Psychotherapy: Theory, Research and Practice*, 15(3), pp. 241–247. Available at https://web-s-ebscohost-com.apollo.worc.ac.uk/ehost/pdfviewer/pdfviewer?vid=0&sid=c47f7f1d-9a6a-477b-8bf1-5e6f5e761ec3%40redis

Hamlin, J. *et al.* (2024) 'Redesigning welcome, induction and transition: A strategic approach and partnership', *Journal of Educational Innovation, Partnership and Change*, 10(1). Available at https://journals.studentengagement.org.uk/index.php/studentchangeagents/article/view/1268

JISC (2024) 'Building digital capabilities framework: The six elements defined'. Available at https://repository.jisc.ac.uk/8846/1/2022_Jisc_BDC_Individual_Framework.pdf

Lizzio, A. (2006) 'Designing an orientation and transition strategy for commencing students: applying the five senses model'. Available at https://studylib.net/doc/5862488/designing-an-orientation-and-transition-strategy-for

Matheson, R. (2018) 'Transition through the student lifecycle', in R. Matheson, S. Tangney and M. Sutcliffe (eds.) *Transition in, Through and Out of Higher Education: International Case Studies and Best Practice*. London: Routledge, pp. 5–16

Morgan, M. (2012) *Improving the Student Experience: A Practical Guide for Universities and Colleges*. Abingdon: Routledge.

Morgan, M. (2023) 'Supporting the student experience: the early transition stages'. Available at https://wonkhe.com/wp-content/wonkhe-uploads/2023/12/Michelle-Morgan_effective-induction-and-onboarding.pdf

NUS (2024) 'NUS – about'. Available at https://www.nus.org.uk/about

Office for Students (2020) 'Mature students'. Available at https://www.officeforstudents.org.uk/for-providers/equality-of-opportunity/effective-practice/mature-students/

UCAS (2020) 'New UCAS insight shows health and social care professions among the most diverse and welcoming – with courses still open for new applications'. Available at https://www.ucas.com/corporate/news-and-key-documents/news/new-ucas-insight-shows-health-and-social-care-professions-among-most-diverse-and-welcoming-courses

Wilkinson, C. (2020) 'Imposter syndrome and the accidental academic: An autoethnographic account', *International Journal for Academic Development*, 25(4), pp. 363–374. https://doi.org/10.1080/1360144X.2020.1762087

Yorke, M. and Longden, B. (2008) 'The first year experience of higher education in the UK'. Available at https://s3.eu-west-2.amazonaws.com/assets.creode.advancehe-document-manager/documents/hea/private/fyefinalreport_0_1568037076.pdf

3 Health and social care in the context of social, demographic and technological change – who cares?

Clive Sealey

The aims of this chapter are to:

- **Outline the key social, demographic and technological changes that have happened over the last 50–60 years**
- **Analyse the effect of these changes on health and social care now and in the future**

Introduction

The last 50–60 years have seen significant changes in the society that we live in which have transformed the way we live, work and play. For example, the reality of family life has changed to include blended families and extended families. Similarly, we now work in very different ways, as exemplified by the growth of flexible working and working from home. For our leisure time, we are now able to choose and do things that would have been unthinkable 50 years ago, such as travelling very long distances in a very short time to experience many different cultures.

There are two important points to note here. Firstly, that these changes have not occurred in isolation from each other, but have and continue to occur in ways that are linked with each other. For instance, the way we live is transforming the way we work (for example, the changed blended family life is relevant to the importance of flexible working); the way we work is transforming the way we play (for example, working from home now means less time travelling to work and more time for leisure); and the way that we play is transforming the way we live (for example, the increased travelling opportunities for leisure has increased our exposure to different cultures and this has changed what we cook and eat).

The second important point is that these changes are having and continue to have an effect on health and social care. Indeed, it would be strange if these significant changes are not having significant effects on health and social care. The chapter outlines in detail how these changes are not only impacting on health and social care now, but also how they have the potential to impact on health and social care in the future. The chapter argues that these changes are being driven by key social, demographic and technological changes occurring in society. The chapter focuses in particular on the effects on health and social care of changes in the family, the increased ageing population and improvements in technologies. This includes a discussion of both positive and negative effects.

This chapter provides you with an understanding of key social, demographic and technological changes occurring in society, and the current and future potential impact of these changes on health and social care.

DOI: 10.4324/9781032619309-4

Social changes

When talking about social changes, we are talking about changes that affect the nature of society. These are changes that affect the way that a society treats those within it, changes that affect the relationships that occur within a society and changes that affect the normal way of doing things in a society. For example, in relation to the way that a society treats those within it, societies can change in terms of how they treat minority groups, as evident from the change that has occurred in relation to more equal treatment of LGBTQ communities (Bristowe *et al.*, 2018). In relation to the changes that affect the relationships that occur within a society, a good example of this is changes in marriage and divorce which has affected the nature of the family (Thompson *et al.*, 2012). And in relation to the normal way of doing things, a good example of this has been the increased number of people going to university, meaning the previous norm for young people of leaving school to go straight into a job is no longer the current norm (Bekhradnia and Beech, 2018).

There have been many social changes over the last 50 years that have specifically affected health and social care. These include changes in income and wealth leading to overall increased social inequality (Bourquin *et al.*, 2022), changes in how and what we eat leading to some improvements in health but also the growth of health conditions such as obesity (Wells *et al.*, 2021), and changes to what we do in our leisure time leading to improved health and social outcomes for some and reduced health and social outcomes for others (Roberts, 2019). However, perhaps a key change that has affected health and social care has been changes in the makeup of the family, and this is detailed below.

Since the 1960s, there has been an increasing diversity of family types. Sixty years ago, the most dominant family type consisted of parents and children living together as a single household unit. This is known as the 'nuclear family' type, as it is a type of family where the nucleus of the family is the male as the 'breadwinner' and the roles of the wife and children built around him. More specifically, the usual expectation in the nuclear family type is that any caring responsibility would fall on women, as a key feature of the nuclear family is that women take on caring responsibilities, while men take on the role of the breadwinner (Sealey, 2023). This notion of a male breadwinner literally refers to the man going out to earn the 'bread' for the family, with bread here meaning money.

However, since then, family types other than the nuclear family type have become more evident, as shown in Figure 3.1.

Figure 3.1 shows that the nuclear family type as represented by '*couple household with children*' was by far the most dominant type of family in the UK 60 years ago. However, this is no longer the case. Instead, it is '*one person households*' which have become the most dominant family type, followed by '*couple households with children*'. There has also been a significant increase in lone-parent households.

There are various reasons for this change such as fewer people getting married, people getting married later, more people co-habiting and an increase in divorce. Whatever the reason, this change means that we can no longer say that the typical family in the UK is the nuclear family type.

The change away from the nuclear family type is significant in the context of health and social care from the fact that in the past, social care needs in particular have been seen as a family responsibility, meaning that it was something that the nuclear family would do. This meant that if and when the need to care for a family member arose either

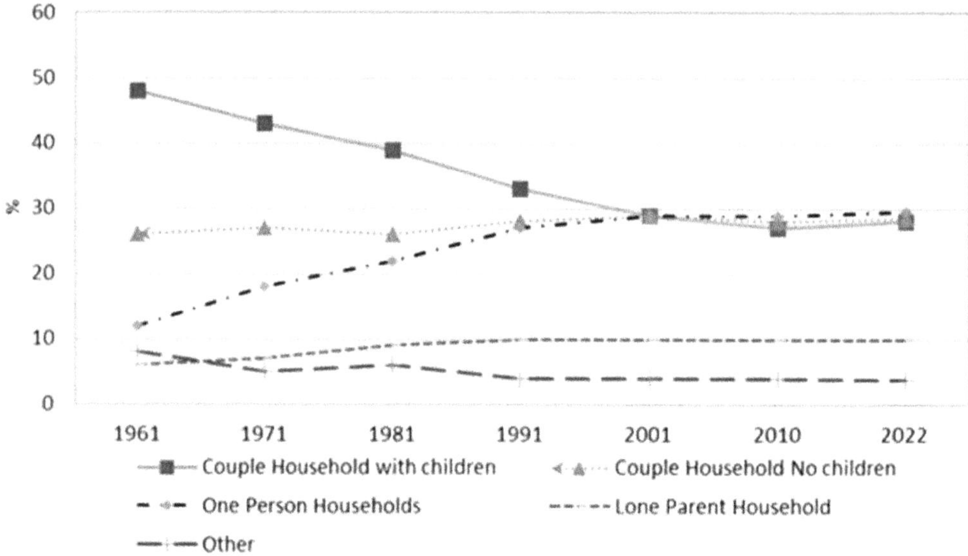

Figure 3.1 Changes in household type in the UK, 1961–2022.

Source: Beaumont (2011: Table 2) and Office for National Statistics (ONS) (2023: Table 7).

as a consequence of illness, disability or old age, the expectation was that nuclear family would provide such care.

Jaspers (2022) has argued that this and other aspects of the nuclear family have been a significant cause of inequality and discrimination for those not living in a nuclear family, meaning that the move away from it is beneficial in many ways. As an example of this, consider that in the past, it was common for unmarried pregnant young girls, and sometimes women, to hand their children over to be taken into care or for 'forced adoptions' to occur where they did not agree voluntarily, due to the stigma that there was around being a single parent (House of Commons and House of Lords Joint Committee on Human Rights, 2022). This event caused significant negative health and well-being issues for both the child and the parent, such as physical trauma, mental health trauma such as anxiety and depression, shame, embarrassment and emotional, physical and sexual abuse (House of Commons and House of Lords Joint Committee on Human Rights, 2022). In this context, it can be argued that the move away from the nuclear family type has had specific beneficial outcomes for health and social care, in terms of limiting the greater stigma and discrimination that other family types, especially lone parents, would have experienced in the past (Mackenzie, 2023). This, in turn, leads to better health and well-being for such family types, which limits the necessity for health and social care. Additionally, for many people, living alone is an active choice which improves their health and well-being in comparison to living together in families and households that cause stress and lead to unhappiness. For example, there is evidence that time alone can lead to feelings of less stress, less pressure and feelings of greater autonomy (Weinstein *et al.*, 2023). In this sense, the move away from the nuclear family type can be viewed positively and beneficial to health and well-being, and very likely leading to less requirement for health and social care for many people.

However, with the continued decline of the nuclear family type, the question of 'who cares?' comes to the fore. In particular, the replacement of the nuclear family type with one person households as the most dominant family type means that there is less possibility of providing care in the family if and when an individual becomes ill. For example, the significant increase in divorce rates since the 1960s, from two divorces per thousand married people in 1960 to a peak of 14 divorces per thousand married people in the 1990s (ONS, 2024), limits the possibility of spousal care, especially in older age when it is more likely to be needed.

Moreover, research shows that those living alone are more likely to suffer from a number of negative health and social care outcomes, such as poor mental health (Chen *et al.*, 2022), dying earlier in younger individuals (Zhao *et al.*, 2022), depression in adults (Mykyta, 2024) and lower life satisfaction (McElroy *et al.*, 2023). This shows that living alone can increase both health care needs and social care needs, which means more health and social care resources required for these and other conditions. As an example, consider the case of an individual living alone who is subject to **detainment/sectioning** (Learning Box 3.1) in a hospital unit as a consequence of a mental health episode or illness. Often, there will be a concern that discharging the individual to living alone will be problematic, for reasons such as an inability to take medication on their own or to care for themself. This means that the individual stays in hospital for longer than would occur if they did not live alone. This not only increases the likelihood that the individual acquires further infections in hospital, and therefore has to stay even longer, but also has a significant financial cost in terms of the cost of the ongoing hospital care (Turner *et al.*, 2016).

This means that a direct consequence of more people living alone is that there is less expectation that the family will provide care and more expectation that care will be provided in other ways. This is most likely to be through the NHS or through local authority provided social care. This presents increasing financial pressures on health and social care in terms of managing resources in the face of increasing demand. This, in turn, increases the pressure on those who work in health and social care to work to ensure that individuals needs are met in the context of limited resources.

Demographic changes

Another key change that has occurred over the last 50–60 years has been demographic changes. Demographic change refers to the way that the size, movement and structure of the population changes. In terms of size, the population can get smaller or larger, such as

> **Learning Box 3.1: Detainment/sectioning of individuals**
>
> Detainment/sectioning refers to where someone is required to stay in a hospital to receive treatment for a mental health condition. This is usually because they are a potential harm to themselves or to others. Detainment/sectioning can only occur after a mental health assessment by an approved mental health professional (AMHP) (see Learning Box 5.1). There are different types of detainment/sectioning, depending on the nature of the harm posed. This is why it is called sectioning, because people can be detained under different sections of the law. Some detainment/sectioning can be voluntary, but others can be compulsory.

when there is an increase or reduction in the number of people being born; in terms of movement, populations can move from one area to another, such as when people immigrate or emigrate between countries and regions; and the structure of populations can change, such as when there is an increase in the number of older or younger people in a population. All of these factors can have significant effects on health and social care, as detailed below.

The key overall change to the UK population over the last 60 years has been its large growth. It has grown from an estimated 52.5 million people in 1960 to just under 68 million people in 2024 (Worldometer, 2024). This is an increase of around 15 million people, or just under 30%. Within this large growth, there are four major demographic factors with the potential to impact on health and social care.

The first is the fact that people are living longer. This is known as increased life expectancy. In 1960, men could expect to live until the age of 68 and women to the age of 73. In 2020, this had increased to the age of 78 for men and the age of 87 for women (ONS, 2022). This means that there are more older people in the population. To exemplify this, consider that in 1981, there were approximately 5.4 million people aged over 65 in England, but in 2021, this number had increased to 10.4 million people aged over 65 in England (Centre for Ageing Better, 2022), which is more than double. The effect of this increased life expectancy is increasing the size of population and changing the structure of the population.

Linked to this is that secondly, less people are dying overall in the population. This is largely in part due to improvements in health and social care for conditions that people would have died of previously. This not only means that people are surviving conditions early on in life that would have previously led to death, such as extremely premature births (Smith *et al.*, 2023), but also that people are living longer with conditions that would have previously led to death, such as cancer, as the survival rate has increased from by 37% for men and 33% for women, despite the fact that cancer rates have increased significantly (Shelton *et al.*, 2024). This is referred to as a falling mortality rate, meaning that people are dying later than they would have previously. The effect of the falling mortality rate is to increase the size of the population.

Thirdly, the number of children being born in the population is falling. This is known as a falling fertility rate. In 1960, the fertility rate in the UK was 2.69 births per woman, meaning that the average woman would have 2.69 children. However, in 2020, the fertility rate in the UK had fallen to 1.56 births per woman (World Bank, 2024). This means that on average, women are giving birth to one less child now than they did 50 years ago. This effect of falling fertility rate is to reduce the size of the population.

Finally, the UK has seen significant increases in net migration since the 1960s. When talking about migration, we need to distinguish between emigration and immigration. Emigration refers to when people leave a country to settle in another country. Immigration refers to when people arrive in another country to live there. The difference between the number of people who emigrate and the number of people who immigrate is what is referred to as *net migration*. For instance, in 1964, there were 211,000 people who immigrated, and 278,000 who emigrated, giving a negative net migration figure of –60,000 people, meaning that 60,000 more people left the UK to live elsewhere than arrived to live in the UK (Statista, 2024). However, in the years since, the net migration figure has largely been positive, meaning more people arriving in the country to live than leaving the country. This is shown in Figure 3.2.

Figure 3.2 shows how the over the last 60 years, the nature of net migration has changed. For much of the period up to the mid-1980s, net migration was negative,

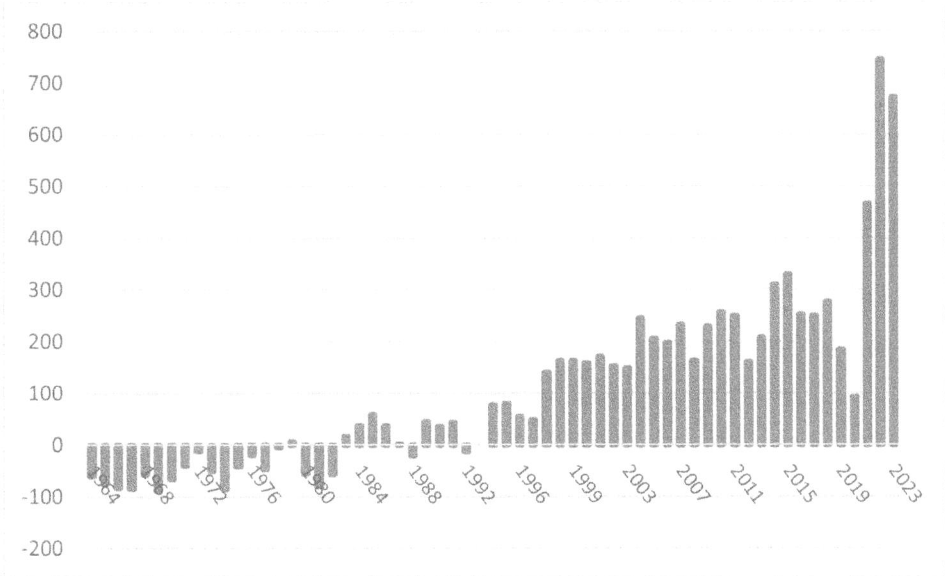

Figure 3.2 UK net migration, 1964–2023.
Source: Statista (2024).

meaning that more people were leaving the UK to live elsewhere than arriving in the UK to live there. However, this started to change in the mid-1980s, when more people started to arrive in the UK to live than leaving the UK to live elsewhere. This positive net migration trend accelerated in the mid-1990s, and has continued since then. In 2022, the net migration figure was positive at 745,000 people, meaning that 745,000 more people arrived in the UK to live there than left to live elsewhere. Net migration can have either a positive or negative effect on the population, but over the last 20 years or so, the trend has been towards positive net migration rather than negative net migration. This has had the effect of increasing the size of the population and changing the structure of the population.

Table 3.1 provides a summary of these main demographic changes and their effect on the population, in terms of resulting in either an increase or a decrease in the population. As Table 3.1 shows, the demographic changes are leading to both increases and decreases in the population. However, most of the changes have led to increases in the population, meaning that overall, the demographic changes are leading to increases in the population. These are the main reasons why since the 1960s, the UK population has increased by 15 million people as detailed above, and is projected to increase to approximately 74 million by 2036 (ONS, 2024a).

For health and social care, the immediate implication of an increasing population is an increase in demand for health and social care services. This leads to the similar question identified in relation to social change posed above of 'who cares?'. This is especially evident in relation to the increased life expectancy, which is leading to more older people in the population. It is in older age that people tend to need and use more health and social care than at other ages (Sealey, 2015), and so this change will likely lead to increased

Table 3.1 Main demographic changes in the UK over the last 20 years

Demographic change	*Explanation*	*Effect on population*
Increased life expectancy	People are living longer	• Increase in size of the population • Changing the structure of the population
Falling mortality rate	Less people in the population are dying	• Increase in size of the population
Falling fertility rate	Less children are being born in the population	• Decrease in size of the population
Increased net migration	More people coming to live in the UK than leaving the UK to live elsewhere	• Increase in the size of the population • Changing the structure of the population

demand for health and social care. Additionally, an increase elderly population will likely lead to increases in the amount of ill-health and disability in the population, such as heart conditions, cancer and diabetes (Government Office for Science, 2016), which also increases the need for health and social care.

The falling mortality rate also likely increases the demand for health and social care, as it creates a need for resources for health and social care conditions that did not previously exist. A good example of this is in relation to premature live births, which is defined as where a baby is born before 37 weeks gestation. According to Hand (2017), when the NHS was launched in 1946, the survival rates for premature babies were very low and no baby born less that 2lbs 3oz survived. However, improvements in health mean that the chances of survival following a premature birth have increased and continue to increase. These improvements have required health resources greater than that previously provided, such as the need for one-to-one neonatal nursing care. Additionally, babies born prematurely are more likely to have ongoing social care needs, either in the form of a severe disability (such as lung disease), a moderate disability (such as a visual or hearing impairment) or a mild disability (such as a squint or requiring glasses) (Tommy's, 2023). At the other end of the age spectrum, the growth in dementia, which is typically a disease of old age, has required the need for both health and social care services that are 'dementia friendly' (Innes *et al.*, 2021). A report for the Alzheimer's Society (Wittenberg *et al.*, 2019) estimates that the total cost of dementia care in the UK is £34.7 billion, with an expectation that this will rise to £94.1 billion by 2040. Additionally, it is social care costs which are the most significant component of these costs.

Both the increased life expectancy and falling mortality rate are changes that are increasing the demand for health and social care services. On the other hand, the falling fertility rate, is a change that is decreasing the demand for health and social care. This is because it reduces the population, thereby reducing the need for services. However, a more specific effect that the falling fertility rate has is limiting the number of people in the workforce, thereby limiting the health and social care workforce at a time when increased life expectancy and falling mortality rates are increasing the need for health and social care workforce (Gietel-Basten *et al.*, 2022). For example, consider where a falling fertility rate means that in a given year, 10,000 less babies are born. This means that there are less people who grow up to be adults and therefore enter the labour market as employees, including health and social care employees, at a time of

Learning Box 3.2: Health tourism

Health tourism refers to the claim that non-UK nationals deliberately travel to the UK specifically to receive health treatments on the NHS. For example, there have been claims that people with cancer have specifically travelled to the UK to receive treatment, and that pregnant mothers have likewise come to the UK to give birth. The claim of health tourism lies in the fact that emergency NHS treatment is free to all, regardless of nationality. While there has been some evidence of deliberate health tourism, the evidence is that it accounts for a very small amount of NHS spending, at 0.3% (The Medic Portal, 2024). As a consequence of these claims, there were changes in legislation to charge non-insured individuals for their non-emergency treatment. It should be noted that the majority of medical professional bodies such as the British Medical Association oppose these charges on the grounds that they are disproportionate and can lead to the spread of disease. Additionally, according to the Department of Health, it is expatriate UK nationals who are the biggest participants of health tourism (Graham, 2016).

increased demand. This means that a smaller number of health and social care workers are available to support the increased health and social care need, which is likely to lead to either to lower quality of care as less workers are required to care for more people with more complex needs, and/or stress, anxiety and burnout in the health and social care workforce.

The increased net migration means an overall increase in the population, which means an overall increase in demand for health and social care services. However, the overall effect of this on health and social care is disputed (Varga-Silva *et al.*, 2022). On the one hand, there is the argument that the use of health services such as hospitals and GP practices leads to longer waiting times for GP appointments and treatments, especially leading to **health tourism** (Learning Box 3.2).

On the other hand, there is the observation that many migrants work in health and social care, meaning that they fill the skills gap that is evident in both. It should also be noted that most migrants are of working age (meaning aged between 16 and 64), and so younger than the general population, which means that they are more likely to be working than the general population and therefore contributing to the health and social care in the form of taxes (Varga-Silva *et al.*, 2022). They are also more likely to be fitter than the general population, meaning that they are less likely to require health and social care than the general population (Goldberg, 2023).

Migrants have also been important in filling vacancies in health and social care, with an estimate that migrants make up 17% of the NHS staff (Goldberg, 2023), which is much higher than the proportion of migrants in the population as a whole. In the absence of such migrants, it is likely that the number of employees in health and social care would be much less, which would result in significant gaps in care for service users and additional working pressures for employees of health and social care. This means that overall, the increase in migrants provides specific benefits to health and social care that limits some of the negative effects of the other demographic changes.

Technological changes

As detailed above, a key demographic change has been the falling mortality rate, meaning that less people are dying than previously. This change has occurred from a variety of factors, such as improvements in food security and diet, improvements in public health such as better sanitation and improvement in public security such as less violence in society. Another key factor in relation to this is improvements in health and social care technology which not only means that people are surviving conditions at birth that they would have died from previously, but that people are living longer with conditions that they would have preciously died from earlier, as detailed above. Perhaps more significantly is the potential that technology provides for individuals to not just live longer but to improve the quality of life for those living with conditions that would previously have been chronic and life limiting, such as diabetes in relation to health (Mills, 2019), or autism in relation to social care (Valencia *et al.*, 2019).

With the development of Artificial Intelligence (AI), the likelihood is that technology will at least continue to play an important role in health and social care, if not an increasing role, and the government have prioritised the continued use of technology as important to health and social care in the future (Department of Health and Social Care, 2021). For example, some social care providers are already using AI chatbots to generate care plans or writing meeting notes (Institute for Ethics in AI, 2024). This highlights how technology will also likely be important to health and social care in the future.

We can define technology in relation to health and social care as any device or procedure that is specifically designed to improve health and social care outcomes. This definition allows us to acknowledge that both big technological changes and small technological changes are important to health and social care, as the focus is usually on big technological changes. For example, big technological changes in health like dialysis machines, MRI scanners and DNA sequencing have all been important big changes, but so have small changes such as improvements in hand washing, the development of portable monitoring equipment such as for blood pressure and the use of video conferencing to conduct appointments. Similarly, there have been big technological changes in social care such as the development of wheelchairs and mobility scooters, the use of telecare for consultations and the use of alarm-receiving centres for people living at home but susceptible to falls. There have also been small technological changes such as wearable devices like smart watches, devices to enable independent living such as those that control lights and other devices in the home, and even the development of apps to deal with issues such as loneliness.

The examples of technology provided above enable us to identify three key perceived benefits of technology to health and social care. The first is that it improves practice by making it easier to do things than it would have been previously, and in this sense empowers service users in particular towards living independently rather than in living in institutions (NHS Confederation, 2023). Using the example of devices that enable independent living such as those that control lights and other devices in the home, this enables service users to be in control of what they do and when they do it, meaning that they are more independent for themselves rather than being dependent on others to do things for them. This leads on to a second benefit of technology, that of making things quicker than they would normally be, meaning that it leads to more efficient use of resources (Maguire *et al.*, 2018). Using the example of wearable devices above, these provide information that can be downloaded and analysed much quicker than the manual inputting of the information, and this means that the time saved can be used to provide health and social care to other service users. Finally, the use of such technologies can be cheaper than the alternative (Wardle, 2024). For example, the use of mobility scooters to enable people to get out and about on their own is cheaper than providing a permanent carer to ensure that the service user gets out and about.

These benefits are not independent of each other but can occur together, as making things easier can also make things quicker which can also make things cheaper. They can also be seen as helping to solve some of the issues previously identified in relation to social and demographic changes. For instance, the issue of loneliness identified as a consequence of social changes may be less of a problem in a world where people are more connected with each other through technology, such as through the use of apps (Zamir *et al.*, 2020). The issue of the increased demand for health and social care as a consequence of demographic changes may also be less challenging where technology reduces the cost of care and so frees up more money and resources to provide care to more people (Lolich *et al.*, 2019). For example, it is estimated that individuals not taking their medication costs £900 million per year in England alone, but the use of apps to remind people to take their medication has been evidenced to improve compliance and therefore reduce cost to health and social care (Armitage *et al.*, 2020). If we refer back to the example earlier of the sectioned patient who remains in hospital due to concerns about whether medication would be taken, this is an example of where technology in the form of apps could be a solution to the problem.

It should be noted here that the use of technology in health and social care requires consideration of specific issues that may limit its potential use. For instance, technology is not cost free, meaning that it can be quite expensive for either the service user or the provider, and this can limit the possibility of its use. For example, a mobility scooter can vary in price from £800 to £5,000, which may be too expensive for some. This itself can lead to what The Academy of Medical Sciences (2020) term the 'digital divide', meaning an unequal access to technology that leads to inequalities in care between groups based on their ability to afford the technology. This digital divide may be evident in what we consider as commonplace technologies, such as smartphone access or superfast broadband, which would lead to a digital divide in many ways.

Additionally, in promoting the use of wearable technologies such as smart watches or using video conferencing for consultations, there is likely to be less physical contact between the service user and health and social care professionals. The importance of physical contact is well known in terms of its generally positive effect on health and well-being (Heatley Tejada *et al.*, 2020), as was especially shown during the COVID-19 pandemic (Hasenack *et al.*, 2023). In specific relation to health and social care, a lack of physical meetings can lead to a lack of social connections, which, in turn, is linked to both negative physical health conditions such as coronary heart disease, stroke, early mortality and malnutrition, as well as mental health conditions such as depression in young and adult populations, social anxiety, psychosis, dementia and cognitive impairment in later life and late life suicidal ideation (Morina *et al.*, 2021). More specifically, a lack of physical contact can lead to increased loneliness, which has already been identified above as a major issue arising from social changes. This would significantly limit the beneficial outcomes of technology.

As stated above, the expectation is that the use of technology will continue to increase in health and social care, especially AI-related technology. AI-related technology can benefit health and social care in specific ways, such as responding to queries from individuals

(Ayers *et al.*, 2023). However, AI is limited in terms of its accuracy of information for specific conditions (Bir Yücel *et al.*, 2024), and where a high level of physical contact and critical thinking skills are important, which is relevant in much of health and social care occupations (Moulds and Horton, 2023). This means that while AI might complement health and social care practice, it is unlikely to replace it.

Summary

This chapter has outlined the key social, demographic and technological changes that have happened over the last 50–60 years. It has analysed the significant effect these changes are having on health and social care in both positive and negative ways, and are likely to continue to do so in the future.

A key point to take away from the chapter is that these changes should not be seen as separate from each other but as interlinked with each other. By this, it is meant that we cannot separate changes in the family from demographic changes, and we cannot separate demographic changes from changes in technology. Indeed, it is typically the case that the changes feed into each other, as evident from the example of how the increase in single-person households can and has occurred from the fact that people are living longer, which, in turn, is occurring from improvements in health and social care.

For health and social care, the key issue that these changes pose is the question of 'who cares?'. This is because the changes have not only disrupted traditional patterns of care, but introduced new care requirements. There is the potential for technology to answer this question to some extent through making care easier, quicker and cheaper. However, the adoption of such technology to caring requires a critical and careful consideration of its effect on the outcomes for service users now and in the future.

References

Armitage, L.C., Kassavou, A. and Sutton, S. (2020) 'Do mobile device apps designed to support medication adherence demonstrate efficacy? A systematic review of randomised controlled trials, with meta-analysis', *BMJ Open*, 10(1), p. e032045. Available at https://doi.org/10.1136/bmjopen-2019-032045

Ayers, J.W. *et al.* (2023) 'Comparing physician and artificial intelligence chatbot responses to patient questions posted to a public social media Forum', *JAMA Internal Medicine*, 183(6), p. 589. Available at https://doi.org/10.1001/jamainternmed.2023.1838

Beaumont, J. (2011) (London) Households and Family. Social Trends 41. Office for National Statistics. Available at https://link.springer.com/content/pdf/10.1057/st.2011.5.pdf (Accessed 28 February 2024).

Bekhradnia, B. and Beech, D. (2018) *Demand for Higher Education to 2030*. HEPI Report 105. Oxford: Higher Education Policy Institute. Available at https://www.hepi.ac.uk/wp-content/uploads/2018/03/HEPI-Demand-for-Higher-Education-to-2030-Report-105-FINAL.pdf (Accessed 28 February 2024).

Bir Yücel, K. *et al.* (2024) 'Can artificial intelligence provide accurate and reliable answers to cancer patients' questions about cancer pain? Comparison of chatbots based on ESMO cancer pain guideline', *Memo - Magazine of European Medical Oncology*. [Preprint]. Available at https://doi.org/10.1007/s12254-023-00954-6

Bourquin, P., Brewer, M. and Wernham, T. (2022) *Trends in Income and Wealth Inequalities*. The IFS. Available at https://doi.org/10.1920/re.ifs.2022.0228

Bristowe, K. *et al.* (2018) 'Recommendations to reduce inequalities for LGBT people facing advanced illness: ACCESSCare national qualitative interview study', *Palliative Medicine*, 32(1), pp. 23–35. Available at https://doi.org/10.1177/0269216317705102

Centre for Ageing Better (2022) *The State of Ageing 2022*. London: Centre for Better Ageing. Available at https://ageing-better.org.uk/summary-state-ageing-2022 (Accessed 4 March 2024).

Chen, T.-Y. *et al.* (2022) 'Living alone is associated with a higher prevalence of psychiatric morbidity in a population-based cross-sectional study', *Frontiers in Public Health*, 10, p. 1054615. Available at https://doi.org/10.3389/fpubh.2022.1054615

Department for Health and Social Care (2021) *People at the Heart of Care: adult social care reform white paper*. Available at: https://www.gov.uk/government/publications/people-at-the-heart-of-care-adult-social-care-reform-white-paper (Accessed: 8 September 2025).

Gietel-Basten, S., Rotkirch, A. and Sobotka, T. (2022) 'Changing the perspective on low birth rates: Why simplistic solutions won't work', *BMJ*, 379, p. e072670. Available at https://doi.org/10.1136/bmj-2022-072670

Goldberg, E. (2023) 'Is immigration harming the NHS?'. Available at https://www.nhsconfed.org/articles/immigration-harming-nhs (Accessed 4 March 2024).

Government Office for Science (2016) *Future of an Ageing Population*. GS/16/10. London: Government Office for Science. Available at https://assets.publishing.service.gov.uk/media/5d273adce5274a5862768ff9/future-of-an-ageing-population.pdf (Accessed 4 March 2024).

Graham, G. (2016) *FactCheck: Does health tourism cost the NHS billions?, Channel 4 News*. Available at https://www.channel4.com/news/factcheck/factcheck-health-tourism-cost-nhs-billions (Accessed 7 March 2024).

Hand, J. (2017) 'Premature Birth and the NHS', *People's History of the NHS*, 26 March. Available at https://peopleshistorynhs.org/encyclopaedia/premature-birth-and-the-nhs/ (Accessed 4 March 2024).

Hasenack, B. *et al.* (2023) 'Longing for touch post-COVID-19: Current observations and future directions', *Scientific Reports*, 13(1), p. 22131. Available at https://doi.org/10.1038/s41598-023-49113-1

Heatley Tejada, A., Dunbar, R.I.M. and Montero, M. (2020) 'Physical contact and loneliness: Being touched reduces perceptions of loneliness', *Adaptive Human Behavior and Physiology*, 6(3), pp. 292–306. Available at https://doi.org/10.1007/s40750-020-00138-0

House of Commons and House of Lords Joint Committee on Human Rights (2022) *The Violation of Family Life: Adoption of Children of Unmarried Women 1949–1976*. HC 270/HL 43. London: House of Commons. Available at https://committees.parliament.uk/publications/23076/documents/169043/default/ (Accessed 29 February 2024).

Innes, A., Smith, S.K. and Bushell, S. (2021) 'Dementia friendly care: Methods to improve stakeholder engagement and decision making', *Journal of Healthcare Leadership*, 13, pp. 183–197. Available at https://doi.org/10.2147/JHL.S292939

Institute for Ethics in AI (2024) *Oxford Statement on the responsible use of generative AI in Adult Social Care*. Available at https://www.oxford-aiethics.ox.ac.uk/oxford-statement-responsible-use-generative-ai-adult-social-care (Accessed 11 March 2024).

Jaspers, E., van der Lippe, T. and Evertsson, M. (2022) 'Gender inequality, households, and work', in K. Gërxhani, N. de Graaf, and W. Raub (eds.) *Handbook of Sociological Science: Contributions to Rigorous Sociology*. Edward Elgar Publishing, pp. 176–195. Available at https://doi.org/10.4337/9781789909432

Lolich, L. *et al.* (2019) 'Embracing technology? Health and Social Care professionals' attitudes to the deployment of e-Health initiatives in elder care services in Catalonia and Ireland', *Technological Forecasting and Social Change*, 147, pp. 63–71. Available at: https://doi.org/10.1016/j.techfore.2019.06.012

Mackenzie, J. (2023) '"I had to work through what people would think of me": Negotiating "problematic single motherhood" as a solo or single adoptive mum', *Critical Discourse Studies*, 20(1), pp. 88–105. Available at https://doi.org/10.1080/17405904.2021.1997775

Maguire, D. *et al.* (2018) *Digital Change in Health and Social Care*. London: Kink's Fund. Available at https://www.kingsfund.org.uk/insight-and-analysis/reports/digital-change-health-social-care (Accessed 7 March 2024).

McElroy, E. *et al.* (2023) 'Living alone and mental health: Parallel analyses in UK longitudinal population surveys and electronic health records prior to and during the COVID-19 pandemic', *BMJ Mental Health*, 26(1). Available at https://doi.org/10.1136/bmjment-2023-300842

Mills, J. (2019) 'Digital health technology in palliative care: Friend or foe?', *Progress in Palliative Care*, 27(4), pp. 145–146. Available at https://doi.org/10.1080/09699260.2019.1650420

Morina, N. *et al.* (2021) 'Potential impact of physical distancing on physical and mental health: A rapid narrative umbrella review of meta-analyses on the link between social connection and health', *BMJ Open*, 11(3), p. e042335. Available at https://doi.org/10.1136/bmjopen-2020-042335

Moulds, A. and Horton, T. (2023) *What Do Technology and AI Mean for the Future of Work in Health Care?* London: The Health Foundation. Available at https://www.health.org.uk/publications/long-reads/what-do-technology-and-ai-mean-for-the-future-of-work-in-health-care (Accessed 7 March 2024).

Mykyta, L. (2024) 'National Health Statistics Reports, Number 199, February 15, 2024', (199). Available at https://www.cdc.gov/nchs/data/nhsr/nhsr199.pdf (Accessed 29 February 2024).

NHS Confederation (2023) *Patient Empowerment: What Is the Role of Technology in Transforming Care?* London. Available at https://www.nhsconfed.org/publications/patient-empowerment-what-role-technology-transforming-care (Accessed 7 March 2024).

Office for National Statistics (2022) *Mortality in England and Wales.* London: Office for National Statistics. Available at https://www.ons.gov.uk/peoplepopulationandcommunity/birthsdeathsandmarriages/lifeexpectancies/articles/mortalityinenglandandwales/pastandprojectedtrendsinaveragelifespan (Accessed 29 February 2024).

Office for National Statistics (2023) 'Families and households'. Available at https://www.ons.gov.uk/peoplepopulationandcommunity/birthsdeathsandmarriages/families/datasets/familiesandhouseholdsfamiliesandhouseholds (Accessed 28 February 2024).

Office for National Statistics (2024) *Divorces in England and Wales: 2022.* London: ONS. Available at https://www.ons.gov.uk/peoplepopulationandcommunity/birthsdeathsandmarriages/divorce/bulletins/divorcesinenglandandwales/2022 (Accessed 29 February 2024).

Office for National Statistics (2024a) *National population projections: 2021-based interim.* Available at https://www.ons.gov.uk/peoplepopulationandcommunity/populationandmigration/populationprojections/bulletins/nationalpopulationprojections/2021basedinterim (Accessed 4 March 2024).

Roberts, K. (2019) 'A future for UK leisure studies: Back to work', *International Journal of the Sociology of Leisure*, 2(3), pp. 239–253. Available at https://doi.org/10.1007/s41978-018-0020-z

Sealey, C. (2015) *Social Policy Simplified: Connecting Theory with People's Lives.* Basingstoke, Hampshire: Palgrave Macmillan.

Sealey, C. (2023) *Applying Social Policy to Criminal Justice Practice: What Every Practitioner Should Know.* Bristol: Policy Press.

Shelton, J. *et al.* (2024) '25 year trends in cancer incidence and mortality among adults aged 35-69 years in the UK, 1993-2018: Retrospective secondary analysis', *BMJ*, 384. Available at https://doi.org/10.1136/bmj-2023-076962

Smith, L.K. *et al.* (2023) 'Effect of national guidance on survival for babies born at 22 weeks' gestation in England and Wales: Population based cohort study', *BMJ Medicine*, 2(1). Available at https://doi.org/10.1136/bmjmed-2023-000579

Statista (2024) *UK long-term migration figures 2023, Statista.* Available at https://www.statista.com/statistics/283287/net-migration-figures-of-the-united-kingdom-y-on-y/ (Accessed 29 February 2024).

The Academy of Medical Sciences (2020) *Technology for sustainable health and social care.* Available at: https://acmedsci.ac.uk/more/news/technology-for-sustainable-health-and-social-care (Accessed: 8 September 2025).

The Medic Portal (2024) *Health Tourism.* Available at https://www.themedicportal.com/application-guide/medical-school-interview/nhs-hot-topics/health-tourism/ (Accessed 7 March 2024).

Thompson, G. *et al.* (2012) *Olympic Britain-Social and Economic Change since the 1908 and 1946 London Games.* London: House of Commons Library.

Tommy's (2023) *Premature birth statistics.* Available at https://www.tommys.org/pregnancy-information/premature-birth/premature-birth-statistics (Accessed 4 March 2024).

Turner, A.J., Nikolova, S. and Sutton, M. (2016) 'The effect of living alone on the costs and benefits of surgery amongst older people', *Social Science & Medicine (1982)*, 150, pp. 95–103. Available at https://doi.org/10.1016/j.socscimed.2015.11.053

Valencia, K. *et al.* (2019) 'The impact of technology on people with autism spectrum disorder: A systematic literature review', *Sensors (Basel, Switzerland)*, 19(20), p. 4485. Available at https://doi.org/10.3390/s19204485

Varga-Silva, C., Sumption, M. and Walsh, P. (2022) *Briefing: The Fiscal Impact of Immigration to the UK*. Oxford: The Migration Observatory. Available at https://migrationobservatory.ox.ac.uk/resources/briefings/the-fiscal-impact-of-immigration-in-the-uk/ (Accessed 4 March 2024).

Wardle, C. (2024) 'How can telehealth reduce health costs?'. Available at https://www.theaccess-group.com/en-gb/blog/hsc-how-can-telehealth-reduce-health-costs/ (Accessed 7 March 2024).

Weinstein, N. *et al.* (2023) 'Balance between solitude and socializing: Everyday solitude time both benefits and harms well-being', *Scientific Reports*, 13(1), p. 21160. Available at https://doi.org/10.1038/s41598-023-44507-7

Wells, J.C.K. *et al.* (2021) 'The future of human malnutrition: Rebalancing agency for better nutritional health', *Globalization and Health*, 17(1), p. 119. Available at https://doi.org/10.1186/s12992-021-00767-4

Wittenberg, R. *et al.* (2019) *Projections of Older People with Dementia and Costs of Dementia Care in the United Kingdom, 2019–2040*. CPEC Working Paper 5. London: London School of Economics and Political Science. Available at https://www.alzheimers.org.uk/sites/default/files/2019-11/cpec_report_november_2019.pdf (Accessed 4 March 2024).

World Bank (2024) *World Bank Open Data, World Bank Open Data*. Available at https://data.worldbank.org (Accessed 29 February 2024).

Worldometer (2024) *U.K. Population (2024) - Worldometer*. Available at https://www.worldometers.info/world-population/uk-population/ (Accessed 29 February 2024).

Zamir, S. *et al.* (2020) 'Intergroup "Skype" quiz sessions in care homes to reduce loneliness and social isolation in older people', *Geriatrics*, 5(4), p. 90. Available at https://doi.org/10.3390/geriatrics5040090

Zhao, Y. *et al.* (2022) 'Living alone and all-cause mortality in community-dwelling adults: A systematic review and meta-analysis', *eClinicalMedicine*, 54. Available at https://doi.org/10.1016/j.eclinm.2022.101677

4 Understanding health for health and social care practice

Lisa Mauro-Bracken

The aims of this chapter are to:

- **Outline different definitions of health**
- **Detail factors that influence definitions of health**
- **Outline the beneficial implications of understanding health for health and social care practice**

Introduction

Health is a fundamental aspect of human life, influencing our ability to live fully and achieve our potential. However, defining health is not straightforward. It is a complex concept due to its broad nature, which is influenced by numerous interconnected factors such as physical, mental, and social well-being. Examples of physical well-being include activities that help the person to feel energetic, able to handle daily tasks and to function. Mental well-being includes practices and habits that foster a sense of belonging, reduce stress, and develop resilience and coping mechanisms (Ni *et al.*, 2020). Social well-being looks at social connectedness through building positive relationships, spending time with friends and family or networking, and creating meaningful interactions (Holt-Lunstad, 2024).

Definitions of health have evolved over time in response to changing social, cultural, and political contexts (Blaxter, 2010). What one society considers healthy may differ significantly from another. For example, in some societies, being slim is considered a sign of good health, while in other societies, larger bodies are consider a sign of good health. This shows that there is no singular definition of health (Huber *et al.*, 2016) Concepts and definitions of health will both differ across diverse contexts, such as cultural, social, and professional settings (van Druten *et al.*, 2022). Therefore, health is influenced by a multitude of factors and cannot be fully understood without considering these various aspects and identifying a clear definition for practitioners and individuals to work within.

This chapter aims to provide a better understanding of health as a way to improve practice. It outlines different definitions of health and considers the implications of these definitions. The chapter identifies issues that influence the definitions of health, such as historical factors, subjective and objective factors, the multidimensional nature of health, and the individual's perspective of health. The chapter outlines the beneficial effects that understanding health can provide for health and social care practice.

DOI: 10.4324/9781032619309-5

Key definitions: Disease, illness and well-being

Before focusing on definitions of health specifically, it is essential to establish clearly what we mean by disease, illness, and well-being, as each of these terms carries distinct meanings that shape our understanding of health.

Disease

Disease refers to a specific pathological condition that affects the structure or function of an organism, often characterised by recognisable signs and symptoms. It is typically diagnosed through medical evaluation and may have underlying biological, genetic, or environmental causes (Walker and Rogers, 2018). Disease can range from acute conditions, such as infections or injuries, to chronic illnesses like diabetes or heart disease. Disease tends to relate to physical dimensions and definitions of health and is seen as objective or measurable (Walker and Rogers, 2018). Disease is a concept that links health to clinical medicine with a focus on what is wrong with the individual (Schramme, 2023). When including disease in the definition of health, it is seen as a negative definition and links to terms such as harm, dysfunction, lack of balance and need for treatment (van der Linden and Schermer, 2022; Marmot *et al.*, 2010).

Illness

Illness, however, includes the subjective experience of feeling unwell or experiencing distress, whether physical, emotional, or mental. Illness can also be viewed in terms of functional impairments that affect an individual's ability to perform daily activities (van der Linden and Schermer, 2022). It involves cognitive representations that influence how individuals perceive and manage their health conditions (Lau, 1997). This means illness reflects an individual's perception and experience of their health and may include symptoms that impact daily functioning. Unlike disease, illness may not always have clear biomedical origins and can be influenced by factors such as social, cultural, and psychological contexts. Therefore, it is important to consider the context in which illness occurs and its impact on a person's quality of life (Walker and Rogers, 2018).

Well-being

Well-being extends beyond health and encompasses overall quality of life, satisfaction, and fulfilment in various aspects of life. It includes physical, emotional, social, and cognitive dimensions, reflecting an individual's sense of happiness, purpose, and contentment (Aked *et al.*, 2008). Well-being can be influenced by factors such as personal relationships, socioeconomic status, environmental conditions, and access to resources and opportunities (Naidoo and Wills, 2022). It focuses on a positive state, creating equilibrium or balance, and is closely linked to mental health, with positive well-being contributing to lower levels of stress and anxiety (Holt-Lunstad, 2024). The role of community and social support is also significant, as strong social networks can enhance an individual's sense of belonging and security (Holt-Lunstad, 2024). Furthermore, engaging in meaningful activities and having a sense of autonomy are crucial for maintaining high levels of well-being (Naidoo and Wills, 2016).

Definitions of health

An important part of understanding health is defining what we mean by health. However, this is not easy, as health has been defined in various ways over time, ranging from the absence of disease to a focus on well-being. Below is an outline of some ways that health has been defined.

Health as absence of illness or disease

This definition focuses on the physical aspects of health and the absence of pathological conditions, such as disease, injury, or pain. Health here is seen as a negative, with emphasis on the lack of symptoms and the absence of medical conditions as an indicator of good health (Svalastog *et al.*, 2017; Williams, 1983). This perspective is often used in medical contexts where the primary goal is to diagnose and treat diseases. However, this definition has been critiqued for being too narrow and not accounting for the broader aspects of health (Blaxter, 1990). Huber *et al.* (2016) propose a more dynamic concept of health, emphasising the ability to adapt and self-manage care in the face of social, physical, and emotional challenges. Van der Linden and Schermer (2022) also argue that health and disease should be viewed as practical and context-specific concepts, rather than seeking a rigid definition.

Health as a resource and strength

Seedhouse (1986) offers a broader definition of health, viewing health as the foundation for achieving one's potential. He argues that health is not just about the absence of disease but also about having the resources to achieve personal goals and live a fulfilling life. This view emphasises the ability to perform daily activities, to function, and to maintain physical resilience even in the presence of minor ailments. This approach aligns with the concept of health as a dynamic and positive resource that supports overall well-being (Naidoo and Wills, 2022). Additionally, Huber *et al.* (2016) support this perspective by highlighting the importance of resilience and resourcefulness in maintaining health. Van Druten *et al.* (2022) further emphasise that health concepts need to be specified for different contexts, suggesting that a general health definition may not be applicable in all healthcare practices and that having a wider conceptual view may enable practitioners to adapt to different circumstances.

Health as physical, mental and social well-being

The World Health Organization (WHO, 1948) defined health as 'a state of complete physical, mental, and social well-being and not merely the absence of disease or infirmity'. The definition sees health as a broad concept that emphasises mental and social factors as well as the absence of disease. Schramme (2023) argues that this definition highlights the comprehensive nature of health, as opposed to seeing health only as an absence of disease. Schramme (2023) also explains that this definition does not imply that individuals must achieve perfect health, but rather it highlights the importance of striving for a balanced state of well-being that encompasses various dimensions of life. This holistic view acknowledges the interconnectedness of various dimensions of health and the importance of a balanced approach to well-being (Blaxter, 2010). Svalastog *et al.* (2017)

also highlight the evolving nature of health definitions, emphasising the impact of digital knowledge landscapes on individual and collective understandings of health.

The idea of health as complete well-being has been critiqued as unrealistic and unattainable especially in the context of chronic diseases and ageing populations (Huber *et al.*, 2016). The definition has been seen as idealistic and potentially leads to the perception that almost everyone is unhealthy at some point in their lives (Blaxter, 2010). Further, Svalastog *et al.* (2017) emphasise the need for definitions that are sensitive to cultural differences, which is not explicitly highlighted in the WHO definition.

These definitions highlight that health can be defined in more than one way, from a very narrow definition focused on illness and disease, to a broader definition focused on what an individual can do, to a very broad definition that includes mental and social well-being. Understanding these different perspectives can help in developing more effective health policies and interventions that address the diverse needs of individuals and communities. The more recent attempts to define health highlight the dynamic nature of health and the importance of having a contextual and balanced view when working in health and social care.

Why is the way health is defined important for practitioners?

For practitioners, understanding the way health is defined is essential for several reasons. First, it informs practitioners' approach to care. A narrow definition of health leads to a narrow focus on physical symptoms and treatment. Conversely, a comprehensive definition of health allows practitioners to address not only physical symptoms but also the mental and social aspects of well-being which is beneficial for chronic health conditions (Huber et al. 2016; Blaxter, 1990). Second, it helps practitioners to communicate more effectively with patients. By understanding the different definitions of health, practitioners can better explain health conditions and treatments in a way that resonates with patients' experiences and beliefs (National Library of Medicine with National Institute of Health, 2015; Williams, 1983).

Finally, understanding how health is defined can enhance the effectiveness of health promotion and disease prevention efforts. Understanding the definition of health is crucial for health and care practitioners as it shapes their approach to patient/service user care, influences health policies, and impacts the overall effectiveness of health interventions (Naidoo and Wills, 2022; Dahlgren and Whitehead, 1991).

Factors influencing the definition of health

There are various factors that can influence the way that health is defined. These include historical factors, subjective and objective factors, and the multidimensional nature of health. These are discussed below. By recognising the various factors that influence health, practitioners can develop more holistic and targeted interventions that address the root causes of health issues (Cross, 2020; Ruggeri *et al.*, 2020).

The historical development of health

The word 'health' originates from the old English word 'hælan', which means wholeness, being whole, sound or well (Naidoo and Wills, 2022). The historic development of the word reflects the **holistic nature of health** (Learning Box 4.1), emphasising the importance of being whole and uninjured.

Learning Box 4.1: The holistic nature of health

The holistic nature of health acknowledges that individuals exist within complex systems where various factors interact to influence overall well-being. This approach emphasises the importance of considering the whole person rather than focusing solely on specific symptoms, injury, or conditions.

Holistic health encompasses physical, mental, emotional, social, environmental, and spiritual aspects of wellness (Schramme, 2023). WHO's (1948) definition of health as a complete state of physical, mental, and social well-being is an example of the holistic view of health.

Modern health models, such as the biopsychosocial (Engel, 1977) (see Chapter 8) and socio-ecological models, adopt a systems perspective, viewing biological, psychological, environmental and social factors as interconnected. Recognising health as holistic underscores the need for a balanced approach to care. Key practices involve promoting multidimensional wellness, person-centred care, preventive care, and nurturing mind-body-spirit and environmental connections.

Prior to scientific, medical developments, health was often linked to spiritual and religious beliefs. For instance, Traditional Chinese Medicine (TCM) focused on the balance between *yin* and *yang* energies to maintain health. Similarly, ancient Egyptian medicine combined using herbal and spiritual remedies to treat various conditions (Naidoo and Wills, 2022). **Shamanistic healers, traditional healers, and herbal healers** (Learning Box 4.2) use rituals and herbal remedies to cure illnesses often believed to be caused by evil spirits or divine punishment.

Learning Box 4.2: Healers

Shamanistic Healers are spiritual healers who often enter altered states of consciousness to interact with the spirit world (Smith, 2015). They use rituals, chants, and herbal remedies. Underlying beliefs see illnesses as spiritual imbalances or caused by evil spirits (Smith, 2015). They act as intermediaries between the physical and spiritual worlds.

Traditional Healers use indigenous knowledge passed down through generations to treat illnesses. They employ a combination of rituals, herbal remedies, and sometimes physical treatments (WHO, 2023). Illnesses can be caused by spiritual, physical, or social factors (WHO, 2023). They serve as community health practitioners with a holistic approach to healing.

Herbal Healers specialise in using plants and natural substances to treat. Their methods focus primarily on the preparation and administration of herbal remedies. Underlying beliefs suggest illnesses are treated through the natural properties of plants (National Library of Medicine with National Institute of Health, 2015). They often work within the framework of traditional medicine but focus specifically on botanical treatments.

Around 307 BC in ancient Greece, a Greek physician and philosopher called Hippocrates, often referred to as the 'Father of Medicine', began to use observation, reasoning, and logic to explain disease. He proposed the humoral theory which suggested that health depended on the balance of four bodily fluids: blood, phlegm, yellow bile and black bile (Naidoo and Wills, 2022). This marked a shift from supernatural explanations of disease to natural and observable causes.

These laid the foundation for the development of scientific approaches to health and medicine. For example, during the 18th and 19th centuries, the Enlightenment and the Industrial Revolution significantly influenced the perception of health. The Enlightenment emphasised reason, science, and empirical evidence. This means that observation, experimental and practical evidence was used, leading to advancements in medical knowledge and practices. The Industrial Revolution brought about urbanisation and changes in living conditions, which highlighted the need for public health measures to control infectious diseases. These developments reinforced the idea of health as the absence of disease, as preventing and treating diseases became central to medical practice. This period saw the development of germ theory by Louis Pasteur and Robert Koch, which identified microorganisms as the cause of many diseases (Naidoo and Wills, 2022). This scientific understanding shifted the focus of health from a holistic concept, as seen in ancient Egypt and Greece, to a more disease-centred approach.

In the 20th century, the biomedical model of health became dominant. This model views health primarily in terms of biological factors and emphasises the diagnosis and treatment of diseases. The success of antibiotics, vaccines, and other medical technologies further reinforced this perspective. The biomedical model's focus on disease eradication and management has profoundly shaped modern health and care systems and public health policies.

This very brief history of the development of health highlights that health is not set in stone but changes over time. Health has been defined from religious and spiritual beliefs, from observable causes, from scientific understanding and from biological factors to recognising the broader factors that are part of health. This is important because it means that health is not static but constantly changing, requiring a flexible and adaptive approach to understanding it and managing it.

Individual/lay experiences

Understanding the individual's experiences of health is important to how we provide care and is accepted as a key part to the support we provide today. Williams (1983) discussed this as the lay perspective, suggesting the importance of including these views when providing care for individuals. His research has been further supported by other sources which have explored how individual experiences with health and illness shape personal definitions of health, recognising this as a crucial factor in defining health (Cross, 2020; Lau, 1997). People's personal health journeys, including their experiences with diseases, living with chronic illness, treatments, recovering from an injury and general experience of healthcare systems, can shape one's understanding of health and what it means to be healthy. These individual experiences can lead to diverse and personalised health definitions, highlighting the subjective nature of health. The lay perspective is seen as particularly important when providing a person-centred approach in practice.

Cognitive and psychological factors

The cognitive and psychological factors of health highlight how mental health models and personal experiences with illness significantly influence their health perceptions. Mental health models or cognitive representations of health and illness can vary widely, affecting how individuals understand and manage their health. For example, an individual who has experienced chronic pain may develop a cognitive representation of health that emphasises the absence of pain as a key indicator of being healthy. These representations influence how people perceive, interpret, and respond to health-related information and experiences (Huber *et al.*, 2016; Lau, 1997). Therefore, cognitive and psychological factors are shaped by personal experiences, cultural beliefs, and social contexts. These factors underscore the need for personalised approaches in healthcare and education (Cross, 2020).

Cultural context

Cultural contexts refer to the ways in which traditions, beliefs, and social practices of a society shape and influence understanding and definitions of health and illness. Blaxter (1990, 2010) argues that health definitions are deeply rooted in cultural contexts because different societies have different cultural experiences. For instance, some cultures may prioritise physical health, while others may emphasise mental or spiritual well-being. Blaxter (2010) also notes that cultural differences can lead to varying interpretations of what constitutes health and illness and that in some cultures, health may be seen as a balance between body, mind, and spirit, while in others, it may be viewed more mechanistically. For example, Native American communities view health as a balance between physical, mental, and spiritual elements and will often seek support with illness from a local healer (National Library of Medicine with National Institute of Health, 2015). Dahlgren and Whitehead's (1991) social model of health, often illustrated by the 'rainbow model', highlights the significant role the wider determinants of health play in shaping our definitions, including the cultural contexts as perceived and addressed in various societies. For example, in low-income communities, health may primarily be associated with the ability to work and provide for one's family (Dahlgren and Whitehead, 1991). As we move into a digital society, new knowledge landscapes will further diversify our definitions of health particularly as information is more accessible that may broaden our views of medical and alternative approaches to care (Svalastog *et al.*, 2017). Understanding the historical and cultural contexts of health provides a foundation for exploring how social norms further shape and influence health behaviours and perceptions within different communities.

Economic factors

Economic factors, including access to healthcare, income levels and employment status, significantly influence health definitions and outcomes. Naidoo and Wills (2016) argue that economic disparities can lead to health inequities, where individuals from lower socioeconomic backgrounds may have different health experiences and perceptions compared to those from higher socioeconomic backgrounds. This supports Williams (1983) discussion on how individuals from different socioeconomic backgrounds may have varying access to healthcare resources, which, in turn, affects their health behaviours and attitudes. Marmot *et al.* (2020) further support this point also highlighting that those with higher socioeconomic status often have better access to healthcare services, healthier food options, and opportunities for physical activity, leading to a more positive outlook on health. Research has identified that individuals from lower socioeconomic backgrounds may face barriers to accessing care, resulting in a more reactive approach to health.

Social norms

Social norms are the mainly unwritten rules that guide human behaviour by encompassing three key aspects: what we do, what we believe others do, and what we believe others approve of and expect us to do (UNICEF, 2021). They are learned from an early age and these societal expectations and standards can influence what is considered healthy or unhealthy. For example, the ideal body image promoted by the media can affect individuals' perceptions of their own health and may lead to issues such as body dysmorphia or eating disorders. In contrast, a medical professional will use specific tools to manage the weight element and assess health/non-health based on the body measurements rather than a subjective idea of body image. Thus, understanding the role social norms play in decision making, behaviour and a community's functioning can inform how to make changes that improve health.

Scientific advancements

Scientific advancements continuously reshape our understanding of health. New medical discoveries and technologies also redefine what is considered healthy. For example, the development of vaccines has changed the perception of infectious diseases and their impact on health. Svalastog *et al.* (2017) and van der Linden and Schermer (2022) discuss how technological advancements, such as telemedicine and health apps, as well as new medical technologies and treatments have impacted how health is monitored and managed. They highlighted that scientific developments have led to context-specific definitions of health and a continuously evolving understanding of health and disease.

Environmental factors

The environment in which individuals live can also impact their health. Factors such as pollution, climate change, and access to green spaces can influence physical and mental well-being (Ni *et al.*, 2020). Van der Linden and Schermer (2022) emphasise the importance of considering the environmental context when defining health, as it affects individuals' ability to function and thrive. For instance, exposure to air pollution has been linked to respiratory and cardiovascular diseases, highlighting the need for clean air to maintain good health (Coughlin *et al.*, 2020). Climate change poses additional risks, such as increased frequency of extreme weather events, which can lead to injuries, mental health issues, and disruptions in healthcare services (Marmot *et al.*, 2020). Addressing these environmental determinants is crucial for promoting holistic health and well-being.

Political factors and institutional influences

Political decisions and policies can shape health definitions and access to healthcare. Government policies on healthcare funding, public health initiatives, and health education can influence how health is perceived and managed within a society. Van Druten *et al.* (2022) highlight that political contexts can affect health promotion strategies and the prioritisation of health issues, such as for example abortion or smoking. The World Health Organization's (1948) definition has significantly influenced global health policies and initiatives, promoting a comprehensive view of health. Institutional definitions, like that of the WHO, play a crucial role in shaping public health agendas and policies, emphasising the importance of a holistic approach to health.

Multidimensional nature of health

Health is not just one thing but is affected by lots of different factors. When we consider definitions of health, it is important to understand the various ways that these factors can influence the health of individuals, families, communities and societies. This is what is meant by the multidimensional nature of health. The multidimensional nature of health is important in three ways.

Firstly, it enables us to consider health in a wide sense, and not just a physical sense, and this can be important for individuals. For example, if we just consider health as referring to physical health, we could not consider someone experiencing loneliness as per the social dimension as having a health issue, even though we know that loneliness can have a serious effect on health. Secondly, although these dimensions are presented separately, they should be seen as linked together, as a change in one dimension can affect another. For example, a change in physical health, such as having a broken leg, can affect mental health in terms of how the person feels about their immediate context. Thirdly, these dimensions are not set in stone but can change over time, in terms of importance and number. For example, Svalastog *et al.* (2017) suggests it is important to reflect on the impact of digital technology and how our digital society has introduced new dimensions to the concept of health. The availability of health information online and the rise of digital health tools have transformed how people perceive and manage their health. This digital landscape adds another layer of complexity, as individuals now have access to a vast array of health-related information and resources, which can influence their understanding and behaviours.

These factors highlight that health is influenced by a complex interplay of historical, individual, cognitive and psychological, cultural, economic, social, scientific, environmental and political, and multidimensional contexts. Understanding these influences is crucial for developing a comprehensive an inclusive definition of health that can guide effective health practice and policy that cater to diverse populations and evolving societal needs. By considering these various influences, we can better appreciate the complexity of health and work towards more effective health promotion and care strategies.

The beneficial effects of understanding health for health and social care practice

Understanding different definitions, factors and dimensions perspectives of health allows health and social care practitioners to tailor their approach to meet the specific needs of the individual. This can lead to better practice and outcomes in a number of ways.

Increasing cultural competence in health and social care practice

Cultural competence and curiosity are crucial in health and care practice. Naidoo and Wills (2022) argue that healthcare providers must be aware of and respect the cultural beliefs and practices of their patients. This involves not only understanding cultural differences but also integrating this knowledge into care plans, asking questions in a sensitive way and responding openly to difference. For example, a practitioner might incorporate traditional healing practices into a treatment plan for a patient who values holistic medicine, thereby enhancing the patient's comfort and adherence to the treatment.

Improving access to health and social care

Health and social care practitioners recognising and addressing the socioeconomic barriers that affect their patients' health means that they can advocate for policies that improve access to healthcare for underserved populations (Scriven *et al.*, 2017). Additionally, they can provide resources and support to help patients overcome barriers, such as connecting them with community services or offering sliding scale fees for medical services. Improving health literacy is a key component of effective healthcare practice. Seedhouse (1986) highlights the importance of educating patients about their health conditions and treatment options. This point is echoed in several other sources which highlight the transformative impact of patient education on healthcare outcomes (Scriven *et al.*, 2017). Huber *et al.* (2016) further state the importance of educating and informing patients about their options as this better equips the management of their health and to actively participate in their care. Therefore, practitioners who use clear, simple language and visual aids ensure that patients understand their health information. By empowering patients with knowledge, healthcare providers can help them make informed decisions and engage in healthier behaviours.

Developing more effective care and treatment plans

A holistic approach to health ensures that practitioners consider all aspects of well-being. Naidoo and Wills (2016) argue that focusing solely on physical symptoms can lead to incomplete care. For instance, a patient with chronic pain may also suffer from depression or anxiety, which can exacerbate their physical condition. By considering mental and social factors, practitioners can develop more effective care and/or treatment plans that address the root causes of health issues. Understanding the definition of health helps practitioners provide culturally competent, sensitive and appropriate care. As mentioned above, different cultures have varying beliefs about health and illness. For example, some cultures may prioritise traditional healing practices over modern medicine which may impact how a person responds to disease, seeks healthcare and engages with treatment and/or support (WHO, 2023). Naidoo and Wills (2022) highlight the importance of respecting these beliefs and integrating them into care plans. This approach not only improves satisfaction but also enhances adherence to treatment. Being aware of these various factors requires that practitioners receive support, training and awareness on how to respond to diverse beliefs and behaviours.

Designing comprehensive health and social care policies for practice

By considering the broad definition of health, practitioners can design interventions that are more comprehensive and impactful. Understanding the impact of health inequalities and the importance of responding to the various factors that impact access, adherence, and health-seeking behaviours assists practitioners to respond more effectively to the needs of the individuals and communities with whom they work. Health definitions influence health policies and resource allocation. Numerous reports such as by Marmot *et al.* (2010, 2020) have identified how socioeconomic factors affect health outcomes and access to care. This discussion continues to inform decisions and impacts the overall health status of society. Further, health interventions are more effective when they consider the multidimensional, complex nature of health. Scriven *et al.* (2017) emphasise the need for interventions that address physical, mental, and social well-being. For example, community health programmes that provide education, social support, and access to healthcare services can significantly improve health outcomes. Policymakers who understand the broad definition of health can create policies that address social determinants of health, such as poverty, education, and housing. This leads to more equitable health outcomes and reduces health disparities.

Enhancing health literacy and patient empowerment in practice

Health literacy is the ability to understand and use health information to make informed decisions. Lau (1997) highlighted the importance of health literacy in achieving better health outcomes. Coughlin *et al.* (2020) further emphasise this point stating that health literacy is crucial for understanding and acting on health information. They note that low health literacy is associated with poorer health outcomes, higher rates of hospitalisation, and increased use of emergency care. Improving health literacy can empower individuals to make informed health decisions, adhere to treatment plans, and engage in preventive health behaviours, ultimately leading to better health outcomes. This discussion continues in health promotion and health research as an important aspect of care and the response individuals have to treatment and care plans.

Practitioners who understand the broad definition of health can communicate more effectively with individuals, helping them understand their conditions and treatment options. This empowers individuals to take an active role in their health management giving them the knowledge and tools to manage their health. Practitioners who adopt the perspective that health is a resource can encourage engagement in healthy behaviours, such as regular exercise, balanced nutrition, and stress management. This proactive approach leads to better long-term health outcomes.

Increasing collaboration with other health and social care practitioners to limit the social determinants of health (SDH)

Social determinants of health are the conditions in which people are born, grow, live, work, and age. Svalastog *et al.* (2017) discuss how these factors influence health outcomes. Practitioners who understand the broad definition of health can identify and address social determinants, such as income, education, and social support, by working with other health practitioners, social services and community organisations. This holistic approach can help reduce health disparities and improve overall health. Engaging with the community is essential for addressing social determinants of health with van Druten *et al.* (2022) highlighting the importance of community-based initiatives that promote health and well-being. Practitioners can partner with community organisations to provide education, resources, and support. This collaborative approach can lead to more sustainable health improvements and stronger community ties.

Summary

Health is a complex, multidimensional concept that encompasses many factors. It is influenced by a range of factors, including cultural beliefs, social norms, individual experiences, and scientific advancements. Various definitions of health exist, from the traditional biomedical model to more holistic approaches.

Understanding these different perspectives on health is crucial for health practitioners. It allows them to provide more personalised and effective care, communicate better with patients, and develop more holistic health promotion and disease prevention efforts. By considering the various dimensions and definitions of health, practitioners can better support individuals in achieving their full potential and living fulfilling lives.

Personalised care involves tailoring health and care to meet the unique needs of each individual. Through understanding these different perspectives on health, practitioners can develop personalised care plans that are more effective and respectful of the patient's values and preferences. Your perspective on health profoundly impacts how you think about health, influencing their behaviours, attitudes, and overall approach to well-being. Personal experiences, cultural background, socioeconomic status, and education all play a role in shaping these perspectives. For practitioners, understanding these individual perspectives is crucial for providing personalised, culturally competent, and effective care. By addressing the unique needs of each individual, enhancing health literacy, and engaging with the community, practitioners can improve health outcomes and promote overall well-being highlighting the importance of a holistic and individualised approach to practice, involving collaborative, integrated care that develops treatment plans that align with an individual's values and lifestyle.

References

Aked, J., Marks, N., Cordon, C. and Thompson, S. (2008) 'Five Ways to Well-being. A report presented to the Foresight Project on communicating the evidence base for improving people's well-being'. Available at https://neweconomics.org/2008/10/five-ways-to-wellbeing (Accessed 20 February 2025).

Blaxter, M. (1990) *Health and Lifestyles*. London: Tavistock/Routledge.

Blaxter, M. (2010) *Key Concepts Health*. 2nd edn. Cambridge: Polity.

Coughlin, S.S., Vernon, M., Hatzigeorgiou, C. and George, V. (2020) 'Health literacy, social determinants of health, and disease prevention and control', *Journal of Environment and Health Sciences*, 6(1), p. 3061. Available at: https://pmc.ncbi.nlm.nih.gov/articles/PMC7889072/ (Accessed 20 January 2025).

Cross, R. (2020) 'Understanding the importance of concepts of health', *Nursing Standard*, 35(12), pp. 61–65. Available at https://journals-rcni-com.apollo.worc.ac.uk/nursing-standard/evidence-and-practice/understanding-the-importance-of-concepts-of-health-ns.2020.e11539/full (Accessed 10 July 2024).

Dahlgren, G. and Whitehead, M. (1991). *Policies and Strategies to Promote Social Equity in Health*. Stockholm: Institute for Futures Studies. Available at https://core.ac.uk/download/pdf/6472456.pdf (Accessed 20 January 2025).

Engel, G. L. (1977) 'The need for a new medical model: A challenge for biomedicine', *Science*, 196(4286), pp. 129–136. Available at https://doi.org/10.1126/science.847460 (Accessed 20 July 2024).

Holt-Lunstad, J. (2024) 'Social connection as a critical factor for mental and physical health: Evidence, trends, challenges, and future implications', *World Psychiatry*, 23, pp. 312–332. Available at https://doi-org.apollo.worc.ac.uk/10.1002/wps.21224 (Accessed 1 February 2025).

Huber, M. *et al.* (2016) 'Towards a 'patient-centred' operationalisation of the new dynamic concept of health: A mixed methods study', *BMJ Open*, 6(1), p. e010091. Available at https://doi.org/10.1136/bmjopen-2015-010091 (Accessed 15 February 2025).

Lau, R.R. (1997) 'Cognitive representations of health and illness', in D Gochman (ed.) *Handbook of Health Behaviour Research*, Vol. 1. New York: Plenum.

Marmot, M. *et al.* (2010). *Fair Society, Health Live*. Available at https://www.instituteofhealthequity.org/resources-reports/fair-society-healthy-lives-the-marmot-review (Accessed 15 November 2024).

Marmot, M., *et al.* (2020). *Health Equity in England: The Marmot Review 10 Years On. Institute of Health Equity*. Available at https://www.health.org.uk/reports-and-analysis/reports/health-equity-in-england-the-marmot-review-10-years-on-0 (Accessed 15 November 2024).

Naidoo, J. and Wills, J. (2016) *Foundation of Health Promotion*. London: Elsevier.

Naidoo, J. and Wills, J. (2022) *Health Studies*. 4th edn. London: Palgrave Macmillan.

National Library of Medicine with National Institute of Health (NLM-NIH) (2015) *Native Voices: Native Peoples' Concepts of Health and Illness*. Available at https://www.nlm.nih.gov/nativevoices/exhibition/healing-ways/index.html [Accessed 25 January 2025].

Ni, M.Y. *et al.* (2020) 'Determinants of physical, mental and social well-being: A longitudinal environment-wide association study', *International Journal of Epidemiology*, 49(2), pp. 380–389. Available at https://doi.org/10.1093/ije/dyz238 (Accessed 15 February 2025).

Ruggeri, K., Garcia-Garzon, E. and Maguire, Á *et al.* (2020) 'Well-being is more than happiness and life satisfaction: A multidimensional analysis of 21 countries', *Health and Quality of Life Outcomes*, 18, p. 192. Available at https://doi.org/10.1186/s12955-020-01423-y (Accessed 20 December 2024).

Schramme, T. (2023) 'Health as complete well-being: The WHO definition and beyond', *Public Health Ethics*, 16(3), pp. 210–218. Available at https://academic.oup.com/phe/article/16/3/210/7232444 (Accessed 20 December 2024).

Scriven, A., Morgan, G. and Woodall, J. (2017) *Ewles and Simnett's Promoting Health: A Practical Guide*. 7th edn. Edinburgh: Elsevier.

Seedhouse, D. (1986) *Health: The Foundations for Achievement*. Chichester: John Wiley and Sons.

Smith, D. (2015). Shaman. In *The Canadian Encyclopedia*. Retrieved from https://www.thecanadianencyclopedia.ca/en/article/shaman (Accessed 1 December 2024).

Svalastog, A.L. *et al.* (2017) 'Concepts and definitions of health and health-related values in the knowledge landscapes of the digital society', *Croatian Medical Journal*, 58(6), pp. 431–435. Available at https://doi.org/10.3325/cmj.2017.58.431 (Accessed 15 June 2024).

UNICEF (2021) Defining social norms and related concepts [Online]. Available at https://www.unicef.org/media/111061/file/Social-norms-definitions-2021.pdf. (Accessed 10 January 2025).

van der Linden, R. and Schermer, M. (2022) 'Health and disease as practical concepts: Exploring function in context-specific definitions', *Medicine, Health Care and Philosophy*, 25, pp. 131–140. Available at https://doi.org/10.1007/s11019-021-10058-9 (Accessed 15 June 2024).

van Druten, V.P. *et al.* (2022) 'Concepts of health in different contexts: A scoping review', *BMC Health Services Research*, 22(1), p. 389. Available at https://doi.org/10.1186/s12913-022-07702-2 (Accessed 15 June 2024).

Walker, M. and Rogers, W. (2018) 'A new approach to defining disease', *Journal of Medicine and Philosophy*, 43, pp. 402–420. Available at https://doi.org/10.1093/jmp/jhy014 (Accessed 1 February 2025).

WHO (2023) *Traditional medicine has a long history of contributing to conventional medicine and continues to hold promise*. Available at https://www.who.int/initiatives/who-global-traditional-medicine-centre (Accessed 20 November 2024).

Williams, R. (1983) 'Concepts of health: An Analysis of lay Logic', *Sociology*, 17(2), pp. 185–204.

World Health Organization (1948) *Constitution of the World Health Organization*. Available at https://www.who.int/about/governance/constitution (Accessed 15 July 2024).

5 Understanding mental health for health and social care

Clive Sealey

The aims of this chapter are to:

- **Outline the current context of mental health**
- **Define key mental health definitions and distinctions**
- **Describe key health and social care practice issues relevant to mental health legislation, diagnosis, stigma and treatment**

Introduction

Within health and social care, the dominant focus has historically been on physical health and trying to heal physical health problems, as outlined in Chapter 4. It is only recently that the importance that mental health has to wider health has been recognised. We now know that having good mental health is very important to what we can do from day to day and our wider relationships with friends, family and the community we live in. Put simply, if we are experiencing positive mental health, we are able to do so many more things that make us feel better and enable us to live our lives as fully as possible, and therefore positively contribute to society at all stages of life. To paraphrase UNICEF (2021: 16), we know that mental health is a positive asset that enables children to thrive in families, teenagers to experience the joys of adolescence with friends, young adults to have the confidence to meet inevitable challenges and families to bond and attach with each other. Additionally, Fusar-Poli *et al.* (2020) outline how good mental health enables individuals to work productively and fruitfully, adapt to changes in life and maintain healthy lifestyles and also to prevent illness. All of these are core aims of health and social care, which means that focusing on mental health is beneficial to health and social care practice.

This chapter presents key issues for health and social care in relation to mental health. It starts by explaining the current context of mental health as a way to contextualise its significance to health and social care. It then outlines two key definitions of mental health and explores the significance of these definitions. This is followed by detailing the importance of distinguishing between mental health, mental illness and mental disorder. It then describes key mental health legislation and diagnoses that you are likely to come across in practice. This leads on to a discussion of the significant of mental health stigma. The chapter concludes with a brief outline of key mental health treatments.

The current context of mental health

As described above, mental health has become more prominent recently, and this has occurred for several reasons. Firstly, over the last 30 years or so, the number of people

DOI: 10.4324/9781032619309-6

Table 5.1 Change over time in diagnosed mental health issues or disorders across the population

	% change	*Trend*
Young people (Gilbert and Mallorie, 2024)	9.7% to 11.2% (1999–2017)	↑
Adults (Baker and Kirk-Wade, 2024)	15.5% to 18.9% (1993–2014)	↑
Men (Baker and Kirk-Wade, 2024)	12% to 14% (1993–2014)	↑
Women (Baker and Kirk-Wade, 2024)	19% to 23% (1993–2014)	↑

diagnosed with mental health illnesses or disorders has increased across the population, as shown in Table 5.1.

Table 5.1 shows that for young people, adults, men and women, the trend has been an upward increase in diagnosed mental health issues and disorders. This means that one in four adults and one in 10 children experience mental illnesses (NHS England, 2025), and mental health problems represent the largest single cause of disability in the UK (NHS England, 2025a). Additionally, Collins *et al.* (2023) argue that there are also lots of mental health illnesses that are undiagnosed or underdiagnosed, suggesting that the true level of mental health illness is higher than we know. This means that throughout the population, the trend is one of increased mental health needs, especially from older people in the form of dementia and depression, and younger people in the form of depression and anxiety (McKee *et al.*, 2021). The number of people with mental health conditions was increasing before the COVID-19 pandemic, but since then it has been increasing faster, with mental health conditions becoming more common between the ages of 16 and 64 (Latimer *et al.*, 2025). This is exemplified by the fact that mental health issues are the leading reason for people being long-term sick off work (CIPD, 2023). As a consequence of this, while in 2011 the costs of dealing with mental health issues were estimated at £105 billion (HM Government and Department of Health, 2011), a more recent report has estimated that the cost of dealing with mental health problems has risen to £118 billion (McDaid and Park, 2022). Finally, an IPSOS (2024) survey identified mental health as the health problem that people in Britain worry most about, ahead of cancer and obesity (IPSOS, 2024). This is the first time that this has happened, which reflects the increasing concern about mental health within the population. Together, this highlights that more people are experiencing and concerned with mental health issues than previously, which is a trend that is likely to continue. It also means that mental health has become more important to health and social care practice than previously.

Mental health definitions

There is no universally accepted definition of mental health (Manwell *et al.*, 2015). Below are two of the most widely referred definitions of mental health:

> A state of mental well-being that enables people to cope with the stresses of life, realize their abilities, learn well and work well, and contribute to their community.
>
> World Health Organization (2022)

> Mental health is a state of mind characterized by emotional well-being, good behavioural adjustment, relative freedom from anxiety and disabling symptoms, and a capacity to establish constructive relationships and cope with the ordinary demands and stresses of life.
>
> American Psychological Association (2018)

These definitions have three important similarities which we can identify as important features of mental health:

- Mental health as a *state* – this refers to having conscious intentions beliefs, desires and emotions to what we are doing at a particular time. For example, if we choose to do something, we need to be consciously aware of what, why and how we are doing it, as this signifies a good state of mind.
- Mental health as *coping with the stresses of life* – this refers to mental health as the ability to do ordinary everyday things on a day-to-day basis; it does not have to be signified as having a major emotional breakdown. For example, if someone is not able to cope in their everyday work, this could be a sign of mental distress, and should be treated as such before it becomes a more significant problem. This means that where an individual is not able to do this, this could be a sign of mental distress.
- Mental health as focused on *well-being* – this refers to mental health as not just about the absence of disease, but is also about a range of other factors that can affect how a person feels on a day-to-day basis, what they are able to do and whether they are able to contribute to society. Factors that can affect our well-being include relationships, friendships, social status, income, education and the environment, and these need to be taken into consideration when considering the mental health of an individual. For example, while a person may be physically well, they may be suffering from bullying, and this can affect their mental health.

The last point has become more relevant in recent years from the recognition that trying to strictly separate mental health and physical health is unrealistic. This is from a realisation that physical health impacts on mental health and mental health impacts on physical health. For example, consider the circumstances of someone with a physical health condition that restricts their mobility. This can affect them physically, such as their ability to socialise, work, exercise and undertake personal care. When this occurs, this can lead to loneliness, isolation and lack of self-worth, all of which can lead to mental illness such as depression. Or consider the circumstances of someone with a mental health illness that affects their ability to go out, such as anxiety. This can lead to reduced mobility and lack of exercise, both of which can affect their physical health.

From a health and social care perspective, this means that we need to be aware that even though mental health conditions visibly occur and affect the mind, there are various other physical, emotional, psychological and social factors that can also cause and affect mental health, and these factors may present themselves in minor or major ways.

Mental health distinctions

People often use *mental health*, *mental disorders* and *mental illness* in the same way to mean the same thing, but in the field of mental health they mean very different things, and they have very different implications. The difference between the three terms is explained below.

Mental health

Mental health is a general term that refers to the feelings, thoughts, emotions and state of mind that we experience on a daily basis. These experiences can be both good, meaning having positive experiences of mental health, or poor, meaning where a person is struggling to cope, but the key point here is that mental health is something that we all experience on a day-to-day basis, either personally or socially through friends or families. For example, you may have achieved all the things you wanted to do in a day, or you may have had a tough day at work or college, either of which can affect your feelings, thoughts, emotions and state of mind. You may have been on a good night out socialising with friends, or had an argument with friends, either of which can affect your feelings, thoughts, emotions and state of mind. Or you may have heard some good news from a family member, or not speaking to a family member, either of which can affect your feelings, thoughts, emotions and state of mind. There is no specific reason why this is the case, it can be something as simple as the weather that can change a person's mental health. These factors can also be things within our control, or things outside of our control, such as something heard on the news. The key point is that we are all likely to experience both good and poor mental health from time to time, and these experiences are usually short-term and can change very quickly based on our everyday experiences, but do not affect our ability to do normal everyday things. Examples of potential mental health problems include psychological issues such as anger, irritation, euphoria or sadness, and physical symptoms such as headaches and tummy aches, sleep disturbances and changed eating patterns. This is the most common type of mental health issue that an individual experiences.

Mental illness

A mental illness occurs when having poor mental health occurs over a long period of time and/or with such intensity that it affects the person's ability to do the things that they would normally do on a daily basis. For example, if someone hears bad news, this can lead to poor mental health, but when this poor mental health means that they are unable get out of bed, go to work, socialise or do hobbies, this is when it becomes a mental illness. Depending on the severity, care can be provided in the community by family or friends, or as outpatient care. Examples of potential mental illnesses include anxiety, depression, self-harm, phobias and substance misuse.

Mental disorder

A mental disorder is when a mental illness becomes so severe that an individual is unable to care for themselves or others that depend on their care, and can also become a danger to themselves or others. This means that they may need their care provided by mental health professions such as psychiatrists, mental health nurse or psychologist either in the community or at an institutional setting. Examples of mental disorders include schizophrenic and delusional disorders; mood (affective) disorders, including depressive, manic and bipolar forms; neuroses, including phobic, panic and obsessive–compulsive disorders; behavioural disorders, including eating, sleep and stress disorders; and personality disorders.

These three terms can be expressed on a line in terms of severity, known as a spectrum, as shown in Figure 5.1.

Figure 5.1 shows the mental health spectrum from 0 to 100. 0 represents no mental health conditions and 100 represents the most severe mental health conditions. As Figure 5.1 shows, mental health refers to the lowest level of mental health conditions, mental illness refers to the next level of conditions and mental disorder is the highest level of conditions. The key difference is that while mental health refers to issues that can occur in everyday life that are not usually serious enough to be diagnosable, mental illnesses and mental disorders specifically refer to diagnosable mental health conditions. So we need to be careful how we use these terms.

Mental health legislation

The importance of the distinction above between mental health, mental illness and mental disorder becomes apparent when we consider relevant mental health legislation.

Mental Health Acts 1983/2007

The *Mental Health Act 1983* and the *Mental Health Act 2007* are usually referred to as *Mental Health Act 1983 [2007]*, as the 2007 Act is essentially an amendment of the 1983 Act. The purpose of these Acts is to set out the assessment, treatment and rights that are available for diagnosed mental disorder. This means that the Act only applies where an individual has been diagnosed by a mental health professional as having a mental health disorder. It does not apply for everyday mental health issues or mental illness, as these are covered in general legislation.

The key points from the Acts are:

- Only an **Approved Mental Health Practitioner** (**AMHP**) (Learning Box 5.1) can diagnose a mental health disorder. An AMHP be a psychiatric nurse, social worker, occupational therapist or clinical psychologist.

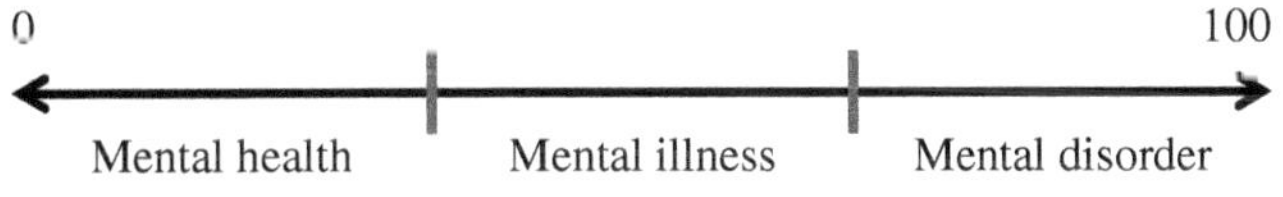

Figure 5.1 The mental health spectrum.

Learning Box 5.1: Approved Mental Health Practitioner and Independent Mental Health Advocate

An Approved Mental Health Practitioner, often referred to as an AMHP, refers to professional who have been trained and certified to assess whether an individual has a mental disorder, as defined by the Mental Health Act 1983[2007]. This means that only an AMHP can determine if a person needs to be detained/sectioned.

When a person is sectioned, they are entitled to have an Independent Mental Health Advocate, often referred to as IMHA. The IMHA person is responsible for ensuring that the sectioned person is treated fairly and their rights are met. They can help people understand what they are being told by mental health professionals and represent their views. They can also help if someone wants to appeal against their sectioning to a Tribunal.

- Treatment for mental disorders can include medicinal treatments, psychological treatments therapies, social treatments (these are explained in more detail later in the chapter), or **detainment/sectioning of individuals** (Learning Box 3.1).
- People diagnosed with a mental disorder have rights, such as the right to an **Independent Mental Health Advocate (IMHA)** (Learning Box 5.1).

When an AMHP makes a diagnosis of a mental disorder, they can determine the appropriate treatment for it. If the mental disorder is serious to the extent that the safety of the individual is at risk, then the AMHP can decide that the person needs to be detained for treatment, which is often termed sectioning. If the person agrees that they need to be sectioned, this is called a voluntary sectioning, but if they do not agree, they can be sectioned against their will. During a period of sectioning, an individual can be assessed further and treated. The treatment can be against their will, such as having drugs administered. The key point here is that sectioning only applies to severe mental health disorders; it does not apply to general mental health issues or diagnosed mental illnesses.

Equality Act 2010

Under the *Equality Act 2010*, an individual with a diagnosed mental health condition is considered to have a disability. This gives them a protected characteristic, meaning that they are legally protected from discrimination based on their mental health condition (see Chapter 15). This is relevant when considering the possibility impact of stigma as detailed below.

Human Rights Act 1998

This is not a specific mental health legislation, but its importance is that it applies human rights to everyone, including those with mental health conditions. These include *Article 2* the right to life, *Article 3* freedom form inhumane and degrading treatment and *Article 5* right to liberty and security.

Mental Capacity Act 2005

The *Mental Capacity Act 2005* provides safeguards for those who may lack capacity due to a mental health condition. It defines the circumstances in which someone may lack capacity, what should be to establish if this is the case, and how care should be done provided in such circumstances.

Mental health illnesses and disorders

The most authoritative classifications of mental health illnesses and disorders are the World Health Organization (WHO, 2022) *International Classification of Diseases 11th Revision* (typically referred to as *ICD-11*) and the American Psychiatric Association (2022) *Diagnostic and Statistical Manual of Mental Disorders* (typically referred to as *DSM-5-TR*). This provides a list of different symptoms for each condition to help diagnose specific illness and disorders. When someone is diagnosed as having an illness or disorder, the likelihood is that the diagnosis has been done by referring to the symptoms in one of these manuals. These are the primary manuals that doctors and other mental health professionals use.

It should be noted that both *ICD11* and *DSM-5-TR* are mainly focused on adult mental health, but they nevertheless do allow for the consideration of similar child and adolescent mental health conditions. It should also be noted that while both *ICD 11* and *DSM-5-TR* do identify specific symptoms to decide a mental health diagnosis, individuals can actually experience symptoms differently from these guides, as a consequence of human biology and social context particularly the family.

Below is a brief outline of commonly diagnosed mental health illnesses and disorders.

Depression

Depression is estimated to affect up to 15% of the population in high-income countries, and 11% of the population in low-income countries (Lim *et al.*, 2018). In the UK, this would translate to up to 10 million people. According to *ICD 11* and *DSM-5-TR*, depression occurs when an individual experiences varying degrees of low mood and loss of enjoyment of activities that they would normally enjoy for most of the day, for nearly every day for a period of at least two weeks, together with other symptoms, including depressive thinking, pessimism about the future, suicidal ideas and biological symptoms such as early waking, weight loss and reduced appetite. It is important to note that it is common to feel depressed as people's mood changes from hour to hour and from day to day, as sadness can be a normal passing human condition. However, when this feeling of depression is persistent over time, this could signify depression.

Anxiety

Anxiety is the constant anticipation of a threat, when that threat does not exist or is exaggerated. Anxiety can be a normal response to unusual circumstances as an essential emotion protecting us from danger, and can even help us to function. For example, think of the last minute rush to hand in assignments if you are a student, or meet deadlines, or even get to school and work on time and run for the bus. However, when anxiety remains constant and is out of proportion to the circumstances, it is a sign of mental distress (Van der Kolk, 2015). Anxiety is not just one condition but is a series of conditions, such as generalised anxiety disorder, phobias, panic disorder, post-traumatic stress disorder and obsessive–compulsive disorder.

Eating disorders

An eating disorder is where an individual controls their intake of food to cope with feelings and other situations. This can be through eating too little, eating too much and/or excessive concern with weight or body shape, or avoiding certain foods and/or restricting the amount of food eaten overall. Examples of common eating disorders are anorexia nervosa, bulimia and binge eating disorder, but usually a person's symptoms do not exactly fit the symptoms of any specific eating disorder. This is known as other specified feeding or eating disorder (OSFED). Eating disorders tend to occur most typically during adolescence (NHS England, 2023).

Psychosis

Psychosis is where an alteration to a person's perception, thoughts, mood and behaviour occurs to the extent that the person has a problem realising what is real and what is not real (Mind, 2024). Its symptoms can include confused and disturbed thoughts (such as rapid or constant speech, or switching from one topic to another), hallucinations (usually in the form of voices) or delusions (such as that other people, objects or things are being controlled by others). The most common age for psychosis to occur is between the ages of 18 and 25, but it can sometimes occur before 18, and this is known as early onset psychosis (EOP). The two main forms of psychotic illness are schizophrenia and bipolar affective disorder.

Substance misuse

Substance misuse refers to the use of any chemical substance, in amounts which or with the intention of harm to themselves or others. The intention of harm, which can include evidence of dependence, is a significant for a diagnosis. Substances can include alcohol, caffeine, pain medication and illicit drugs. Getting drunk is not substance misuse, it becomes substance misuse when this occurs to the extent that it is causing significant physical and social harm.

Neuro-developmental conditions

Neuro-developmental conditions refer to where there is late or non-development of the brain or spinal cord. This late development can be in the womb or after birth. The terminology can refer to conditions, disorders and difficulties and is interchangeable. The most common are attention deficit hyperactivity disorder (ADHD) (sometimes referred to as hyperkinetic disorder), conduct disorder (CD) and autistic spectrum disorder (ASD).

Self-harm

NHS (2023) defines self-harm as when somebody intentionally damages or injures their body. This can include *physical* (i.e. hitting yourself or things and cutting yourself), *neglectful* (i.e. excessive alcohol or illegal drug use or having repeated unsafe sex) and *emotional* (i.e. having repeated negative thoughts) self-harm. Young women are particularly susceptible to self-harm as compared to young men (NHS, 2016). Reported instances of self-harm very likely underestimate the true extent of self-harm, as people do not always report it but prefer to keep it hidden (NICE, 2022), due to its stigmatisation, leading to guilt and shame (Aggarwal *et al.*, 2021). Taking instances of self-harm seriously as a practitioner is important as there is evidence of a clear link between self-harming and suicide or suicidal thoughts, such as a 30–50-fold risk of suicide following self-harm in the year after presentation at hospital (NICE, 2022).

Suicidal behaviour

Suicidal behaviour refers to death or harm by an individual with the intent to end their life (Centers for Disease Control and Prevention, 2024). Suicide is often the result of overwhelming feelings rather than an explicit wish to die, as suicide attempts provide an active response to triggers acting as stressors. Reasons given might include an argument with a close friend or family member or failing exams. Suicide attempts can be about a last sense of control over feelings of helplessness with the corresponding relief then experienced. People under 20 have the lowest suicide rate of all ages, but among men aged 20–34, suicide is the leading cause of death in England (Baker, 2024). More specifically, in contrast to depression, males have higher suicide rates than females for all age groups (Baker, 2024). There continues to be ongoing stigma and shame and often negative attitudes towards those who attempt suicide (Pitman *et al.*, 2016).

This list of commonly diagnosed mental health diseases and disorders is very limited in terms of scope, as there are many others not listed. For instance, in *DSM-5-TR*, there are 306 identified mental health diagnosis. However, one thing that the list does highlight is the breadth and range of mental health illnesses and disorders, as well as the similar breadth and range of its causes, ranging from neurological, to psychological to social, which is something that is important to be aware of as a health and social care practitioner. This is also an important consideration when thinking about treatment.

Mental health stigma

From the description of mental health illnesses and disorders above, one issue that is evident is the significance of stigma. Stigma has been a recurring issue in relation to mental health, whereby historically someone living with a mental health issue was treated as either 'mad, bad or sad' (Appignanesi, 2009). Mad in terms of being seen as a danger to themselves, bad in terms of being a danger to society, and sad in terms of being seen as living outside the norms of society. This stigma towards mental health has lessened from what it previously was but still exists, and this has significant implications for health and social care practice. Stigma acts as a barrier to accessing treatment and care (Kular *et al.*, 2019), as people are less likely to ask for help, which can lead to a reluctance to seek help and subsequently a worsening of mental health (Knaak *et al.*, 2017). It is also relevant to highlight that mental health professionals can also have and exhibit stigmatising attitudes and behaviours towards mental illness (Jauch *et al.*, 2023), which can have significant negative consequences for individuals. As a health and social care practitioner, it is important to have an awareness of the possibility that stigma has affected the mental health experience of an individual, and also to be aware of possible stigmatising attitudes that may affect the care that you provide. It is also important to be aware that discriminatory treatment based on stigma is illegal, as detailed above.

Learning Box 5.2: Eugenics

Eugenics refers to trying to change the genetic characteristics of a population by only allowing those with the most desirable characterises to reproduce. Underpinning eugenics is the belief that certain 'undesirable' or 'negative' characteristics, such as lack of intelligence, deviance, disease, race and mental ill health, should be genetically bred out of a population. This would mean that such 'undesirable' people would not be allowed to have children, through either voluntary or forced sterilisation. In the UK, eugenics was never officially adopted as government policy, but in some countries, such as Germany, Sweden, China and the US, it was carried out officially by governments (Wilson, 2025).

Mental health treatments

Historically, the treatment of mental health conditions focused on either locking people away from the rest of society in asylums, punishing certain mental health behaviours by making them a criminal offence such as suicide or subjecting people with mental health conditions to painful and debilitating medical treatments such as lobotomies (cutting away a part of the brain) or even eugenics (Learning Box 15.2). This means that those with mental health conditions were often viewed very negatively in society, which contributed to the stigma associated with having a mental health condition.

However, more recently, there has been a move away from such care towards three main types of treatment for mental health: medicinal treatments, psychological treatments and social treatments.

Medicinal treatments

Medicinal treatments, also known as pharmacological treatments, involve the use of medication to treat mental health illnesses and disorders. This occurs from an underlying belief that mental health conditions occur from a chemical imbalance in the brain, which the prescribed medication is intended to rebalance. This can either increase or decrease the number of certain chemicals in the brain, which changes the way that brain cells communicate with each other, in order to improve mood, behaviour or thinking. Well-known medication includes antidepressants, the most common of which is *fluoxetine*, more usually known as *Prozac*; anti-anxiety medication such as *benzodiazepines* and *tranquilizers*; stimulants to treat hyperactive behaviour such as ADHD, the most common of which is *methylphenidate*, usually known as *Ritalin*; antipsychotics to treat psychosis, the most common of which are *clozapine* and *olanzapine*; and mood stabilisers to treat bipolar disorder and mania, the most common of which are *lithium* and *valproate*.

For some mental health conditions, medicinal treatments are highly effective and relevant. However, as a health and social care practitioner, it is important to note that medicinal treatment does not cure the mental health condition, they simply stabilise the mood of the individual which makes the condition more manageable, enabling the person to manage living with the condition. This means that medication can be required to be taken for a long time. This is relevant from the fact that medication usually has side effects associated with them, which can be minor or major, such as insomnia, sexual problems, nausea, depression, drowsiness, weight gain, loss of appetite and heart problems among others. This means that it is also important to be aware of the side effects of medication that service users use.

Psychological treatments

Psychological treatments rely on the personal contact between the person needing help and a trained professional. Psychological treatments aim to improve and mental health condition by focusing on changing an individual's thinking, emotions and behaviours through using a specific theory to support this change (Arnberg *et al.*, 2013). The theory outlines that the mental health condition occurs from a specific way of thinking, feeling or behaving, and so changing these can improve the mental health condition. *NHS Talking Therapies* (previously *Improving Access to Talking Therapies*) is an example of psychological therapies within health and social care.

There are four main types of psychological treatments:

- *Person-centred/humanistic theories* – the core belief of these treatments is that individuals have the capacity to do the right thing, and that providing them with the right environment enables them to self-reflect and come up with solutions themselves. This means that the role of the therapist is to provide the environment that enables this change to occur.
- *Psychodynamic treatments* – the core focus of these treatments is how the unconscious processes of the mind affect what we do without us even knowing this. The psychodynamic approach aims to uncover these unconscious processes, through uncovering childhood and the feelings, memories, beliefs and fantasies that occurred during this time, as a way to explain current mental health issues so that we are better able to manage them.
- *Systemic treatments* – the core focus of these treatments is on understanding how wider relationships affect behaviour, rather than just on an individual's thoughts and feelings. The individual is seen as part of a wider system that affects their mental health. The aim of the intervention is to introduce new ideas and perspectives that help the individual to see how mental health conditions occur due to problems with relationships, which enables them to avoid blaming themselves or others as the cause of problems.
- *Cognitive behavioural therapy treatments* – the core focus of these treatments is enabling individual to unlearn negative behaviours. The treatments are built out of the notion that all human behaviour is learnt, which includes behaviours that cause mental health conditions. The intervention works by observing what people actually do, not what they say they do or imagine that they do, and noting how this behaviour leads to distress. Once this is observed, negative behaviours can be stopped and positive behaviours can be reinforced, to create positive mental health.

From a health and social care perspective, it is important to note that psychological treatments typically occur over a long period, and also require a certain level of cognition on the part of the individual to work. Also, the psychological treatments above have been presented individually as if they are practised in isolation, but often they are combined to provide a more comprehensive treatment programme.

Social treatments

As identified above, social issues can play a key role in the development of mental health conditions, with issues such as loneliness, poverty, bullying, relationships, family and culture all having the potential to do so. For example, at the core of loneliness is not having friends, which is not a medical issue but is a social issue that can have a significant effect on mental health, such as leading to anxiety and depression (Mann *et al.*, 2022). In the past, when presented with social issues as such, there could be a tendency on the part of medical professionals to prescribe medication, especially in the case of depression and anxiety.

There is now much more focus on providing social treatments for the social causes of mental health issues, such as through **social prescribing** (Learning Box 8.1). Examples of this can include:

- group activities such as crafting and cinema clubs to reduce loneliness;
- walking groups to improve low activity levels and reduce the effect of long-term conditions;
- outdoor activities and exercise, including gardening or swimming to reduce anxiety and improve well-being

(Rice, 2023)

A key reason for this change is the realisation that people with mental health illnesses and disorders can live fulfilling lives without the need for medicalised treatments in asylums or hospitals, as long as there is social support from relevant professions (Turner *et al.*, 2015), and also friends, family and the community that they live in. Social support is seen as an important aspect of enabling people with mental health conditions to live in their community, and this has reduced the stigma around mental health, although not totally eliminated it. This shift has highlighted the importance of the social context to improving mental health, in terms of emphasising that mental health issues can often be decreased or resolved with good systems of social support in place.

From a health and social care perspective, this highlights that it is important to consider the possibility of social causes of mental health conditions, as effective treatment can require identifying relevant social activities.

Summary

The positive benefits of mental health make it an important focus for health and social care. However, over the last 30 years or so, the number of people diagnosed with mental health illnesses or disorders has increased across the population, which is a trend that is likely to continue. There is also a growing awareness that even though mental health conditions visibly occur and affect the mind, there are various other physical, emotional, psychological and social factors that can also cause and affect mental health, and these factors may present themselves in minor or major ways. It is crucial to understand the distinction between mental health, mental illnesses and mental disorders, especially as this has legal implications in law. Diagnosed mental health conditions identify the breadth and range of its causes, ranging from neurological, to psychological to social, which is something that is important to be aware of as a health and social care practitioner. As a health and social care practitioner, it is also important to have an awareness of the impact that stigma can have on the mental health experience of an individual, and also to be aware of possible stigmatising attitudes that may affect the care that you provide. When considering treatment for mental health illnesses and disorders, it is important to consider whether medicinal, psychological or social treatments, or a combination of these, are the most appropriate to treat the condition, in order to ensure the positive benefits of mental health occur and are sustained.

References

Aggarwal, S., Borschmann, R. and Patton, G.C. (2021) 'Tackling stigma in self-harm and suicide in the young', *The Lancet Public Health*, 6(1), pp. e6–e7. Available at: https://doi.org/10.1016/S2468-2667(20)30259-0

American Psychiatric Association (ed.) (2022) *Diagnostic and statistical manual of mental disorders: DSM-5-TRTM. Fifth edition, text revision.* Washington, DC: American Psychiatric Association Publishing.

American Psychological Association (2018) *APA Dictionary of Psychology*. Available at https://dictionary.apa.org/mental-health (Accessed 11 March 2025)

Appignanesi, L. (2009) *Mad, Bad, and Sad: A History of Women and the Mind Doctors*. 1st edn. Erscheinungsort nicht ermittelbar: W. W. Norton & Company, Incorporated.

Arnberg, F.K. *et al.* (2013) 'Recent randomized controlled trials of psychological interventions in healthcare: A review of their quantity, scope, and characteristics', *Journal of Psychosomatic Research*, 75(5), pp. 401–408. Available at https://doi.org/10.1016/j.jpsychores.2013.08.019

Baker, C. (2024) *Suicide Statistics*. London: House of Commons Library. Available at https://commonslibrary.parliament.uk/research-briefings/cbp-7749/ (Accessed 5 November 2024).

Baker, C. and Kirk-Wade, E. (2024) *Mental health statistics: prevalence, services and funding in England*. Number CBP-06988. Available at https://researchbriefings.files.parliament.uk/documents/SN06988/SN06988.pdf (Accessed 11 March 2025).

Centers for Disease Control and Prevention (2024) *Facts about suicide, suicide prevention*. Available at https://www.cdc.gov/suicide/facts/index.html (Accessed 13 March 2025).

CIPD (2023) *Health and wellbeing at work*. Available at https://www.cipd.org/globalassets/media/knowledge/knowledge-hub/reports/2023-pdfs/8436-health-and-wellbeing-report-2023.pdf (Accessed 11 March 2025).

Collins, B. *et al.* (2023) 'Investigating the impact of undiagnosed anxiety and depression on health and social care costs and quality of life: Cross-sectional study using household health survey data', *BJPsych Open*, 9(6), p. e201. Available at https://doi.org/10.1192/bjo.2023.596

Fusar-Poli, P. *et al.* (2020) 'What is good mental health? A scoping review', *European Neuropsychopharmacology*, 31, pp. 33–46. Available at https://doi.org/10.1016/j.euroneuro.2019.12.105

Gilbert, H. and Mallorie, S. (2024) *Mental health 360: prevalence, The King's Fund*. Available at https://www.kingsfund.org.uk/insight-and-analysis/long-reads/mental-health-360-prevalence (Accessed 11 March 2025).

HM Government and Department of Health (2011) *No health without mental health*. London: Department of Health. Available at: https://assets.publishing.service.gov.uk/media/5a7c348ae5274a25a914129d/dh_124058.pdf (Accessed: 13 December 2023).

IPSOS (2024) *Ipsos Health Service Report 2024*. Paris: IPSOS. Available at: https://www.ipsos.com/en/ipsos-health-service-report (Accessed: 23 September 2024).

Jauch, M., Occhipinti, S. and O'Donovan, A. (2023) 'The stigmatization of mental illness by mental health professionals: Scoping review and bibliometric analysis', *PLOS ONE*, 18(1), p. e0280739. Available at https://doi.org/10.1371/journal.pone.0280739

Knaak, S., Mantler, E. and Szeto, A. (2017) 'Mental illness-related stigma in healthcare: Barriers to access and care and evidence-based solutions', *Healthcare Management Forum*, 30(2), pp. 111–116. Available at https://doi.org/10.1177/0840470416679413

Kular, A. *et al.* (2019) 'Stigma and access to care in first-episode psychosis', *Early Intervention in Psychiatry*, 13(5), pp. 1208–1213. Available at https://doi.org/10.1111/eip.12756

Latimer, E., Ray-Chaudhuri, S. and Waters, T. (2025) *The role of changing health in rising health-related benefit claims*. The IFS. Available at https://doi.org/10.1920/re.ifs.2025.0012

Lim, G.Y. *et al.* (2018) 'Prevalence of depression in the community from 30 countries between 1994 and 2014', *Scientific Reports*, 8(1), p. 2861. Available at: https://doi.org/10.1038/s41598-018-21243-x

Mann, F. *et al.* (2022) 'Loneliness and the onset of new mental health problems in the general population', *Social Psychiatry and Psychiatric Epidemiology*, 57(11), pp. 2161–2178. Available at https://doi.org/10.1007/s00127-022-02261-7

Manwell, L.A. *et al.* (2015) 'What is mental health? Evidence towards a new definition from a mixed methods multidisciplinary international survey', *BMJ Open*, 5(6), p. e007079. Available at https://doi.org/10.1136/bmjopen-2014-007079

McDaid, D. and Park, A.-L. (2022) *The economic case for investing in the prevention of mental health conditions in the UK*. London: Mental Health Foundation. Available at: https://www.mentalhealth.org.uk/sites/default/files/2022-06/MHF-Investing-in-Prevention-Full-Report.pdf (Accessed: 13 December 2023).

McKee, M. *et al.* (2021) 'The changing health needs of the UK population', *The Lancet*, 397(10288), pp. 1979–1991. Available at https://doi.org/10.1016/S0140-6736(21)00229-4

Mind (2024) *What is psychosis?* Available at: https://www.mind.org.uk/information-support/types-of-mental-health-problems/psychosis/about-psychosis/ (Accessed: 7 November 2024).

NHS (2016) *Adult Psychiatric Morbidity Survey: Survey of Mental Health and Wellbeing, England, 2014*. Available at: https://digital.nhs.uk/data-and-information/publications/statistical/adult-psychiatric-morbidity-survey/adult-psychiatric-morbidity-survey-survey-of-mental-health-and-wellbeing-england-2014 (Accessed: 6 November 2024).

NHS (2023) *Why people self-harm, nhs.uk*. Available at https://www.nhs.uk/mental-health/feelings-symptoms-behaviours/behaviours/self-harm/why-people-self-harm/ (Accessed 6 November 2024).

NHS England (2023) 'Mental Health of Children and Young People in England, 2023: Wave 4 follow up to the 2017 survey'. Available at: https://digital.nhs.uk/data-and-information/publications/statistical/mental-health-of-children-and-young-people-in-england/2023-wave-4-follow-up/data-sets (Accessed: 7 November 2024)

NHS England (2025) *Adult and older adult mental health*. Available at https://www.england.nhs.uk/mental-health/adults/ (Accessed 11 March 2025).

NHS England (2025a) *Mental health*. Available at https://www.england.nhs.uk/mental-health/ (Accessed 11 March 2025).

NICE (2022) *Self-harm is everyone's business, NICE says in new draft guideline | NICE*. Available at: https://www.nice.org.uk/news/articles/self-harm-is-everyone-s-business-nice-says-in-new-draft-guideline (Accessed: 6 November 2024).

Pitman, A.L. *et al.* (2016) 'The stigma perceived by people bereaved by suicide and other sudden deaths: A cross-sectional UK study of 3432 bereaved adults', *Journal of Psychosomatic Research*, 87, p. 22. Available at https://doi.org/10.1016/j.jpsychores.2016.05.009

Rice, B. (2023) *The Missing Link. Social Prescribing for Children and Young People*. London: Barnados. Available at https://www.barnardos.org.uk/sites/default/files/2023-10/report-missing-link-social-prescribing-children-young-people.pdf (Accessed 10 October 2024).

Turner, J. *et al.* (2015) 'The history of mental health services in modern England: Practitioner memories and the direction of future research', *Medical History*, 59(4), pp. 599–624. Available at https://doi.org/10.1017/mdh.2015.48

UNICEF (ed.) (2021) *On My Mind: Promoting, Protecting and Caring for Children's Mental Health*. New York, NY: UNICEF (The state of the world's children, 2021). Available at https://www.unicef.org/media/114636/file/SOWC-2021-full-report-English.pdf (Accessed 18 March 2025).

Van der Kolk, B.A. (2015) *The Body Keeps the Score: Mind, Brain and Body in the Transformation of Trauma*. London: Penguin Books.

WHO (2022) *Mental health*. Available at https://www.who.int/health-topics/mental-health (Accessed 19 September 2024).

Wilson, P. (2025) *Eugenics - Social Darwinism, sterilization, eugenicists, Britannica*. Available at https://www.britannica.com/science/eugenics-genetics/Popular-support-for-eugenics (Accessed 10 March 2025).

6 Legislation/laws guiding health and social care practice

Clive Sealey and Lisa Porter

The aims of this chapter are to:

- **Define what legislation/law is**
- **Explain the importance of legislation/law to health and social care**
- **Outline important health and social care practice behaviours and guiding legislation/ law**

Introduction

Before starting this chapter, it is important to understand the difference in meaning between *legislation* and *law*, as these two words are often confused. The difference is that there is no difference, they both mean the same thing! They are the equivalent of using either elevator or lift, car or automobile, apartment or flat. Some people prefer to use one word, others prefer to use another. Similarly, legislation and law mean the same thing, and both terms are used in this chapter and book to mean the same thing. Using one over the other is usually down to a style preference, and this is the case in this chapter.

One minor difference between legislation and law is in its grammar. Legislation is what is known as a non-count noun, meaning that you never apply an 's' to make it plural as it has no plural form, meaning that it is always spelt legislation, never legislations. In contrast, law is a count noun and can be singular or plural, so it can be law or laws.

Table 6.1 shows a list of recent legislation in the UK, and a key focus of each.

From Table 6.1, we can identify some key features of legislation (or law!). The first is that when people talk about legislation, they only tend to think about laws in relation to crime as per the *Police and Crime Sentencing Act 2022, Domestic Abuse Act 2021*, *Protection from Sex Based Harassment In Public Act 2023* and *Firearms Act 2023*. However, Table 6.1 shows that laws do not just relate to crime, they relate to almost everything that we do in our everyday life. For example, legislation affects the age that we can do certain things, such as the age we can get married (*Marriage and Civil Partnership Act 2022*), and administer certain substances in our bodies (*Botulinum Toxin and Cosmetic Fillers Act 2021*), as well as the age at which we can smoke, drink and drive.

Legislation also affects what we cannot do, such as being able to go to school, go to college and go to university, as there are laws that give us the rights to do these. Legislation also affects the quality of our lives, such as the quality of the water that we drink (*Water (Special Measures) Act 2023*), the quality of our housing (*Social Housing Regulation Act 2023*), the quality of medicines and medical devices (*Medicines and Medical Devices Act 2021*), the price that we pay for certain goods (*Energy Prices Act 2022*), our

DOI: 10.4324/9781032619309-7

Table 6.1 Recent UK legislation

Legislation	*Key focus*
Water (Special Measures) Act 2025	Regulating water companies
Leasehold and Freehold Reform Act 2024	Banning and/or regulating the use of leasehold for houses and flats
Protection from sex-based harassment in Public Act 2023	Making harassment, alarm or distress in public because of that person's sex a criminal offence
Online Safety Act 2023	Regulating internet service
Firearms Act 2023	Regulation and use of guns and ammunition
Child Support (Enforcement) Act 2023	Enhancing the enforcement child maintenance payments
Social Housing Regulation Act 2023	Regulating social housing
Employment (Allocation of Tips) Act 2023	Ensuring that tips, gratuities and service charges paid by customers are allocated to workers
Energy Prices Act 2022	Regulating energy prices
Marriage and Civil Partnership (Minimum Age) Act 2022	Setting a minimum age for marriage and civil partnership
British Sign Language Act 2022	Recognising British Sign Language as a language
Skills and Post-16 Education Act 2022	Banning the use of essay mills in further and higher education
Down Syndrome Act 2022	Meeting the needs of people with Down Syndrome
Police, Crime, Sentencing and Courts Act 2022	Making new criminal offences and amending sentencing and court procedures
Health and Care Act 2022	Updating existing health and social care laws
Domestic Abuse Act 2021	Defining domestic abuse, and length of sentencing for domestic abuse offences
Botulinum Toxin and Cosmetic Fillers (Children) Act 2021	Banning the use of botulinum toxin and cosmetic fillers for under 18 years old
Medicines and Medical Devices Act 2021	Making safety regulations on medicines and medical devices
Education (Guidance about Costs of School Uniforms) Act 2021	Limiting the costs of school uniforms

employment (*Employment (Allocation of Tips) Act 2023*), and regulates our use of the goods and services *(Internet Safety Act 2023)*. Legislation also enhances our rights in certain areas (*Child Support (Enforcement) Act 2023*), and ensure that the needs of specific groups are met (*British Sign Language Act 2022*; *Down Syndrome Act 2022*), and how we should treat service users (*Health and Care Act 2022*).

It is very unlikely that none of the laws above affect you in some way or other, it is more likely that many of these laws do affect you directly, even if it is just the *Skills and Post-Education Act 2022*, which means that you are not allowed to use essay mills to write your assessments on your course! This shows that legislation is comprehensive in nature, affecting all aspects of our everyday life, even if we do not realise this to be the case. As well as affecting what we do in everyday life, legislation also affects what we can or cannot do in practice. This means that knowing what the law is and how this affects what we can do as practitioners is very important for health and social care practitioners, and this is the focus of this chapter.

The chapter starts with a discussion of what legislation is. It does this by identifying and discussing the purpose of legislation, and providing a simple definition of legislation. The chapter then discusses the importance of legislation for health and social care, as this may not always be apparent. The chapter concludes by briefly linking ten key health and social care practice behaviours to key legislation. The focus is on detailing how these legislation affect health and social care practice.

What is legislation/law?

As mentioned above, when people think of legislation/law, they tend to think of crime and the parts of the legal system that investigates, prosecutes and punishes crime, such as the police, the courts and prison. This tends to lead to a thought that the primary function of the law is sanctions and punishment. However, while sanctions and punishment are important parts of the law, they are not its primary function. Actually, the primary function of a law is to guide behaviour in a certain way. As an example, consider the law on wearing seatbelts. This law is not primarily there to punish those who do not wear seatbelts, but it is primarily there to get people to wear seatbelts in the first place. The punishment for not wearing seatbelts occurs from not doing what the law is guiding you to do, i.e. not wearing a seatbelt. Similarly, when considering health and social care laws, the primary reason they exist is to guide behaviour, not to punish bad behaviour. So, for example, laws on safeguarding are there to guide behaviour on safeguarding in a certain way. This means that the first thing we can say about laws is that their primary purpose is to guide behaviour in a certain way.

Another important aspect of law relates to who makes them. Laws are unique from general everyday rules in that most laws have to be followed by everyone that they apply to. For example, everyone who drives a car has to follow the rules of the driving as well as the rules for having a car. However, not all rules have to be followed. For example, if your neighbour made a rule that you cannot park in front of their house, you would know that we could ignore this rule as it has no standing and there would be punishment for ignoring the rule. However, if the government made a law that said that you could only park a car in front of your own house, we would know that we would have to follow it because it was made by the government. From this, we can define laws as rules made by the government or government institutions.

These two aspects of law allow us to provide a simple definition of law as *rules made by government or government institutions to guide behaviour in a certain way.*

Who makes legislation/law?

The definition above outlines that legislation is made by government or government institutions. The two main organisations that do this are Parliament and the law courts.

Parliament

Parliament is where most legislation is made. Parliament refers to two Houses, the House of Commons and the House of Lords. The House of Commons is made up of Members of Parliament (MPs), who are wholly elected during a general election by the general population. The House of Lords is made up of Lords who are appointed by the government, elected by other Lords or who inherited their place. Most legislation starts in the

Learning Box 6.1: Criminal law v Civil law

Criminal law refers to where a crime has been committed and the law has been broken. Civil law refers to where there is a dispute between people. For example, consider where two people are involved in a car accident. If the reason for the accident was because the person was driving dangerously, this is against the law and would be a criminal offence, and so be the responsibility of the criminal justice system. However, if the accident was caused accidently, then any claim would be a dispute between the two individuals, and be the responsibility of the civil justice system. Issues like divorce, debt and contracts are civil issues. A key difference is that while responsibility for bringing criminal law to court is the responsibility of the police, the responsibility for bringing civil law to court is the individual's. Also, while the penalty for breaking criminal law can be quite severe and include prison, for civil law the penalty is less severe and is usually financial.

House of Commons. Legislation has to be agreed by both Houses of Parliament for it to become law, but it is the House of Commons that has the final say on whether legislation becomes law. This is because it is the part of Parliament that is wholly elected by the general population. Once a legislation is passed by Parliament, it is referred to as an Act. Most legislation is made by Parliament.

Law courts

The law courts are where legal cases are held. This can include **criminal cases and civil cases** (Learning Box 6.1). They are overseen by either trained judges (as in the case of Crown, Appeals, Civil, Tribunal and Supreme courts) or volunteers from the local community known as Magistrates (as in the case of Magistrate courts).

The purpose of the law courts is to ensure that the law is being followed, and where this is not the case to impose punishment or sanctions. Law courts do not directly make laws, but their judgements can lead to changes in the law. This decision then sets what is known as a precedent that must be followed by other judges unless there is good reason not to do so. Where this occurs, this is known as case law. Very little legislation is made by the law courts in the form of case law. This is discussed in more detail below.

Different types of legislation/law

Parliament and law courts make different types of legislation, which can be defined as direct and indirect legislation, as shown in Table 6.2.

Table 6.2 shows the four main types of legislation: primary legislation, secondary legislation, central government guidance and case law. The first three of these are made by Parliament and last is made by the law courts. Legislation that Parliament makes is called direct legislation. Legislation that the law courts make is called indirect legislation. As Table 6.2 shows, most legislation is direct legislation, including most health and social care legislation. But it should become apparent later on in the chapter why it is important for you to know that both types of legislation exist. The four types of legislation are discussed below.

Table 6.2 Different types of legislation

	Direct legislation	*Indirect legislation*
Parliament • *House of Commons* • *House of Laws*	• Primary legislation • Secondary legislation • Central government guidance	
Law Courts • *Magistrates court* • *Crown court* • *Appeal courts,* • *Civil court* • *Supreme Court* • *Tribunals*		• Case law

Primary legislation

Primary legislation is the main type of legislation. It refers to legislation that is passed by Parliament. The aim of primary legislation is to set out the broad principles and rules of the law, saying what the law does. For example, if you wanted to create a law to build more hospitals, you would first create a primary legislation giving you the power to do this, e.g. *Building of Hospitals Act 2025*. This is another reason why it is called primary legislation. The easy way to identify primary legislation is that it ends with *Act*, such as the legislation detailed above and in Table 6.1.

Secondary legislation

Secondary legislation follows on from primary legislation. It provides the detail of how the primary legislation will work. To go back to our example above, having created the primary legislation giving the power to build more hospitals, the secondary legislation would detail how this is to be done, such as, for example, stating where they would be built, how they would be funded and who would build them. While primary legislation is called Acts, secondary legislation are called Statutory Instruments (SI), with the title being the year and its number creation order, e.g. *SI 2025/605*.

There are three key important points relevant to secondary legislation. The first is that many more of these are created than primary legislation (Mills, 2024). For example, in 2024, 25 Acts were created, while about 3,500 SIs were created. The second is that SI have to be linked to a piece of primary legislation, they cannot be created on their own. And thirdly, while primary legislation is created by Parliament, secondary legislation is created by Ministers in the government of the day.

Central government guidance

Sometimes, the government will provide specific guidance on how an issue or topic should be specifically addressed and undertaken. This is usually when the topic is complex or there is some controversy about the topic. This is because the primary and secondary legislation is not detailed enough and there may be variations in how people interpret it. For example, our Act stated that more hospitals can be built and our SI determined where they would be built, how they would be funded and who would build them. The government may also provide guidance on the size of the hospitals, the number of rooms and the type of facilities. In actual fact, such a guidance document does exist as the *Health Building Note 00-01 General design guidance for healthcare buildings* (Department of Health, 2014). The aim of guidance is to ensure that there is a clear and uniform approach to the issue in question.

There are two main types of guidance, statutory guidance and non-statutory guidance. Statutory guidance is the guidance that must be followed unless there is very good reason not to do so. An example of health and social care statutory guidance is the *Working together to safeguard children* (HM Government, 2024), which sets out the guidance on the safeguarding of children which professionals must follow, unless they have good reason not to do so. Non-statutory guidance is the guidance that can be followed, but does not have to be, there is much more discretion on whether to do so for individuals. An example of non-statutory health and social care guidance is *Gender Questioning Children* (Department of Education, 2023) which sets out guidance for schools and colleges in relation to gender identity which professionals can follow if they choose to do so. In essence, the crucial difference between statutory and non-statutory guidance is that statutory guidance must be followed, while non-statutory guidance can be followed.

Case law

Case law is when changes in the way the law is applied occur as a consequence of court judgements by judges. Sometimes a court makes a decision in a case that interprets the law in a certain way, or people go to court to challenge the law, and if they win the case, the outcome of the case becomes the new way that the law is interpreted. A good example of this occurred in relation to criminal records check for working with children and vulnerable adults. Currently, criminal records checks are called Disclosure and Barring Service (DBS) checks. Previously, they were called Criminal Records Bureau (CRB) checks. When they were CRB, this required individuals to disclose all convictions that they had received, regardless of its relevance to the role. So, for example, if someone had been convicted of criminal damage, they had to disclose this, even if not relevant to the role they were applying for. This was challenged in court by a 21-year-old individual who had been convicted of stealing bikes when he was 11. This conviction was disclosed when he applied for a CRB check for a part-time job at a local football club aged 17 and for a university course in sports studies when 19, and as a consequence, he was denied these roles. He challenged the requirement to disclose all convictions, even those not relevant to the role. In the case, the judge agreed with him that this was a breach of his right to privacy under the *Human Rights Act 1998*. Subsequently, CRB changed to DBS, with the requirement that only relevant convictions needed to be disclosed. This is an example of how a court case directly led to a change in the law.

Figure 6.1 shows how the four different types of legislation are hierarchically linked to each other. It shows that primary legislation is at the top of the hierarchy, hence the term primary legislation. Secondary legislation occurs from primary legislation, and guidance occurs from secondary legislation. Case law is separate as it is made by judges, but it affects how primary, secondary and guidance legislation is made.

The importance of legislation for health and social care

In the Introduction, we outlined how legislation is important to almost everything that we do. It affects, want we can do, what we cannot do, the quality of our lives and how

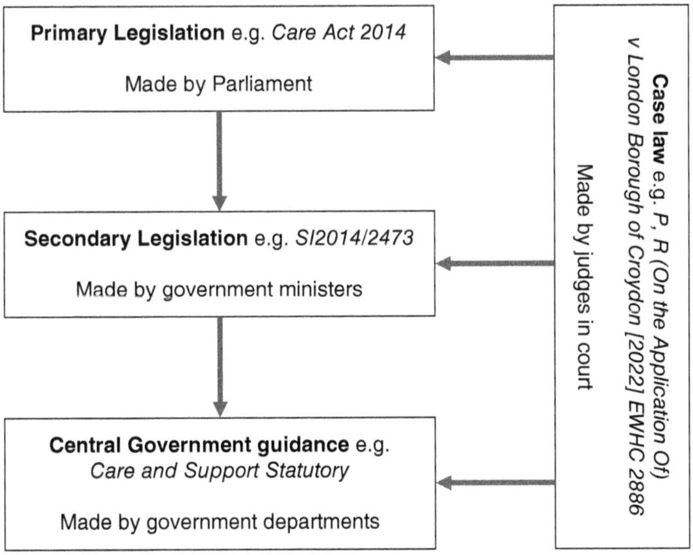

Figure 6.1 Simplified diagram of the link between four different types of legislation.

we work. To consider why we need legislation, we only need to consider what would happen if there was no legislation in these areas. So, for example, if there was no legislation affecting when we could smoke, drink or drive, this could mean that anyone at any age could do these activities – consider what the possible consequences of this could be. If there was no legislation enabling us to go to school, go to college or go to university, this could mean not having the right to these – consider what the possible consequences of this could be. If there was no legislation for quality of food that we eat, the quality of water that we drink or the quality of our employment, this could mean we would not be sure how good these would be – consider what the possible consequence of this could be. And in specific relation to health and social care, if there was no legislation detailing how we safeguard service users, the quality and standards of care that we are expected to provide or how we should treat service users, this could mean any standard of care would be acceptable – consider what the possible consequences of this could be. This reinforces the point that the key focus of legislation is to guide behaviour so that individual acts in specific ways.

Hopefully, reading the above paragraph has given you food for thought as to the importance of health and social care legislation. We can summarise four key ways in which legislation guides behaviour in health and social care:

1 Health and social care legislation guides behaviour to give individuals the right to access health and social care services to meet needs that they have
2 Health and social care legislation guides behaviour so that the things we do are safe and appropriate based on our age, competency and experiences, which protects both the individual and society
3 Health and social care legislation guides behaviour to enable us to go do things in the expectation that they are safe to do so
4 Health and social care legislation guides behaviour to enable us to receive a basic standard of care when we need care

The last of these reasons is particularly relevant to health and social care, as typically when we need health and social care, we are least able to consider the standard of care that we are receiving. For example, if we consider someone going into a care home with dementia, it is likely that they are not able to direct to the home what care they should be receiving and how good it should be. They will very likely depend on the care home meeting these standards as a matter of course. It is here that legislation can enable this to be, through primary legislation which states that all care homes should be inspected to ensure that the care home is meeting minimum standards of care, secondary legislation to detail who should carry out the inspection, guidance on how the inspection should be carried out and case law to ensure that this is all done in a way that is legal.

Ten important health and social care practice behaviours and guiding legislation

As discussed above, the key focus of health and social care legislation is to guide behaviour. The chapter now briefly outlines important behaviours for health and social care practice, and legislation that guides these behaviours. These are behaviours and that you will very likely come across in practice. This provides only a limited outlined; more detailed outlined should be accessed from the other chapters in this book or from other sources.

It is important to know here that while some of the health and social care legislation outlined in this chapter apply to all of the UK (England, Scotland, Wales and Northern Ireland together), not all of them do, and there may be a different legislation that applies to England, Scotland, Wales and Northern Ireland. For example, the *Care Act 2014* only applies in England, and different legislation applies in Wales and Scotland. This is because of **devolution and devolved matters** (Learning Box 6.2). Most health and social care is devolved and the different legislation that apply are shown in the Tables 6.3–6.13. However, due to space limitation, the discussion that follows only relates to legislation in England.

Providing access to health care

This is devolved legislation, as shown in Table 6.3

> **Learning Box 6.2: Devolution and devolved matters**
>
> Devolution refers to where there are different laws that apply in different parts of a nation, as opposed to the same law applying in all parts of the nation. The nation of the United Kingdom (UK) is made up of four separate countries, England, Scotland, Wales and Northern Ireland. There are some laws that apply to all these countries, meaning that you will be treated the same in each of these countries. For example, data protection legislation is the same in all parts of the UK. However, there are some laws that are different depending on which part of the UK you are in. For example, someone applying to university in England is entitled to different levels of funding from someone going to university in Scotland, Wales and Northern Ireland. This is because higher education is a devolved matter, meaning that the different countries can make their own laws on it. Health and social care are mainly devolved matters, meaning that the law is different in the different countries (Greer, 2016).

Table 6.3 Providing access to healthcare legislation

Country	*Legislation*
England	*National Health Service Act 1946*
Wales	• *National Health Service Act 1946* • *National Health Service (Wales) Act 2006*
Scotland	*National Health Service (Scotland) Act 1978*
Northern Ireland	*Health and Social Care (Reform) Act (Northern Ireland) 2009*

The NHS in England and Wales was set up in 1948 through the *National Health Service Act 1946*. This Act provided access to a range of new health services based on three key principles:

1 NHS services should be provided to all of the population (universality)
2 NHS services should be free at the point of delivery
3 NHS services should be based on clinical need, not the ability to pay.

These principles still largely guide NHS services, although some of these principles are not fully followed today, such as principle 2, as some services such as dental services are not wholly free. However, they still largely guide practice in relation to NHS services, meaning that they guide the expectation of both practitioners and service users.

Providing access to social care

This is devolved legislation, and there are different legislation for adults and children in relation to accessing social care, as shown in Tables 6.4 and 6.5.

The *Children Act 1989* places a duty on local authorities to provide services for children in need in their area. This means that local authorities have a legal duty to provide

Table 6.4 Legislation for children

Country	*Legislation*
England and Wales	*Children Act 1989*
Scotland	*Children (Scotland) Act 1995*
Northern Ireland	*Children (Northern Ireland) Order 1995 (SI 1995/755 (N.I. 2)*

Table 6.5 Legislation for adults

Country	*Legislation*
England	*Care Act 2014*
Wales	*Social Services and Well-being (Wales) Act 2014*
Scotland	*Community Care and Health (Scotland) Act 2002*
Northern Ireland	*Health and Social Care Act (Northern Ireland) 2022*

social care where someone under 18 is at risk of poor health and social development, such as neglect or domestic abuse in the family, or because they are disabled. There is the expectation that local authorities will intervene to ensure that such children's needs are met, such as through taking children into care.

The *Care Act 2014* (CA2014) is the main social care legislation for adults in England. It is devolved legislation. In Wales, the *Social Services and Well-being (Wales) Act 2014* is the main legislation. In Scotland, there is no single law which is similar to the *Care Act 2014*, instead a range of different laws underpin Scottish access to social care, including the *Public Bodies (Joint Working) (Scotland) Act 2014* and *Carers (Scotland) Act 2016*. There is no equivalent legislation in Northern Ireland.

The CA2014 aims to ensure that local authorities provide care and support primarily to adults who need social care – it only applies to children in very limited circumstances. In the *Act*, an 'adult' is anyone over the age of 18. An individual can request an assessment of their care needs which the local authority has to carry out if the individual appears to have needs for care and support, or the local authority has a legal duty to an assessment of the care needs of adults who appears to have needs for care and support. The assessment determines if the adult:

1 Has needs arising from a physical or mental impairment or illness.
2 Is unable to achieve two or more specified outcomes in their daily life due to these needs.
3 Experiences a significant impact on their well-being as a result.

If the assessment identifies that the adult has care and support needs, then the local authority is required to provide information, advice or service to enable the identified needs to be met.

Safeguarding

This is devolved legislation, and there is different legislation for children and adult safeguarding, as shown in Tables 6.6 and 6.7.

In England, the local authority, police and Integrated Care Board are responsible for safeguarding children. They are required to work together and with other relevant agencies, such as schools and voluntary organisations. Their responsibility is to co-ordinate

Table 6.6 Safeguarding children legislation

Country	*Legislation*
England	• *Children Act 1989* • *Children Act 2004* • *Children and Social Work Act 2017* • *Working together to safeguard children (statutory guidance)*
Wales	• *Children Act 2004* • *Social Services and Well-being (Wales) Act 2014*
Scotland	*Police and Fire Reform (Scotland) Act 2012* *Children's Hearings (Scotland) Act 2011.*
Northern Ireland	*Children (Northern Ireland) Order 1995 (Statutory Instrument)*

Table 6.7 Adult safeguarding legislation

Country	*Legislation*
England	*Care Act 2014*
Wales	*Social Services and Well-being (Wales) Act 2014*
Scotland	*Adult Support and Protection (Scotland) Act 2007*
Northern Ireland	*No specific safeguarding legislation (Montgomery and Joyce, 2017)*

and ensure the effectiveness of safeguarding work, and to make necessary arrangements to ensure children are safeguarded.

The *Care Act 2104* established safeguarding adults as a statutory duty, meaning that it is a legal requirement for local authorities and healthcare providers to protect vulnerable adults at risk of abuse or neglect. Local authorities have to take steps to prevent abuse or neglect and work together with other bodies such as the police and NHS to create joint safeguarding strategy. Where abuse and neglect occur, they have to carry out reviews to establish what happened.

Equality

There is a single legislation that covers most countries, as shown in Table 6.8.

The *Equality Act 2010* (EA2010) focuses on promoting equality in two ways. The first is to protect individuals from discrimination, and the second is to ensure that reasonable adjustments at work are provided for disabled people.

Protection from discrimination

The EA2010 makes it unlawful to **discriminate** (Learning Box 6.3) against people if they have one of nine protected characteristics. These nine protected characteristics are:

- age
- disability
- gender reassignment
- marriage and civil partnership
- pregnancy and maternity
- race
- religion or belief
- sex
- sexual orientation.

Table 6.8 Equality legislation

Country	*Legislation*
England, Wales and Scotland	*Equality Act 2010*
Northern Ireland	*No specific promoting equality legislation*

Learning Box 6.3: Discrimination

Discrimination is when an individual or group is not treated equally compared to other individual or groups. This can include where men are treated better than women, which would be sex discrimination, or where one ethnic group is treated better than another, which would be race discrimination. Discrimination can include denial of access to services, lower level of provision of services, lower quality of services and limiting scope of services provided. There are two main types of discrimination. Direct discrimination is where an action specifically targets an individual or group, such as not allowing all women to join a club. Indirect discrimination is where an action does not specially target an individual or group but disproportionately affects that group. For example, a rule that requires all employees to stay in the office until a certain time would indirectly discriminate against those with caring responsibilities. While direct discrimination is always illegal, indirect discrimination can in some circumstances be justified.

The EA2010 gives these nine protected characteristics protection against discrimination at work, in education, as a consumer, when using public services, when buying or renting property, as a member or guest of a private club or association. These protections against discrimination apply when both provide care or receive care.

Ensuring reasonable adjustments

The EA2010 outlines that employers are required to make reasonable adjustments in the workplace where an employee has a recognised disability. Reasonable adjustments refer to adjustments or changes that an organisation is required to make in order to remove or reduce the effect of a person's disability. This can include both physical and social adjustments. For example, for a service user who uses a wheelchair, a physical adjustment would be ensuring that ramps are available so that they are able to access buildings, while a social adjustment could include transport for the wheelchair so that they can get to assessments or meetings.

Human rights

There is a single legislation for human rights across the UK, as shown in Table 6.9.

Table 6.9 Human rights legislation

Country	*Legislation*
England	*Human Rights Act 1998*
Wales	
Scotland	
Northern Ireland	

Table 6.10 Data protection legislation

Country	*Legislation*
England, Wales, Scotland and Northern Ireland	*Data Protection Act 2018* *UK General Data Protection Regulation (UK GDPR)*

The *Human Rights Act 1998* (HRA1998) sets out specific rights and freedoms that individuals have to services, goods and treatment. It has 16 Articles that set these out. This includes fundamental rights such as the right to life, freedoms such as the right to free speech and services such as the right to education. The HRA1998 applies to all public authorities, including health and social care providers. The key aspect of the HRA1998 is the ability to take the government to court if your rights have been breached. Key Articles of the HRA1998 that are relevant to health and social care are Article 1: *Right to life*; Article 8: *Respect for your private life and family, home, correspondence* and Article 14: *Protection from discrimination in relation to Articles of the Act.*

Data protection

Data protection legislation covers all countries, as shown in Table 6.10.

The legislation is aimed to ensure that *personal data* is used lawfully, fairly, transparently, specifically, limitedly, accurately, appropriately and timely. Personal data is any data that can identify a person such as name, address, phone number and bank account details. Personal sensitive data such as health, genetic and biometric data, and data that reveals racial and ethnic origin, political opinions, religious or ideological convictions or trade union membership has to be handled in special ways as compared to other personal data. A person has the right to see the personal data that an organisation, company or business has on them. This means that care has to be taken when handling such data, especially when sharing data. Working in health and social care is working with sensitive data on a daily basis, and so understanding and compliance with data protection legislation are very important.

Mental health

Mental health legislation is devolved, as shown in Table 6.11.

The *Mental Health Act 1983* and *Mental Health Act 2007* are usually abbreviated as *MHA 1983 [2007]*, as the 2007 Act is an amendment of the 1983 Act. The Acts apply to both adults and children. The key point is that they only apply for those with a diagnosed mental disorder, not for general mental health issues (see chapter 5). They inform

Table 6.11 Mental health legislation

Country	*Legislation*
England and Wales	• *Mental Health Act 1983* • *Mental Health Act 2007*
Scotland	*Mental Health (Care and Treatment) (Scotland) Act 2003*
Northern Ireland	*Mental Health (Northern Ireland) Order 1986*

Table 6.12 Mental capacity legislation

Country	*Legislation*
England and Wales	• *Mental Capacity Act 2005* • P v Cheshire West and Chester Council and P and Q v Surrey County Council [2014*]*
Scotland	*Adults with Incapacity (Scotland) Act 2000*
Northern Ireland	*Mental Capacity Act (Northern Ireland) 2016*

the assessment, treatment and rights of people with a mental disorder. It details how and who should assess for a mental disorder, what should happen in the event of a diagnosis of a mental disorder and provides safeguards to ensure that treatment is fairly and correctly applied.

Mental capacity

Mental capacity legislation is devolved, as shown in Table 6.12.

Lacking mental capacity refers to the inability to make decisions based on the information provided, and to relate what your decision is. This can be short term or long term, and can occur at any age, but is usually associated with illnesses such as dementia, mental disorders and age. When this occurs, the MCA2005 determines who can make decisions for you and what treatment is relevant. Sometimes treatment involves depriving someone of their liberty. However, the MCA2005 provides safeguards when this occurs called Deprivation of Liberty Safeguards (DoLS). In case law, the decision in case *of* P v Cheshire West and Chester Council and P and Q v Surrey County Council [2014] by the Supreme Court provided important clarification when and how this should occur.

Regulation of health and social care organisations

The regulation of health and social care organisations is devolved, as shown in Table 6.13.

Regulation of health and social care organisations is aimed to ensure that the care that health and social care organisations provide is safe, effective, caring, responsive and well-led (see Chapter 7). The Care Quality Commission is responsible for ensure this. It does this by inspecting health and social care organisations and monitoring their care. It can take action where this is not the case.

Table 6.13 Health and social care organisations legislation

Country	*Legislation*
England	*Health and Social Care Act 2008*
Wales	*Regulation and Inspection of Social Care (Wales) Act 2016*
Scotland	*Regulation of Care (Scotland) Act 2001*
Northern Ireland	*Personal Social Services (Quality, Improvement and Regulation) (Northern Ireland) Order 2003*

Regulation of health and social care professionals

There are lots of different health and social care professional, such as doctors, social workers, psychiatrists and care works. For this reason, there is no single piece of legislation that covers them all, there are lots of different legislation, too numerous to list here. Regulation is designed to ensure that health and social care professionals provide care that is competent, behave correctly towards service user and provide the same level of care to all. This is important to enable trust between health and social care professionals and health and social care service users. See Chapter 7 for more detail on this.

Summary

Legislation/law affects us all in our everyday life in comprehensive ways, affects what we can/cannot do, our quality of life and enhances our rights. We can simply define legislation *as rules made by government or government institutions to guide behaviour in a certain way*. This definition enables us to see that the main aim of legislation is to guide us to behave in certain ways, and only to enforce punishment when we do not act in specified ways, and also that legislation is made in certain ways by certain government institutions, namely Parliament mostly and the law courts occasionally. This is highly relevant to health and social care, as this is typically provided when the individual is least able to voice their wishes and feelings. The principles and legislation outlined here are ones which you will very likely come across in your practice, and so are important to have knowledge of.

References

Department of Education (2023) *Gender Questioning Children - non-statutory guidance*. London: Department of Education. Available at: https://consult.education.gov.uk/equalities-political-impartiality-anti-bullying-team/gender-questioning-children-proposed-guidance/supporting_documents/Gender%20Questioning%20Children%20%20nonstatutory%20guidance.pdf.

Department of Health (2014) *Health Building Note 00-01: General Design Guidance for Healthcare Buildings*. London: Department of Health.

Greer, S.L. (2016) 'Devolution and health in the UK: policy and its lessons since 1998', *British Medical Bulletin*, 118(1), pp. 16–24. Available at: https://doi.org/10.1093/bmb/ldw013.

HM Government (2024) *Working together to safeguard children*. Available at https://www.gov.uk/government/publications/working-together-to-safeguard-children--2 (Accessed 30 January 2025).

Mills, A. (2024) 'Judicial review challenges to secondary legislation in England and Wales: Courting controversy', *Statute Law Review*, 45(1), p. hmae010. Available at https://doi.org/10.1093/slr/hmae010

P v Cheshire West and Chester Council and P and Q v Surrey County Council (2014) Available at https://www.supremecourt.uk/cases/uksc-2012-0068 (Accessed 5 March 2025).

7 Regulation in health and social care

Improving the quality of care?

Clive Sealey

The aims of this chapter are to:

- **Analyse the functions and purposes of regulation in health and social care**
- **Examine the processes of regulation for health and social care**
- **Consider whether regulation can improve the quality of care**

Introduction

When we think about why individuals use and need health and social care, we can see that it is primarily to improve the quality of their lives. This can refer to major improvements or minor improvements in their life. For example, consider that when people access GP services, go to A&E, use care homes and access mental health services, they do so because their quality of life is somewhat diminished to greater or lesser extents, and they require care to improve it. So we can say that when people access these and other health and social care services, they do so in the expectation that it will improve the quality of their lives.

However, there are a number of issues that can affect the care that they receive. The first is the volume of health and social care activities that occur. Table 7.1 shows the number of people receiving health and social care services in England for the time periods shown.

What Table 7.1 highlights is the vast number of health and social care activities that occurs in any given period. A specific issue here is how to ensure that such a large volume

Table 7.1 Health and social care activity statistics (England)

Health and social care activity	*Number of people*
Urgent and Emergency Care: January 2024	2.1 million people (NHS England, 2024)
Elective treatment: January 2024	1.6 million people (NHS England 2024)
GP appointments: January 2024	33.5 million people (Fraser *et al.*, 2024)
Adult social care support: 2022–23	Over 1 million people (NAO, 2023)
Number of adult care home residents: 2022–23	372,035 people (ONS, 2023)
Children's social care referrals: 2022–23	640,430 people (Samuel, 2023)

DOI: 10.4324/9781032619309-8

Learning Box 7.1: The Francis Report

The Francis Report (2013) examined the unnecessary deaths of patients at Stafford NHS Hospital over a period of time. The Report focussed on how inadequate care had contributed to these deaths, and why managers at the hospital had ignored warnings about what was happening. The Report argued specifically that a lack of fundamental standards for healthcare was a cause of the deaths, and made recommendations related to ensuring that patients receive fundamental standards of care to when going to hospital.

of activities is all of good quality to improve the lives of individuals. If providing good quality care was the only concern that professionals have to worry about, this would not be so much of a concern. However, we know that health and social care is a field of many pressures and issues. These include financial pressures, staffing pressure and workload pressures. We have learnt that when health and social care operates within such pressures and issues, it is often quality of care that suffers and is reduced (Farr and Cressey, 2015). For example, **The Francis Report** (Francis, 2013) (Learning Box 7.1) detailed that a cause of the significant failings identified as occurring at Mid-Staffordshire NHS Hospital Trust in between 2005 and 2009 was because of care professionals focussing on issues such as meeting targets at the expense of ensuring quality of care. This shows that despite its importance, professionals can overlook quality of care and undermine its importance in significant ways.

Additionally, this high volume of health and social care activity inevitably places a strain on the ability of professionals to provide good quality care. For example, the increasing number of people requiring adult social care support has led to long waiting lists and lack of staff, which in turn have affected the quality of care (NAO, 2023). Similarly, Tamburello (2023) has observed that there are staffing issues in nursing care that have led to high patient ratios and where this occurs, it can ultimately lead to reduced quality of care. This shows that staffing issues can work to overwhelm the focus on quality of care.

Together, this shows that good quality of care is not something that is guaranteed to happen in health and social care. The pressures and issues within social care can combine to limit the quality of care in various ways. The significance of this is that where quality of care is affected, this can lead to significant risks for service users. At the most extreme, this risk of harm can be a matter of life and death, such as in relation the care provided in A and E or for terminal health conditions such as cancer. However, even where this risk of harm appears minor, it can have significant effects on individuals' lives. For example, while someone being bullied online may seem a relatively minor harm, we know that it can lead to even greater harm in the absence of social support care to cope with it (Castaño-Pulgarín *et al.*, 2022).

One way to try to ensure that care is of good quality is through the use of regulation. This chapter analyses the functions and purposes of regulation to explain the role that regulation serves within the context of health and social care. It then examines the processes of regulation for health and social care to provide an understanding of how it works. This will include key bodies involved in the process of regulation. Finally, the chapter provides a critical analysis of the process of regulation to consider whether regulation can improve the quality of care.

What is regulation?

At its simplest, regulation can be described as laws and guidelines that define and enforce the competencies, behaviours and attitudes of health and social care professionals (Kreutzberg *et al.*, 2019).

The first key aspect of health and social care regulations is that they are made up of laws and guidelines. As discussed in Chapter 6, laws are rules that have been made by government that determine what we can and cannot do within society. While only government can make laws, guidelines can be made by anyone. However, guidelines in relation to health and social care are usually made by organisations that have been given that power through a law. This is known as **statutory regulation** (Learning Box 7.2). Because these guidelines usually occur from statutory regulation, professionals must follow them. Together laws and guidelines combine to determine what health and social care professionals can and cannot do in their practice. This is the essence of regulation.

What are the benefits of regulation to health and social care?

Regulation can often be viewed negatively by those working in health and social care, as it can seem that it disrupts care and imposes an unnecessary and complicated burden on practice (Oikonomou *et al.*, 2019), meaning that it may be viewed negatively and narrowly by those who are subject to regulatory oversight. However, we can identify three key benefits of regulation to health and social care: clarifying what quality of care means, improving trust between professionals and service users, and improving outcomes.

Clarifying what quality of care means

Defining what we mean by quality of care is not easy, because defining 'quality' is not easy. There are many definitions of healthcare quality which focus on different things, ranging from patient welfare, professional knowledge, health outcomes, access to care

> **Learning Box 7.2: Statutory regulation**
>
> Statutory regulation is where there is a legal requirement for an individual to register with a professional regulatory body before they can work in certain professions. Not doing so is a criminal offence. It is also a criminal offence for someone to use a professional title when they are not registered with the regulated body. So, for example, an individual cannot call themselves a nurse, unless they are registered as a nurse, and an individual cannot call themselves a social worker unless they are registered as a social worker. Employers are legally required to check that a person who they employ is registered with the appropriate regulatory body. There are 34 statutory regulated health and social care professions, as shown in Tables 7.2 and 7.3.

and safe care (Busse *et al.*, 2019). This makes it difficult to understand what to focus on when trying to achieve quality of care. For example, consider when you go to the cinema. There are many elements that could affect the quality of your experience, such as how good the film is, how expensive the snacks are, how comfortable your seating is, how good your view of the screen is and so on. Similarly, when talking about care, there are lots of things that could affect the quality of your care, such as how long it takes to receive care, whether the care is effective, how long the care takes, how you are treated when you receive the care and so on. This is because care is not a product but a service, and a service is something that is unique to an individual, and so defining it is not easy.

Crucially, the factors of care above are all factors that are essentially outside the control of service users, and this leads to the question of who should determine what quality is, in terms of whether it should it be practitioners of care or service users of care. For example, research has highlighted that what nurses are required to do in practice does not always match up to patients' values and concerns (Farr and Cressey, 2015). This contradiction means that what a practitioner may view as quality care may not be viewed the same as what a service user views as quality care. This means that lots of time and energy could and has been spent on arguing what quality of care is and how it should be met.

Regulation helps us to move beyond such arguments and towards a definition of quality, as it sets a standard for care that acts as a baseline for quality. There is now a shared single view of quality in relation to care across health and social care. This has been agreed by the National Quality Board (2021), which consists of members from numerous health and social care organisations, such as NHS England, NHS Digital, the Care Quality Commission, the UK Health Security Agency, the National Institute for Health and Care Excellence, the Office for Health Improvement and Disparities, the Department of Health and Social Care, Healthwatch England and the Health Services Safety Improvement Body. The definition provided by the National Quality Board states that quality care should be:

- Safe
- Effective
- Positively experienced
- Well-led
- Sustainably resourced
- Equitable

This definition helps both practitioners and service users to have greater clarity in understanding whether or not quality is achieved. For example, if regulation says that a marker of quality of care is that all care homes are deep cleaned every six months, this sets a standard which has to be met. This limits disagreement between professionals and service users about whether a service is achieving quality of care, meaning that less time is spent on arguing what quality care is and more time can be spent on actually trying to achieve it.

Improving trust between professionals and service users

It is important to remember however that most individuals who use health and social care are not experts in the care that they receive. The experts are those who provide the care. This means that in accessing care, individuals are trusting that the care that they receive will be of sufficient quality to improve their lives (McKee *et al.*, 2023). This trust is important as using health and social care can involve a significant amount of risk of harm for individuals.

Trust is not just relevant to health and social care. It is relevant to all transactions that we make in our everyday life. For example, when buying a car, we use our judgement to decide whether we trust that the person selling us the car is honest in their dealings with us. Similarly, when buying food, we use our judgement to judge whether we can trust that the food is safe to eat. However, the nature of requiring health and social care presents unique issues in relation to trust. For instance, while people may be in good health when buying most other goods and services, this is not the case in relation to health and social care. Indeed, by its very nature, the health and/or social care of these requiring care is impaired in some way. This means that their capacity to make judgements on whether to trust the person providing their care is also impaired. Additionally, their ability to judge the quality of care that receive is also impaired, from both the nature of their condition but also due to the sometimes technical and specialised knowledge that is required to provide health and social care.

This means that to solely rely on trust to ensure that health and social care is of good quality is problematic. This is where the regulation of health and social care makes itself relevant. Regulation is simply a way to try to ensure that the quality of health and social care is met regardless of the needs that the individual has. It is a bridge between trust and need, in the sense that its aim is to reassure individuals that they can trust the quality of the care that they receive, regardless of the need that they have. Understanding regulation, then, is an essential component of the care that individuals receive, and so it is essential to understand it.

Improve the quality of care

As stated above, the key aim of health and social care is to improve the lives of individuals. It does this by setting a minimum standard of care for the delivery and supply of services. An important outcome of such a minimum standard is to reduce variation in services, meaning that what is received by one person in one area is the same received by another person, regardless of who they are or where they live. For example, consider where in the absence of regulation, there is variation in what the threshold is for accessing social care. This means that in some areas, people can access social care if they have *moderate* care needs, meaning unable to carry out personal care tasks such as dressing, but in other areas they can only access care if they have *critical* care needs, meaning that there is a risk to their life. From such variation, it is likely that the quality of life for those needing to have critical care needs is diminished in comparison to those only needing to have moderate care needs. However, with the introduction of the regulation in the form of *Care and Support (Eligibility Criteria) Regulations 2015*, this led to increased support for people who had previously been denied care due to such variation (Fernandez *et al.*, 2015), thereby setting a minimum standard of care for all. This improves the overall quality of life for all to a standard higher than that previously.

Additionally, regulation can also work to make the care that individuals appropriate to their needs. For example, regulation exists that requires care to be **person-centred care (PCC)** (Learning Box 7.3), meaning that it is personalised specially to them. This can include care that ensures information is accessible, adjusts the time people go to bed to suit

Learning Box 7.3: Person-centred care (PCC)

Person-centred care is an approach to providing care that is specific to the needs and preferences of the individual, rather than being the same for everyone. The care reflects the different needs, preferences and abilities that individuals have. This requires care that is designed with their involvement and consent, and allows them to have a choice over who provides care and and/or the type of care that is provided. This means that each individual can have a different type of care provided for them.

them, and giving people a choice of what to have for dinner. Prior to the implementation of person-centred care regulation, care focussed predominantly on viewing the patient as a passive recipient of care, with the perspective of the professional taking priority (Fridberg *et al.*, 2022). However, according to Meranius *et al.* (2020) the shift to PCC has identified numerous beneficial outcomes from person-centred care such as improved health and well-being, improved mutual interaction in relationships, improved cost-effectiveness and improved work environment. This is supported by Rosengren *et al.*'s (2021) observation that PCC is associated with shorter hospital stays, lower readmission rates, higher quality of care and satisfaction with healthcare. This highlights how such regulation can lead to improvements in the quality of care.

How does regulation work in health and social care?

Regulation in health and social care operates at two distinct levels. At one level, there is the regulation of professionals who work in health and social care such as nurses, doctors, and social workers. On another level, there is the regulation of the resources and services where care is provided, such as care homes, hospitals and GP practices. This distinction is important to understand as it means that health and social care professional may be subject to different types of regulation from different organisations. This is explained in more detail below.

The regulation of professionals – Profession's regulators

The regulation of professionals refers to how people become professionals and what professionals do. The aim of regulation here is to set and enforce standards in relation to professional behaviour, competence and ethics (Pickett, 2017). There are eight individual healthcare professions regulators and four individual social care professions regulators in the UK, and these are shown in Table 7.2.

In addition to these specific professional regulators, there is also the Health and Care and Professions Council (HCPC), which regulates 15 allied professions as detailed in Table 7.3. The role of the HCPC is effectively to review the work of these regulators, to ensure that they are working effectively.

The most obvious point to make from Table 7.2 is that there are many more regulators of healthcare than there are of social care. This means that healthcare is more highly regulated than social care. A second point is that the HCPC regulates professions across the UK, which means that the regulations are the same regardless of where you live and work

Table 7.2 Individual healthcare and social care professions regulators in the UK

Healthcare professions regulators	*Social care professions regulators*
***The General Chiropractic Clinic* (GCC) – regulates chiropractors**	***Social Work England* (SWE) – regulates social workers in England**
***The General Dental Council* (GDC) – regulates dentists**	*Northern Ireland Social Care Council* (NISCC) – regulates the social care workforce in Northern Ireland only
***The General Medical Council* (GMC) – regulates doctors, including GPs**	*Social Care Wales* (SWC) – regulates the social care workforce in Wales only
***The General Optical Council* (GOC) – regulates dispensing opticians and optometrists**	*Scottish Social Services Council* (SSSC) – regulates the registration of people who work in social services in Scotland only
***The General Osteopathic Council* (GOsC) – regulates osteopaths**	
***The Nursing and Midwifery Council* (NMC) – regulates nurses, midwives, and specialist community public health nurses.**	
***General Pharmaceutical Council* (GPhC) – pharmacists, pharmacy technicians, and pharmacy premises.**	
Pharmaceutical Society of Northern Ireland (PSNI) – regulates pharmacists and pharmacy premises in Northern Ireland	

Source: HCPC (2024)

Table 7.3 Health and care professions council (HCPC) regulated professions in the UK

Art therapists
Biomedical scientists
Chiropodist/Podiatrist
Clinical scientists
Dieticians
Hearing aid dispensers
Occupational Therapists
Operating department practitioners
Orthoptists
Paramedics
Practitioner psychologists
Physiotherapists
Prosthetists/orthotists
Radiographers
Speech and language therapists

Source: HCPC (2024)

in the UK. However, this is not the case for some individual professions as per Table 7.2, with, for example, the regulator for social work in England, SWE, being different from the regulator for social work in Scotland, Wales and Northern Ireland. Additionally, it is noticeable that the names of the regulators in Scotland, Wales and Northern Ireland are different, in that they refer to social care and social services, rather than just social work, meaning that they regulate a wider range of social care professions rather than just social workers as per SWE. This occurs because of **devolution** (Learning Box 6.2).

Additional to this, the Professional Standards Authority (PSA) is a separate independent body that regulates some of the individual health care and social care regulators shown in Table 7.2, as highlighted in bold. It also oversees all of the work of the HCPC in Table 7.3, as also highlighted in bold.

The regulators in Tables 7.2 and 7.3 focus on regulating specific aspects of professional practice, as detailed below.

Competencies

Competencies refer to the skills that professionals have. For example, to become a doctor or social worker, there is regulation in place that says that you are required to undertake specific training to ensure that you acquire the professional skills to carry out these professions. Individuals are not allowed to call themselves professions like a doctor, social worker or occupational therapist unless you meet these professional skills. This means that when an individual visits a doctor or social worker, they are being seen by someone who has met the relevant professional competencies.

Furthermore, to continue to be a professional like a doctor, social worker or occupational therapist, there is regulation in place that requires these professionals to undertake a certain amount of continued professional development (CPD). For example, the Royal College of Physicians (RCP) requires doctors to undertake a minimum average of 50 hours of CPD per year (RCP, 2015), and to continue to practise as a social worker in England, SWE requires social worker to demonstrate one example of CPD in a given year (SWE, 2024). This means that when an individual visits a doctor or social worker, the person is still able to meet these competencies despite how long previously they have qualified. This is important because improvements in health and social care can occur very quickly, and without CPD these improvements can overtake and therefore limit the competencies of professionals.

Behaviours

Regulation also focusses on the behaviours of health and social care professionals. This relates to what professionals actually do in practice. The difference between competency and behaviour can be explained by reference to the fact that someone may have professional competence and so have good knowledge of what they are doing, but their practice may be characterised by behaviours such as rudeness, bullying or lack of empathy. When such behaviours occur, they pose a threat to the quality of care that individuals receive (Layne *et al.*, 2019). A regulated professional has to show that they display certain behaviours in practice, such as politeness, honest and respect and empathy.

Attitudes

Finally, professions regulation is also focussed on the attitudes of health and social care professionals. Attitude refers to what we think and how we behave towards individuals (Price, 2015). So for example, society may view some conditions more negatively than others, such as lung cancer caused by smoking or mental health conditions. To do so could lead to stigma towards individuals, which in turn can affect the quality of care that they receive and therefore the effectiveness of the care (Price, 2015). Additionally, it can lead to some service users choosing not to access care that would benefit them, which ultimately limits the potential beneficial outcomes of care (Mannava *et al.*, 2015). Regulation is aimed to ensure that such negative attitudes do not affect professional practice, by setting out clear ways of providing care that all professionals are required to follow, regardless of their beliefs. Regulation can also help professionals to make a decision about care where there is the potential for lots of choice in decision making, as it eliminates some decisions which limits the choices available to professionals (Kaine *et al.*, 2010).

These explanations show that the key focus in health and social care regulation is on what professionals do and how they do it. The aim of regulation is to ensure that the care that professionals provide is of a certain quality and standard not just some of the time, but most if not all of the time. It does this by setting rules and regulation which professionals must follow either to become a professional in the first place or to continue to remain a professional.

Regulation of services – Care Quality Commission (CQC)

As well as specific individuals, there is also regulation of the environment in which health and social care professionals work and the services that they provide. The Care Quality Commission (CQC) is the sole regulator of health and social care services. The responsibility of the CQC involves regulating:

- Providers of healthcare services to people of all ages, including hospitals, ambulance services, clinics, community services, mental health services and other registered locations, including dental and GP practices.
- Providers of social care services for adults in care homes (where nursing or personal care is provided), in the community and in people's own homes.
- Providers of services for people whose rights are restricted under the *Mental Health Act 1983/87*.
- Providers of health and care services for children or young people.

(CQC, 2023)

The list above shows that the role of the CQC is wider than that of individual professional regulators. It covers almost all health and social care services. This means that even if your profession is not regulated by a specific professional regulator, where you work is, and so regulation affects what you do in practice.

The difference between what the professional regulators do and what the CQC does is exemplified by reference to a GP practice. In this context, the GMC as the professional regulator regulates the competencies, behaviours and attitudes of the GPs. The CQC, as the regulator of services, regulates how the GP practice itself operates, in terms of the treatment, care and support care that the GP practice provides. Therefore, CQC regulation is much wider than professions regulation.

To exemplify further, consider if you go into a shop to buy something. There is a distinction between the person who serves you and the environment in which they serve you. The professional regulators regulate the person who serves you in terms of whether they are competent enough to serve you and how they treat you. The CQQ regulate how clean the shop is, how the shop treats you and whether they are providing the services they are supposing to be providing.

The CQC regulates through a sequential and ongoing five-stage process of registering, monitoring, rating, inspecting and action. Firstly, the CQC requires individuals who wish

Learning Box 7.4: Key Lines of Enquiry (KLOEs)

Key lines of enquiry, or KLOEs for short, are the criteria that CQC uses to assess whether every health and social care setting is providing good quality care.
There are five different KLOEs:

- Safe – which refers to protecting individual from harm and abuse
- Effective – which refers to the outcomes that the care is achieving
- Caring – which refers to how staff treat individuals
- Responsive – which refers to how well the service is responding to the changing needs of individuals
- Well-led – which refers to the leadership and management of the service

The CQC rates each of these KLOEs individually as 'Outstanding', 'Good', 'Requires Improvement' or 'Inadequate'. This contributes to the overall rating of the service.

to run health and social care service or who are in charge of such services to register with them. The CQC makes checks to ensure that individuals are 'fit and proper' to run services.
Secondly, once the service is running, the CQC monitors the services to ensure that they are meeting set quality standards. This is done by assessing whether the service is meeting five standards, referred to as **Key Lines of Enquiry (KLOEs)** (Learning Box 7.4). Thirdly, the CQC can also carry out inspections to monitor a service. These inspections are usually periodic and announced in nature. They include speaking to staff and service users, and observing care as it is practised in the service.
Fourthly, once undertaken, the CQC will provide a rating for the service, which will state whether the service is '*Outstanding*', '*Good*', '*Requires Improvement*' or '*Inadequate*'. Where there is concern about a service or a complaint has been made, the CQC can carry out unannounced inspections, meaning that they can turn up at any given time. The CQC have unique powers that give it the right to enter a regulated service at any time, much in the same way as the police do. This is a fairly strong regulatory power that the professional regulators do not have. Additionally, a rating of '*inadequate*' can lead to the CQC requiring a service to be placed in special measures. The aim of special measures is to improve the service with a given time, but if this improvement does not happen, the CQC can cancel its registration, as occurred in the case of Cestrian Care (CQC, 2023a). A cancelled registration means that the provider can no longer provide health and social care services.
The CQC also publishes an annual *State of Care* report, which sets out systematic issues, challenges and improvements within health and social care. This report provides a snapshot of what is working and what is not working in health and social care.
According to Smithson *et al.* (2018), the work of the CQC has had specific positive regulatory impacts on health and social care providers in eight ways. These are:

1 *Anticipatory impact* – meaning providers raising standards in anticipation of monitoring and inspection.

2 *Directive impact* – meaning providers raising standards as a response to directives from the CQC.
3 *Organisational impact* – meaning providers changing the dynamics, leadership, culture, or motivation of their organisation and whistleblowing from the CQC requirements.
4 *Relational impact* – meaning providers having a better relationship with the CQC from having regular contact, which leads to more openness and honesty.
5 *Informational impact* – meaning providers being mindful of the impact of the fact that the CQC publicly publishes information which can affect whether service users choose them.
6 *Stakeholder impact* – meaning providers under pressure from other interested organisation to improve performance due to CQC regulation.
7 *Later impact* – meaning providers using the findings from other CQC reports to improve their practice.
8 *Systematic impact* – meaning providers using the publication of the CQC's State of Care reports to identify recurring issues for improvement in their practice.

This suggests that CQC regulation has had specific beneficial effects for health and social care. However, Smithson *et al.* (2018) also note that the CQC is not an improvement agency. This means that while it does provide direction on whether service should be improved, it does not provide specific expertise on how services could be improved, meaning that it has a limited impact on improving the quality of care. Additionally, it should also be noted that there are some healthcare procedures that neither the CQC nor profession's regulators regulate. The most obvious non-regulated sector is **non-surgical cosmetic surgery** (Learning Box 7.5).

Can regulation improve quality of care?

The evidence highlighted above supports a notion that regulation can improve the quality of care. This evidence is especially evident in relation to the CQC, for which there are 8 ways in which it has had an impact on the quality of services. However, the evidence suggests that regulation alone is not a sustainable way to improve care. For example, regulation can lead to a focus on meeting the regulation requirements, while limiting the care. The assumption of regulation is that in meeting the regulation, the aim of the regulation is met. However, we know that a focus on a target can mean that providers focus solely on this, without considering the wider aspects of what they are doing. So while they may

Learning Box 7.5: Non-surgical cosmetic surgery

Non-surgical cosmetic procedures can be simply defined as those that do not require anaesthetic or an incision of the skin. It can include procedures such as Botox, laser hair removal, tattoo removal, skin lightening and microdermabrasion. While surgical cosmetic procedures are regulated as detailed above, non-surgical cosmetic procedures are neither profession's or CQC regulated. This means that they can be carried out by anyone in any kind of premise, with no guarantee of the quality of the work.

have met the regulation, they may not be understanding that the actual care that they provide may be substandard. As an example of this, consider where the regulation states that all patients in a hospital that no longer require treatment should be discharged as soon as possible. This is from the evidence that such regulation is good for quality of care (Horton and Wood, 2022). However, it may be possible to meet this regulation, but still not improve the quality of care, if the discharge is not properly undertaken, so that the service user is discharged to an inappropriate place (Horton and Wood, 2022). Additionally, Toffolutti *et al.* (2017) have observed that improvements that occur from regulation can often diminish once the regulatory intervention is over. This is where compliance with regulation is done simply as a requirement, referred to as 'gaming' (Bevan and Hood, 2006), rather than wholehearted compliance within the spirit of the regulation.

This highlights, as Kelly *et al.* (2023) state, that regulation by itself does not improve care, meaning that regulation should be seen as just one tool for improving care. Perhaps the most important tool here is ensuring a deeper theoretical understanding of the role that health and social care can play to improving quality of life. Care is not an exact science but is a human trait, meaning that different people will view care differently. However, an understanding of the explicit theoretical foundations that are important to care can improve the care provided (Grol *et al.*, 2007). This is because such a deeper understanding can improve what practitioners do, how they do it and why they do it. It is only when such a deeper understanding is present on an ongoing basis that quality of life is truly and meaningfully improved.

Summary

An essential function of health and social care is to improve the quality of life of individuals. In order to do this, care needs to be of good quality. However, there are many pressures and issues that can limit this, meaning that quality of care is not something that is automatically guaranteed to happen. This is where regulation becomes important to health and social care. Regulation is designed to ensure that quality of care is not overlooked, undermined or overwhelmed in the context of these pressures and issues. Many but not all health and social care professions are subject to statutory regulation, in the form of professions regulation or CQC services regulation. The evidence suggests that regulation can help to clarify what quality of care means, improve trust between professions and service users and improve the quality of care. However, relying on regulation alone is not a sustainable way to improve care. This is because regulation can become focussed on compliance, rather than meaningfully improving care. What is required by health and social care professionals is an understanding of and commitment to the explicit theoretical foundations that are important to care. It is only from such an understanding that quality of care and therefore quality of life is truly and meaningfully improved in a sustainable way.

References

Bevan, G. and Hood, C. (2006) 'What's measured is what matters: Targets and gaming in the English public health care system', *Public Administration*, 84(3), pp. 517–538. Available at https://doi.org/10.1111/j.1467-9299.2006.00600.x

Busse, R., Panteli, D. and Quentin, W. (2019) 'An introduction to healthcare quality: Defining and explaining its role in health systems', in *Improving Healthcare Quality in Europe: Characteristics, Effectiveness and Implementation of Different Strategies [Internet]*. European Observatory on Health Systems and Policies. Available at https://www.ncbi.nlm.nih.gov/books/NBK549277/ (Accessed 13 March 2024).

Care Quality Commission (2023a) *CQC cancels Cheshire care company registration after inspection finds the services inadequate*. Available at https://www.cqc.org.uk/news/releases/cqc-cancels-cheshire-care-company-registration-after-inspection-finds-services (Accessed 2 April 2024).

Care Quality Commission (2023) *Services we regulate*. Available at https://www.cqc.org.uk/what-we-do/services-we-regulate/services-we-regulate (Accessed 2 April 2024).

Castaño-Pulgarín, S. *et al.* (2022) 'Perceived Social SPerceived Social Support and Risk of Cyberbullying in Adolescents: A Systematic Reviewupport and Risk of Cyberbullying In Adolescents: A Systematic Review', *The Qualitative Report* [Preprint]. Available at: https://doi.org/10.46743/2160-3715/2022.5039.

Farr, M. and Cressey, P. (2015) 'Understanding staff perspectives of quality in practice in healthcare', *BMC Health Services Research*, 15(1), p. 123. Available at https://doi.org/10.1186/s12913-015-0788-1

Fernandez, J.-L., Snell, T. and Marczak, J. (2015) *An Assessment of the Impact of the Care Act 2014 Eligibility Regulations*. PSSRU Discussion Paper DP2905. London/Canterbury: London School of Economics/University of Kent. Available at https://www.pssru.ac.uk/pub/5141.pdf (Accessed 2 April 2024).

Francis, R. (2013) *Report of the Mid Staffordshire NHS Foundation Trust Public Inquiry Executive Summary*. London: Stationery Office. Available at https://assets.publishing.service.gov.uk/media/5a7c9bec40f0b65b3de09fde/0898_i.pdf (Accessed 18 March 2024).

Fraser, C., Beech, J. and Mendelhson, E. (2024) *General practice tracker, The Health Foundation*. Available at https://www.health.org.uk/news-and-comment/charts-and-infographics/general-practice-tracker (Accessed 18 March 2024).

Fridberg, H., Wallin, L. and Tistad, M. (2022) 'Operationalisation of person-centred care in a real-world setting: A case study with six embedded units', *BMC Health Services Research*, 22(1), p. 1160. Available at https://doi.org/10.1186/s12913-022-08516-y

Grol, R.P. *et al.* (2007) 'Planning and studying improvement in patient care: The use of theoretical perspectives', *The Milbank Quarterly*, 85(1), pp. 93–138. Available at https://doi.org/10.1111/j.1468-0009.2007.00478.x

HCPC (2024) *Health and social care regulators*. Available at https://www.hcpc-uk.org/about-us/who-we-work-with/other-regulators/health-and-social-case-regulators/ (Accessed 13 March 2024).

Horton, T and Wood, S (2022) *Improving hospital discharge in England: the case for continued focus and support*. Available at: https://www.health.org.uk/news-and-comment/blogs/improving-hospital-discharge-in-england-the-case-for-continued-focus (Accessed: 2 April 2024).

Kaine, G. *et al.* (2010) 'A framework for understanding individual response to regulation', *Food Policy*, 35(6), pp. 531–537. Available at https://doi.org/10.1016/j.foodpol.2010.06.002

Kelly, Y. *et al.* (2023) 'Factors that influence the implementation of (inter)nationally endorsed health and social care standards: A systematic review and meta-summary', *BMJ Quality & Safety*, 32(12), pp. 750–762. Available at https://doi.org/10.1136/bmjqs-2022-015287

Kreutzberg, A. *et al.* (2019) 'Regulating the input: health professions', in *Improving Healthcare Quality in Europe: Characteristics, Effectiveness and Implementation of Different Strategies [Internet]*. European Observatory on Health Systems and Policies. Available at https://www.ncbi.nlm.nih.gov/books/NBK549267/ (Accessed 13 March 2024).

Layne, D. *et al.* (2019) 'Negative behaviors among healthcare professionals: Relationship with patient safety culture', *Healthcare*, 7(1), p. 23. Available at https://doi.org/10.3390/healthcare7010023

Mannava, P. *et al.* (2015) 'Attitudes and behaviours of maternal health care providers in interactions with clients: A systematic review', *Globalization and Health*, 11(1), p. 36. Available at https://doi.org/10.1186/s12992-015-0117-9

McKee, M., Greenley, R. and Permanand, G. (2023) *Trust: The Foundation of Health Systems*. Policy Brief 58. Geneva: WHO. Available at https://eurohealthobservatory.who.int/publications/i/trust-the-foundation-of-health-systems (Accessed 18 March 2024).

Meranius, M.S. *et al.* (2020) 'Paradoxes of person-centred care: A discussion paper', *Nursing Open*, 7(5), p. 1321. Available at https://doi.org/10.1002/nop2.520

National Audit Office (2023) *Reforming Adult Social Care in England*. Session 2023-24 10 November 2023 HC 184. London: House of Commons.

National Quality Board (2021) *A shared commitment to quality for those working in health and care systems*. Available at https://www.england.nhs.uk/wp-content/uploads/2021/04/nqb-refreshed-shared-commitment-to-quality.pdf (Accessed 13 March 2024).

NHS England (2024) *NHS England » Monthly operational statistics – January 2024*. Available at https://www.england.nhs.uk/long-read/monthly-operational-statistics-january-2024/ (Accessed 18 March 2024).

Oikonomou, E. *et al.* (2019) 'Patient safety regulation in the NHS: Mapping the regulatory landscape of healthcare', *BMJ Open*, 9(7), p. e028663. Available at https://doi.org/10.1136/bmjopen-2018-028663

ONS (2023) 'Care homes and estimating the self-funding population, England'. Available at https://www.ons.gov.uk/peoplepopulationandcommunity/healthandsocialcare/socialcare/articles/carehomesandestimatingtheselffundingpopulationengland/2022to2023 (Accessed 18 March 2024).

Pickett, L. (2017) *Professional Regulation in Health and Social Care*. Briefing Paper Number CBP8094. London: House of Commons Library.

Price, B. (2015) 'Understanding attitudes and their effects on nursing practice', *Nursing Standard*, 30(15), pp. 50–60. Available at https://doi.org/10.7748/ns.30.15.50.s51

Rosengren, K., Brannefors, P. and Carlstrom, E. (2021) 'Adoption of the concept of person-centred care into discourse in Europe: A systematic literature review', *Journal of Health Organization and Management*, 35(9), pp. 265–280. Available at https://doi.org/10.1108/JHOM-01-2021-0008

Royal College of Physicians (2015) *CPD for revalidation, RCP London*. Available at https://www.rcplondon.ac.uk/events-and-education/education-and-professional-development/ (Accessed 18 March 2024).

Samuel, M. (2023) 'Child protection enquiry total hits new annual high but proportion finding abuse continues to shrink', *Community Care*. https://www.communitycare.co.uk/2023/10/30/child-protection-enquiry-total-hits-new-annual-high-but-proportion-finding-abuse-continues-to-shrink/, 30 October. Available at https://www.communitycare.co.uk/2023/10/30/child-protection-enquiry-total-hits-new-annual-high-but-proportion-finding-abuse-continues-to-shrink/ (Accessed 18 March 2024).

Smithson, R. *et al.* (2018) *Impact of the Care Quality Commission on Provider Performance. Room for Improvement?* London/Manchester: The King's Fund/University of Manchester. Available at https://assets.kingsfund.org.uk/f/256914/x/3bc00421c8/impact_cqc_provider_performance_2018.pdf (Accessed 2 April 2024).

Social Work England (2024) *What you need to know, Social Work England*. Available at https://www.socialworkengland.org.uk/cpd/what-you-need-to-know/ (Accessed 18 March 2024).

Tamburello, H. (2023) *Impact of Staffing Levels on Safe and Effective Patient Care Literature Review*. London: Royal College of Nursing. Available at https://www.rcn.org.uk/-/media/Royal-College-Of-Nursing/Documents/Publications/2023/February/010-665.pdf (Accessed 18 March 2024).

Toffolutti, V., McKee, M. and Stuckler, D. (2017) 'Evidence points to "gaming" at hospitals subject to national health service cleanliness inspections', *Health Affairs*, 36(2), pp. 355–361. Available at https://doi.org/10.1377/hlthaff.2016.1217

Part 2

Essential knowledge for studying health and social care

8 Key sociological theories for health and social care

Dawn Goodall

The aims of this chapter are to:

- Explain the importance of sociological theory in developing a deeper understanding of health and social care
- Outline different types of sociological theories relevant to health and social care
- Detail how we can use the different 'lens' of sociological theories to provide more effective health and social care

Introduction

Theory is a word that you have very likely used in your everyday conversation. For example, you may say, 'I have a theory about that', when you mean that you are making a guess about something. This also shows the way that you think about something. You can think of any theory as a pair of magnifying glasses. When you put on a pair of magnifying lenses, the world looks one way, and then when you adjust the magnification, it looks different although you are viewing th same thing. In the same way, when you are considering what is happening in a situation, adopting different theories may offer different ways of viewing the same events to create meaning and sense.

This brings us to the importance of understanding how social theories offer very different lenses through which we might observe service users' situations and consider our own attitudes and values within this. Sociological theory helps us understand how individual consciousness forms through social experiences and circumstances. By studying it, we can examine our own norms and perspectives. As we try to interpret the social world and establish different ways we could understand social relations, so we can find more effective ways to respond to the life experience of the people we support.

In this chapter, we identify some important sociological theories for health and social care practice, even though they may seem detached from your practical work in health and social care. Throughout this chapter, we look at ways in which studying social theory supports health and social care practitioners to develop a deeper understanding of the complex interplay between individuals and society, enabling more effective and accountable practice. To do this, we need to embark on a sociological journey through time to see the different ways in which theorists have been attempted to quantify and understand the world in which we live.

DOI: 10.4324/9781032619309-10

The importance of theory

Before explaining the importance of theory, it is important to explain the difference between fact and theory. A fact is something that has been repeatedly confirmed with evidence and can be shown to be true through evidence. For example, in 2000, there were 12 mobile phone subscriptions per 100 people, and in 2023, there were 111 per 100 people in the world (World Bank Group, 2025). This is something that has been measured and established as true. A theory is a belief about something that has not been confirmed with evidence, although there may be some limited evidence to support the belief. For example, to go back to the example of mobile phones, the significant use of mobile phone by teenagers suggests that using this device reduces the time available for activities that benefit cognitive development and academic performance (Röhlke, 2024). The key word here is 'suggests', as this is not something that has been proven with evidence, but it is something that the evidence suggests is a possibility. The essential difference between fact and theory is that a fact is something that is proven, while a theory is something that has not been proven.

Social theory focuses on how human belief and action are products of social influences (Jones and Bradbury, 2018). They help us to make sense of the world around us, especially when significant changes occur. I can exemplify this by referring to the technological changes that have occurred over the last 70 years. Someone arriving here from the 1960s or 1970s would likely find 2025 to be a world of astonishing technological advancements, greater connectivity, and significant cultural shifts. The technological advancements over the past 30 years have had profound implications for communication. Instant messaging and video calls have made communication almost instantaneous, significantly reducing the time it takes to convey messages. This has made it easier to stay in touch with friends, family, and colleagues regardless of geographical distance. Social media platforms have connected people from all over the world, allowing for the exchange of ideas, cultures and information on an unprecedented scale. This global connectivity has fostered a more interconnected and informed society. However, the ease of communication has both positive and negative effects on personal relationships. While it allows for more frequent and convenient interactions, it can also lead to superficial connections and a decrease in face-to-face interactions, potentially impacting the depth of relationships.

The pace of change and the integration of technology into nearly every aspect of our lives offer both exciting possibilities and new challenges. Trying to make sense of these changes and challenges is difficult and complex. Theory helps us to organise this information in ways that highlight patterns, differences, and trends. This is important because it helps us to better understand the world around us. In the absence of theory, we would struggle to understand and explain what we think is happening around us.

Key sociological terms

Before discussing specific sociological theories, there are some key sociological terms that are important to understand.

Socialisation

Socialisation is the process where individuals and/or groups are taught to behave or think in a certain way. For example, children can be taught that going to school is important, boys can be socialised to act play with certain toys and not others, and teenagers can be socialised to act in certain ways when with their friends. There are various groups where socialisation can occur.

- **Family:** Families are often the primary source of health-related norms and values. They influence dietary habits, attitudes towards exercise and approaches to healthcare. For example, children raised in families that prioritise healthy eating and regular medical check-ups are more likely to adopt these practices themselves (Wäsche *et al.*, 2021).
- **Educational Institutions:** Schools and colleges can socialise individuals about important skills, knowledge, and values that they need in society. For example, they can socialise them about the importance of study, the importance of exams, and the importance of certain behaviours.
- **Peer Groups:** Peers can influence behaviours such as smoking, drinking, and drug use. Peer influence can encourage healthy behaviours or pressure others in conforming to risky activities.
- **Mass Media:** Media plays a significant role in shaping public perceptions of health and illness. Campaigns promoting healthy lifestyles or raising awareness about diseases can influence public behaviour and attitudes towards health. For example, in February 2025, the NHS used the media to launch their first ever breast cancer screening campaign to encourage more women to access their mammograms, because they found that 'more than four in ten (46.3%) [of women] invited for the first time don't act on their invitation' (NHS England, 2025).
- **Religion:** Religious beliefs and practices can impact health behaviours and attitudes towards medical interventions. For instance, some religions promote fasting, which can affect dietary habits, while others may have specific views on medical treatments.

Structure v Agency

- **Structure** refers to the set of institutions, customs, laws and traditions that influence what a person can do, for example, family, school and work. Structures MAY be a powerful influence on any decision that an individual makes (even if they don't know it).
- **Agency** refers to the ability of individuals to act independently and make their own choices. Agentic freedom (the extent to which someone CAN do this) is an important consideration when working with service users.

Norms v values

- **Norms** are the unwritten rules and expectations about how people should behave in a particular society or group. They guide everyday behaviour and interactions, ensuring that individuals act in ways that are considered acceptable and appropriate.
- **Values** are deeply held beliefs about what is good, desirable, and important in a society. They serve as the foundation for norms and guide individuals' behaviour and decision-making. Values can vary widely between different cultures and societies. Values underpin norms. For example, if a society values honesty, it will develop norms that encourage truthful behaviour and discourage lying. Similarly, if a society values respect, it will have norms that promote courteous and considerate behaviour.

Norms and values are crucial for maintaining social order and cohesion. They provide a framework for expected behaviour and help individuals understand who they are in society.

Culture

Culture refers to where there is a similarity in individuals in the way that they look, act, or think and/or behave, such as, for example, by nationality (Welsh), by age (teenagers), or by behaviour (Goths). Diverse cultural beliefs and practices can sometimes conflict with mainstream health norms, leading to non-compliance with certain health behaviours. For example, beliefs about death and dying can influence decisions about end-of-life care, such as where in some cultures, considering death and making advance arrangements are considered taboo. Healthcare providers may find it challenging to discuss palliative care options and ensure that patients' wishes are respected. For example, in post-war Japan, 'Death Cafes' opened as a response to what was seen as a 'death-avoidant society' where discussion of the subject was taboo (Ito *et al.*, 2023).

Stigma

Stigma refers to where certain groups are treated unfairly based on a negative attitude towards them, such as, for example, mental illness or HIV/AIDS. This is referred to as stigmatisation. Stigmatisation can discourage individuals from seeking care and adhering to treatment. For example, Hajizadeh *et al.* (2024) found that in most studies when stigmatisation was associated with mental health disorders, there was delayed and decreased use of health services and substandard treatment leading to poorer health outcomes and an increased risk of human rights violations for the affected individuals.

Key sociological theories

There are many different sociological theories, some of which you very likely have come across before. This chapter focuses on three distinct types of social theories and explores the different ways we can understand the way society works and then apply these lenses to health and social care practice. These are:

- **Consensus Theories** (structural, focusing on how societal structures influence behaviour to benefit all)
- **Conflict Theories** (structural, focusing on how societal structures influence behaviour to benefit some)
- **Action Theories** (agentic, focusing on the role of human interpretation in creating society)

Consensus theories

Consensus theories stress societal agreement and shared norms into which it is in everybody's best interest to be socialised.

Social facts – Emile Durkheim

Emile Durkheim is a French sociologist, who founded the Consensus Perspective and Functionalism. His major works include *The Division of Labour in Society* (1893), *The Rules of the Sociological Method* (1895), *Suicide* (1897), and *The Elementary Forms of Religious Life* (1912).

Durkheim introduced the concept of *social facts* to describe the norms, values, and shared ways of acting that exist independently of individuals but shape their behaviour. These social facts exert a moral constraint on individuals, guiding their actions and ensuring conformity to societal expectations. Durkheim's work aimed to uncover these external forces, much like the natural sciences sought to categorise the physical world (May and Powell, 2008). Our shared beliefs and values form a collective conscience, which is essential for social solidarity. This collective conscience ensures that individuals feel part of a larger social collective, aligning their desires with societal goals. It plays a crucial role in maintaining social order and cohesion.

Implications for health and social care

Durkheim's concept of social facts and the collective conscience can provide us with valuable insights into how societal norms and values shape individual behaviour and social order. In health and social care practice, understanding these dynamics is essential for promoting social solidarity, addressing inequalities, and providing culturally sensitive and ethically sound care.

Health and social care practices contribute to social solidarity by promoting shared values and norms related to health and well-being. This includes encouraging healthy behaviours, preventive care, and community support. The collective conscience can sometimes reinforce hierarchical inequalities, as societal norms and values may reflect the interests of dominant groups. Health and social care professionals must be aware of these dynamics and work to address inequalities in access to care and health outcomes.

Health and social care professionals must balance the needs of individuals with the goals of the larger society. This involves respecting individual autonomy while promoting behaviours that benefit the collective. Health and social care professionals often face ethical dilemmas when societal norms conflict with individual rights or well-being. Navigating these dilemmas requires a careful consideration of ethical principles and the collective conscience. For example, decisions about end-of-life care may involve balancing the patient's wishes with societal norms about the sanctity of life and the allocation of healthcare resources.

Durkheim's theories on Consensus and Functionalism underscore the importance of societal structures in shaping individual behaviour. His insights into social facts and the collective conscience remain relevant for understanding the complex interplay between individuals and society. His work highlights the necessity of social cohesion and the role of institutions in maintaining societal stability.

Theory of social action – Talcott Parsons

Talcott Parsons is an American sociologist and a key theoretical figure from the end of World War II to the mid-1960s. His work attempted to synthesise the classical traditions of Durkheim and Weber (more on him later). His major works included *The Structure of Social Action* (1937) and his co-authored work with Edward A. Shils *Toward a General Theory of Action* (1951).

Parson's *Theory of Social Action* argues that social agency is not merely arbitrary actions or total free will but is framed within the patterned structure of relationships that are reproduced through social order and norms. His notion of individual agency is a synthesis of individual actions and social systems.

Parsons' theory was particularly well-suited to the needs of modern capitalism, coinciding with the dominance of the United States as the wealthiest and most powerful country by the 1950s. His arguably most impactful work was his theory of the family, with its gender-specific expressive and instrumental roles. This has been seen as a celebration of American hegemony. Hegemony, a concept from Italian Marxist Antonio Gramsci, refers to the ideological domination of the ruling class for whose benefit all areas of culture and society are organised. In the mid-20th century, the nuclear family, with its specific roles, became the norm by which consideration of alternatives was measured (see Chapter 3). This accepted form of society now appeared natural and inevitable, making it resistant to examination and challenge.

Implications for health and social care

Parsons' approach emphasises the importance of social structures and norms in shaping individual actions. Health and social care practitioners might use this knowledge to understand the ways in which their service users' behaviours are influenced by their social environments, including family dynamics, cultural norms, and societal expectations (Carr *et al.*, 2023). Parsons' theory of the family, with its gender-specific roles, can help practitioners understand the influence of family structures on health behaviours. For example, understanding the role of caregivers within a family can inform strategies for supporting service users and their families in managing health conditions (Ho *et al.*, 2022). Parson's theory also highlights the ways in which social norms and values shape behaviour, and health and social care practitioners can use this understanding to promote healthy behaviours and challenge harmful norms. For instance, Sadeghi *et al.* (2020) explored the ways in which public health campaigns have been designed to shift societal attitudes towards smoking.

Conflict theories

Conflict theories take a different view from consensus theories. Its emphasis is on challenging the idea of a consensus-based society by seeing the idea of consensus as being about maintaining the benefits of society for the few not for everyone, which lead to a conflict of interests. This section focuses on feminist and Marxist social theories.

Feminist social theory

Feminists Accepted by Production Editor [Prabhu Chinnasamy]: argue that the private spheres of domestic life and gender inequality require deeper examination as sites of conflict. They emphasise that the societal roles and experiences of women reveal significant insights into broader patterns of inequality and oppression, contrasting with the previously dominant focus on public institutions.

Where consensus theorists such as Talcott Parsons see the socialisation to gender-specific roles as reflecting 'natural' differences between men and women, feminist theories assert that these are actually the products of socialisation. More importantly, sexist ideologies contained within socially constructed gender roles are internalised from a young age, shaping boys and girls into predefined roles that limit their potential. This perpetuates gender inequality and serves as a form of social control, where the societal position of women is a construct of social, political, and economic forces, rather than a natural phenomenon (May and Powell, 2008).

One crucial aspect of feminism as it developed was the recognition that oppression is not uniform, and experiencing oppression in one form does not preclude one from being an oppressor in another context. There is no automatic sisterhood because experiences of oppression vary widely among women. This critique highlighted that while many middle-class, white feminists focused on shared victimhood, they occupied more privileged and powerful positions compared to most people. For example, White women had the potential to become oppressors, a possibility often not available to Black women. Hence, the term *feminisms* is used to indicate the nuanced nature of the different conflict positions where the intersection of other forms of discrimination may be experienced.

Implications for health and social care

If we recognise gender as a construct of power difference, we can explore how gender roles, norms, and power relations influence health and social care. By observing the effects of gender stereotyping, we can better understand the extent to which the construction of gender may be leading to disparities in clinical practice. A review by Alcalde-Rubio *et al.* (2020) examined interventions designed to overcome or reduce gender bias in clinical practice. They highlight the importance of addressing gender inequities to improve the quality of healthcare. They also noted the 'alarming [absence of] studies of interventions in primary healthcare where the impact of narrowing of gender bias could be greatest' (p. 6). Research by Barr *et al.* (2024: 19) emphasises the need for integrating gender as a social, cultural and structural variable into health research to promote health equity because 'healthcare and biomedical research have predominantly focused on men and male bodies'.

Gender can significantly impact the provision of elderly care due to societal expectations and gender roles. Daughters are more likely to take on the role of primary caregivers for their elderly parents compared to sons, despite this taking a larger toll on their own well-being than their male siblings (Swinkels *et al.*, 2019). This is often due to traditional gender roles that expect women to be more nurturing and responsible for caregiving. Research by Rurka *et al.* (2023) showed that even the gender composition of the siblings could affect the expectations of care provision for elderly relatives. For example, think about the average day in your household and who does what and why. When one of my daughters was ill at school, the school would always call me, despite their father being listed as a contact. That was in the 1990s and early 2000s, but it is something that still largely exists. This is evident from the 2021 Census (ONS, 2023) question, '*Do you look after, or give any help or support to, anyone because they have long-term physical or mental health conditions or illnesses, or problems related to old age?*' which showed that statistically significantly more women were providing unpaid care than males in every age group up to 75–79 years. If we accept the significant impact that being female can have on the provision of elderly care, influenced by societal and cultural gender norms, then we can see how this can affect our practice in health and social care.

Marxist historical materialism

Karl Marx was a German social philosopher who pioneered historical materialism. His theory detailed how society's development into a capitalist society was tied to its relationship with means of production, land, factories, raw materials, and it is often referred to as Marxism. Marx identified capitalist society's division into the bourgeoisie, referring to those who owned the means of production, and the proletariat, referring to those who sold their labour to create profit for others. He advocated for a scientific understanding of capitalism's structures, emphasising the inequitable nature of a modern society based on labour exploitation and surplus value extraction. This means that conflict is intrinsic to capitalism.

The changing social conditions between Marx's writing and the rise of mass media and consumerism led to new variations of Marx's theory. Critical Theory, developed by German neo-Marxist theorists at the Frankfurt School, argued that the expansion of mass production leads to a consumer culture. Conflict theorists scrutinised mass culture's role in diverting the *populus* from underlying societal conflicts and reinforcing capitalist norms. They critiqued the media's promotion of consumerism, employing a concept Marx had termed *commodity fetishism*. Cultural ideas, values and practices become built around consumption, which manipulates people from recognising their 'real needs' by distracting them with 'false' ones, thus keeping the capitalist economy turning. The site of domination in advanced capitalist society had shifted to the realm of culture.

Implications for health and social care

Accepting the viewpoint of Marxist Theory encourages practitioners to recognise and challenge the structural and cultural factors that contribute to health disparities. By understanding how power relations and societal norms influence health outcomes, practitioners can develop more equitable and inclusive care models.

The National Health Service (NHS) in the UK has seen increasing levels of privatisation over recent years. This shift has significant implications for access to healthcare, particularly for low-income populations. Privatisation may lead to cost-cutting measures aimed at maximising profits. This can result in reduced staffing levels and lower quality of care (Goodair and Reeves, 2024). By examining them through the conflict theory lens, you may develop a more critical understanding of the changes you encounter. Using a Marxist analysis, it is the individuals who can only access NHS treatment via long waiting lists who are disproportionately affected by privatisation as they now have less access to essential services at the same level as those who can afford to 'jump the queue'. If private healthcare becomes the standard option for those who can afford it, it may exacerbate and solidify existing health disparities (Institute for Public Policy Research, 2022). Practitioners could use Critical Theory to explore the social determinants of health and the impact of factors like socioeconomic status, race, and gender on their service users' health and well-being. From this awareness, staff may become advocates for systemic change to address these issues.

As well as looking outwards, practitioners can use Critical Theory to reflect on their own biases and the broader societal influences on their practice. This reflective approach can lead to more compassionate and effective care.

Action theories

Thus far in the chapter, we have examined theories which prioritise the effects of structural pressures on the individual in the structure/agency dichotomy, where the impact of social ideas outside of the individual strongly influences the choices and outcomes for people. For Consensus theorists, these structural influences achieve the best for all, as these structures have developed to enable the best outcome for the dominant group. As we delve into Action Theory and explore 'interpretive sociology', our new premise is that understanding the subjective purpose and intent of the agent (person) is essential before an observer can grasp the meaning of any social action.

Interpretative sociology – Max Weber (pronounced Vey-ber)

Interpretative sociology argues that the subject matter of social sciences is fundamentally different from that of natural sciences. This theory prioritises the role of language in socially constructing identity and difference, classifying and grouping objects through shared meanings. The objects of study are individuals whose social action is based on values, ideas and beliefs. Weber posited that *Verstehen* (meaning 'understanding' in German) is the unique method of social sciences. Rather than the world creating the individual, Weber argued that 'The world is as it is because of social action' (Jones and Bradbury, 2018, p. 84). This means that social life cannot be explained by a single factor, but instead, we need to take multiple ideas into consideration because ideas have the power to shape social behaviour and structure. Applying this lens is the belief that human behaviour results from the viewpoint of individual choices and intentions, rather than these being solely determined by social forces.

Various other writers have contributed to this theory. Herbert Blumer (1900–1987) coined the term 'symbolic interactionism' (SI) and emphasised the centrality of the production of shared meanings in human behaviour that are continuously modified through interpretation. In other words, society is the product of individuals and their actions, not the other way round. These theories focus on individual agency rather than constraint by social structures. After all, as individuals, we exercise agentic choice, we give meaning to objects and events, and we act with intent. Goffman's (1959) work on SI looked at how we present ourselves to others, and help us to view social interactions more reflectively. The *Back Stage* is where individuals prepare for interaction, not for public consumption, while the *Front Stage* is where they act out formal roles for others to see. Cooley's (1902) concept of the 'looking-glass self' suggests that we acquire a sense of personal identity only through interaction with others, reflecting on how we believe others perceive us. Mead's (1934) work presents the idea of agency and creation at the social level. The 'I' is the spontaneous, unpredictable element of the self, while the 'Me' is the conformist aspect, reflecting organised aspects of the self. Individuals alternate between 'I' and 'Me' as they participate in society adapting an ever-changing set of roles.

Implication for health and social care

As we discuss the shift from conflict theories to Action Theory such as interpretive sociology, we are emphasising the importance of individual agency over structural constraints. This is evident in the fact that despite significant advancements in health and social care, both patients and health professionals frequently express concerns that healthcare systems often fail to adequately respect the individuality and human dignity of those seeking assistance (Bernsten *et al.*, 2021). Action Theory's focus on individual choices and intentions aligns with the principles of **person-centred care** (Learning Box 7.3) in health and social care. Practitioners are encouraged to understand the unique needs, preferences and goals of each individual, rather than applying a one-size-fits-all approach, so we can focus on people's agency within their situation. By prioritising individual agency, health and social care practitioners can empower service users to take an active role in their own care. This involves recognising and supporting their ability to make informed decisions about their health and well-being (Carroll and Walsh, 2024).

Understanding the subjective purpose and intent of individuals allows practitioners to adopt a holistic approach to care (see Chapter 4). This means considering not just the physical health of clients, but also their emotional, social and psychological needs. Interpretative sociology's emphasis on understanding individual perspectives can enhance cultural sensitivity in practice. Examining the patient perspective on diversity-sensitive care, Lauwers *et al.* (2024) found that shared decision-making, personalised care, and effective and transparent communication were key components for success. By employing an Action Theory lens, health and social care providers can better understand and support the diverse backgrounds and experiences of their clients, leading to more effective and respectful care.

Applying Goffman's theory can help develop a partnership approach that ensures that care plans are tailored to the specific needs and preferences of the individuals, leading to better outcomes. For example, a study into collaborative practice found that the 'patients' roles were conducted not only in healthcare settings but across all aspects of life ...' (Davidson *et al.*, 2024: 3). Recognising the importance of the roles that people employ to make sense of the world could encourage effective collaboration between practitioners and service users.

Cooley's 'looking glass self' concept highlights the importance of understanding how service users perceive themselves through their interactions with you. Health and social care practitioners can use this insight to better understand clients' self-identity and how it influences their health behaviours and choices, and the role these could play in supporting outcomes.

Effective communication is crucial in health and social care, as it helps build trust, convey empathy and ensure that clients feel heard and understood. Blumer's SI emphasises the role of language and social interactions in constructing the service user's identity and the meanings they (and you) make of your time with them. In a recent study of nurses, employing an SI lens, researchers showed that by appreciating the spoken language and the symbolic expressions of patient behaviour, staff they were seeking to comprehend the meanings individuals assign to their experiences in the ward (Mairink *et al.*, 2021).

Mead's 'I' and 'Me' has relevance to social prescribing which is being developed in UK practice. According to Mead, the 'Me' is shaped by societal expectations and interactions. **Social prescribing** (Learning Box 8.1) facilitates integration into the community, helping individuals feel more connected and valued, while Mead's concept of the 'I' represents the individual's response to societal expectations.

Learning Box 8.1: Social prescribing

Social prescribing is a healthcare approach where professionals refer patients to non-medical activities and community services, instead of solely relying on medication or clinical treatments. Patients may be offered activities like exercise classes, creative workshops (such as painting, drawing, or writing), volunteering opportunities, support groups for shared experiences and hobbies like gardening or cookery. According to the Office for Health Improvement and Disparities (2022):

> Recognising that people's health is determined primarily by a range of **social, economic** and **environmental** factors, social prescribing seeks to address people's needs in a holistic way. It also aims to support individuals to take **greater control of their own health** [my emphasis].

Social prescribing empowers individuals to take control of their health and well-being, fostering a sense of agency and personal responsibility. Social prescribing still requires research into its efficacy (Handayani *et al.*, 2025). Applied to the Action Theory lens, social prescribing enhances the agency of service users by connecting them with opportunities that address their social, emotional and practical needs through meaningful social interactions. One approach to understanding the service users' experiences of this pathway could be to apply the theoretical lens of a person's ability to be both I and Me. After all, if we agree with the premise that personal identity is shaped through social interactions, this is a reason to prioritise social support as part of health and well-being. In your interactions with your service users, you can see beyond addressing their immediate needs to facilitating connections with community resources to build a positive self-concept by engaging in community activities and forming meaningful relationships. By applying Mead's theory, social prescribing can be seen as a powerful tool to enhance individual and community well-being through meaningful social interactions and engagement.

Summary

This chapter highlights the importance of considering the role that sociological theories play in enhancing health and social care practices. Understanding these theories could help practitioners address inequalities, promote culturally sensitive care and empower service users.

An understanding of Consensus Theories highlights the influence of family dynamics and social norms on health behaviours. This theory enables health and social care practitioners to understand and use shared norms to promote social solidarity, and encourage healthy behaviours and preventive care in service users to effectively manage health conditions.

An understanding of Conflict Theories enables you to challenge the notion of societal consensus by identifying how societal structures benefit only certain groups. Utilising Feminist theory allows you to examine gender roles and inequalities faced by both service users and caregivers. By emphasising the social construction of gender and its impact on healthcare, practitioners can address gender disparities in clinical practice and support caregivers influenced by traditional gender roles. Applying a Marxist theory lens helps uncover societal divisions and the impact of capitalism on health disparities. A critical understanding of power relations and societal norms empowers practitioners to develop equitable care models and advocate for systemic change.

Finally, an understanding of Action Theories prioritises individual agency and subjective purpose. This perspective encourages understanding of social action through individual choices, intentions and examining the creation of shared meaning through social and practice interactions.

When you take the opportunity to reflect on your practice and the experiences of your service users and their families by applying these different sociological theories, you can adopt a person-centred approach that empowers service users to actively participate in their care. This approach not only considers their unique needs and preferences, but also takes into account the broader societal context in which this care occurs.

References

Alcalde-Rubio, L. *et al.* (2020) 'Gender disparities in clinical practice: Are there any solutions? Scoping review of interventions to overcome or reduce gender bias in clinical practice', *International Journal for Equity in Health*, 19(166), pp. 1–8. https://doi.org/10.1186/s12939-020-01283-4

Barr, E. *et al.* (2024) 'Gender as a social and structural variable: Research perspectives from the National Institutes of Health (NIH)', *Translational Behavioural Medicine*, 14(1), pp. 13–22. https://doi.org/10.1093/tbm/ibad014

Bernsten, G.R. *et al.* (2021) 'Person-centred care (PCC): The people's perspective', *International Journal for Quality in Health Care*, 33(2), pp. 23–26. https://doi.org/10.1093/intqhc/mzab052

Carr, S. *et al.* (2023) 'Service users' experiences of social and psychological avoidable harm in mental health social care in England: Findings of a scoping review', *The British Journal of Social Work*, 53(3), pp. 1303–1324. https://doi.org/10.1093/bjsw/bcac209

Carroll, B. and Walsh, K. (2024) 'Interrogating the effectiveness of service engagement for underserved populations in complex health and social care systems: Towards an equitable engagement strategy', *International Journal for Equity in Health*, 23(197), pp. 1–17. https://doi.org/10.1186/s12939-024-02272-7

Cooley, C.H. (1902) *Human Nature and the Social Order*. New York: Charles Scribner's Sons.

Davidson, A.R. *et al.* (2024) 'Patients' experiences of and roles in interprofessional collaborative practice in primary care: A constructivist grounded theory study', *Primary Health Care Research & Development*, 25(24), p. 9. https://doi.org/10.1017/S1463423624000148

Goffman, E. (1959) *The Presentation of Self in Everyday Life*. New York: Doubleday Anchor Books.

Goodair, B. and Reeves, A. (2024) 'The effect of health-care privatisation on the quality of care', *The Lancet Public Health*, 9(3), pp. 199–206.

Hajizadeh, A. *et al.* (2024) 'How to combat stigma surrounding mental health disorders: A scoping review of the experiences of different stakeholders', *BMC Psychiatry*, 24, p. 782. https://doi.org/10.1186/s12888-024-06220-1

Handayani, N.H., Wanat, M. and Tierney, S. (2025) 'Experiences of social prescribing in the UK: A qualitative systematic review', *British Journal of General Practice*, 75(752), pp. 203–210. https://doi.org/10.3399/BJGP.2025.0179

Ho, Y.C.L. *et al.* (2022) 'The role of the family in health promotion: A scoping review of models and mechanisms', *Health Promotion International*, 37(6). https://doi.org/10.1093/heapro/daac119

Institute for Public Policy Research (2022) *Revealed: A third of adults struggled to access NHS during pandemic, driving many to private healthcare*. Available at https://www.ippr.org/media-office/revealed-a-third-of-adults-struggled-to-access-nhs-during-pandemic-driving-many-to-private-healthcare#:~:text=New%20IPPR%2FYouGov%20polling%20shows,they%20needed%20during%20the%20pandemic (Accessed 1 March 2025).

Ito, K. *et al.* (2023) 'Encouraging death communication in a death-avoidant society: Analysis of interviews with death café organizers', *BMC Health Services Research*, 23(1), p. 944. https://doi.org/10.1186/s12913-023-09967-7

Jones, P. and Bradbury, L. (2018) *Introducing Social Theory*. Medford, Polity Press.

Lauwers, E.D.L. *et al.* (2024) 'The patient perspective on diversity-sensitive care: A systematic review', *International Journal for Equity in Health*, 23(117), pp. 1–18. https://doi.org/10.1186/s12939-024-02189-1

Mairink, A.P.A., Gradim, C.V.C. and Panobianco, M.P. (2021) 'Use of the symbolic interactionism theory', *Journal of Research in Humanities and Social Science*, 9(9), pp. 34–37.

May, T. and Powell, J.S.L. (2008) *Situating Social Theory*. 2nd edn. Maidenhead: McGraw-Hill Education.

Mead, G.H. (1934) *Mind, Self, and Society: From This Standpoint of a Social Behaviorist*. Chicago, USA: The University of Chicago Press.

National Health Service England (2025) *NHS launches first-ever breast screening campaign to help detect thousands of cancers earlier*. Available at https://www.england.nhs.uk/2025/02/nhs-launches-first-ever-breast-screening-campaign-to-help-detect-thousands-of-cancers-earlier/ (Accessed 1 March 2025).

Office for Health Improvement and Disparities (2022) *Guidance social prescribing: Applying all our health*. Available at https://www.gov.uk/government/publications/social-prescribing-applying-all-our-health/social-prescribing-applying-all-our-health (Accessed 19 March 2025).

Office for National Statistics (2023) *Unpaid care by age, sex and deprivation, England and Wales: Census 2021: The provision of unpaid care at country, regional and local authority level and analysis on deprivation with comparisons to Census 2001 and 2011*. Available at https://www.

ons.gov.uk/peoplepopulationandcommunity/healthandsocialcare/socialcare/articles/unpaidcare-byagesexanddeprivationenglandandwales/census2021 (Accessed 1 March 2025).

Röhlke, L. (2024) *Changes in Early Adolescents' Time Use after Acquiring Their First Mobile Phone: An Empirical Test of the Displacement Hypothesis*. Bern, University of Bern, Department of Social Sciences.

Rurka, M.M. *et al.* (2023) 'How do own and siblings' genders shape caregivers' risk of perceiving care-related criticism from siblings?, *Journals of Gerontology: Social Sciences*, 78(3), pp. 520–531. https://doi.org/10.1093/geronb/gbac188

Sadeghi, R., Masoudi, M.R. and Khanjani, N. (2020) 'A systematic review about educational campaigns on smoking cessation', *The Open Public Health Journal*, 13, pp. 748–760. https://doi.org/10.2174/1874944502013010748

Swinkels, J. *et al.* (2019) 'Explaining the gender gap in the caregiving burden of partner caregivers', *Journals of Gerontology: Social Sciences*, 74(2), pp. 309–317. https://doi.org/10.1093/geronb/gbx036

Wäsche, H. *et al.* (2021) 'Family health climate: A qualitative exploration of everyday family life and health', *BMC Public Health*, 21(261). https://doi.org/10.1186/s12889-021-11297-4

World Bank Group (2025) *Mobile cellular subscriptions (per 100 people)*. Available at https://data.worldbank.org/indicator/IT.CEL.SETS.P2 (Accessed 18 March 2025).

9 Core models of health

Lisa Porter and Emily Byrne

The aims of this chapter are to:

- **Outline the principles and relevance of the medical, social, and biopsychosocial models of health**
- **Explain the relevance of these models to healthcare provision**
- **Analyse the strengths and limitations of each model**

Introduction

Working in health or social care can involve many different roles and working alongside a wide variety of professionals. Different professionals may bring different understandings of health with them, which affects the care provided. A medical doctor's focus is on physical healthcare, a psychologist's focus is on psychological health and wellbeing (the mind), and a social worker's main concern maybe the individual and their social environment. This means that care is now influenced by many different and variable perspectives regarding health.

This chapter explores three predominant perspectives or 'models' of health that significantly shape our understanding and approaches to care. These are the *medical model*, the *social model*, and the *biopsychosocial (BPS) model*. Each model of health offers a unique perspective, highlighting different factors that contribute to understanding health and therefore affect the care of individuals. The chapter introduces the reader to definitions of health, as they align with each of the core models of health. Understanding how health is defined and framed is also important for health and social care students because it informs understanding of one's own working practices (and that of others), and aids clarity on what is and what is not relevant to care. Additionally, it enables the student to have a better understanding of the systems and processes within which they are working.

The medical model of health

Rudolf Virchow's work in the 19th century on cell biology laid the groundwork for the medical model perspectives to health and ill-health, particularly his idea that 'every cell stems from another cell' (Porter, 1997). Virchow's work led to an approach that views diseases as the result of internal cellular abnormalities. This in turn revolutionised diagnostics and treatment by focusing on identifying and correcting these physical issues. Virchow's 'biomedical' approach underpins the medical model of health. It aligns with the traditional definition of health in the Western world, whereby health is defined as the

DOI: 10.4324/9781032619309-11

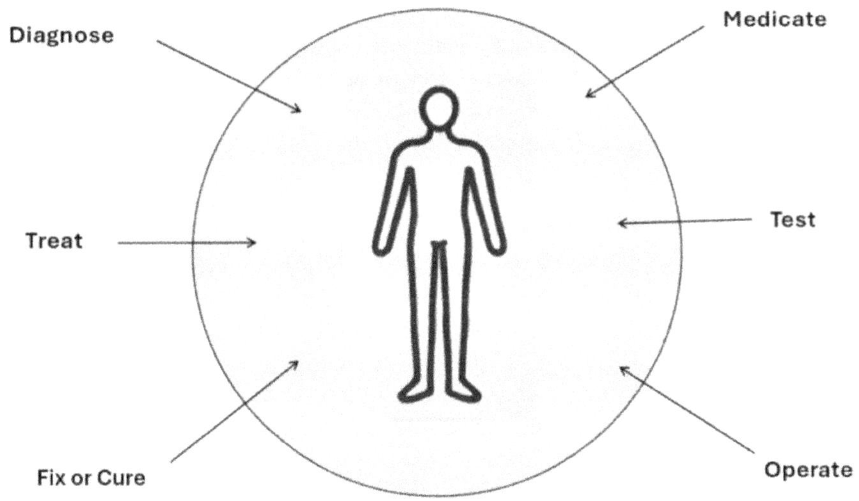

Figure 9.1 The medical model of health.

'absence of disease' (Larsen, 2022). Under this definition, if someone does not show signs of illness, they are healthy, regardless of any aspects of a person's wellbeing which are not considered. The medical model measures health primarily in terms of deficit, focusing on the human body's malfunction due to biological reasons such as disease or illness. An individual experiencing ill-health is labelled as a 'patient', and is perceived as having a problem that requires medical intervention. Figure 9.1 shows the key features of the medical model.

As Figure 9.1 shows, the medical model focuses on physical, sensory, or mental impairments, aiming to restore, improve, or manage these issues. The medical professional is regarded as the expert with the necessary knowledge and skills to 'fix', cure, or alleviate the patient's condition. Typically, the treatment takes place in the medical expert's environment, such as a hospital or clinic, where the professional has access to the necessary tools and resources and where the patient is subjected to various interventions aimed at restoring health or managing the illness (Farre and Rapley, 2017; Wade and Halligan, 2004).

Strengths of the medical model

The medical model has been the most dominant way of viewing health for over a century (Zaks, 2023). The medial model is underpinned by a biomedical approach, which views health and illness as related purely to biological functions. The biomedical has significantly advanced medical science, diagnostics, treatment, and therefore improved healthcare outcomes by providing a clear, structured approach to diagnosing and treating diseases, resulting in significant reductions in morbidity and mortality (Wade and Halligan, 2004). This has driven innovation in medical technology and pharmacology, enabling precise and effective disease management (Farre and Rapley, 2017). By emphasising scientific evidence, a robust framework for medical research and education has been established, advancing preventive medicine, enhancing diagnostic accuracy and reliability (Farre and Rapley, 2017). Furthermore, the focus on physical health has led to substantial improvements in surgical techniques and medical procedures, which have enhanced patient outcomes and recovery rates. It has also supported the development of standardised treatment and evidence-based practice, ensuring consistent and high-quality care across healthcare settings (Shah and Mountain, 2007).

Limitations of the medical model

The limitations of the traditional definition of health became evident during World War 1 between 1914 and 1919. Beyond the risk of being killed in battle, diseases and injuries created many sick and wounded soldiers, necessitating medical treatment and leading to advances in medical knowledge. However, the medical model of health, in only focussing on the absence of disease (Larsen, 2022), failed to acknowledge psychological and stress-related conditions. Traumatised soldiers without physical injuries were often misunderstood, assumed to be feigning illness and denied appropriate care, sometimes being considered malingerers and therefore shot by their own army superiors (Wade and Halligan, 2004). This narrow definition of health did not account for the psychological impacts of war, such as shell shock (now recognised as post-traumatic stress disorder (PTSD) (see Chapter 5). The lack of recognition and care for these conditions highlighted the deficiencies of defining health solely by the absence of disease.

While foundational in modern healthcare, the medical model has significant limitations in explaining all forms of illness. Wade and Halligan (2004) identify three key incorrect assumptions of the medical model. First, that all illness has a single underlying cause. Second, that disease is always the single cause. And third, that the removal of the disease will result in a return to health. These are considered incorrect because many illnesses, particularly those involving mental health, cannot be traced to a single cause. Additionally, the presence of a disease does not always link directly with the experience of illness, and removing the physical signs and symptoms of a disease does not necessarily restore a person's overall health. These limitations suggest that the medical model's simplistic approach oversimplifies the complex way that different factors interact to affect health and illness (Farre and Rapley, 2017).

Critics of the medical model and the biomedical approach that underpins it argue that defining health as simply the absence of disease places undue power in the hands of a medical profession who hold the authority to declare an individual healthy or diagnose illness. Consequently, healthcare resources are predominantly allocated towards physical health issues as defined by medical criteria. The patients' subjective experiences and expertise over their own health and wellbeing are excluded from this approach (Shah and Mountain, 2007). This can be stigmatising, as it implies that those with chronic or untreatable conditions are perpetually 'unhealthy'. The medical model's failure to consider the psychological, social, environmental, and emotional factors involved fails to recognise **the holistic nature of health** (Learning Box 4.1) (Farre and Rapley, 2017; Shah and Mountain, 2007).

Regardless of its limitations, understanding the medical model is essential for health and social care students because it shapes healthcare delivery both in the UK and internationally. In a time of limited resources and great demand, a key benefit of the medical model's approach is quick and effective treatment. Its strengths in supporting diagnosis, treatment, and managing diseases have made it the fundamental basis of healthcare systems worldwide, driving progress in medical science and improving the quality of life for populations (Farre and Rapley, 2017; Shah and Mountain, 2007; Wade and Halligan, 2004). Recognising its strengths and limitations enables healthcare students to build on its benefits while incorporating more holistic approaches that address the full range of factors influencing health.

The social model of health

The issues identified with the medical model during World War 1 identified the need for a different understanding of health. This was because the war significantly increased the population of disabled people, creating hundreds of thousands of disabled ex-service persons and civilians returning to their lives in the UK. These groups were motivated for change, and they organised into campaigning groups from the 1940s, which became charities with clear objectives. Campaigns by ex-service members pressured for rehabilitation, support, and protection, inspiring the disabled population. Within the UK, this led to new legislation, such as the *1944 Disability Employment Act*, and the establishment of the National Health Service (NHS) in 1948, providing a range of services, including much-needed rehabilitation services.

Additionally, following the devastation of World War 2 and the resulting widespread health crises in any countries, there was global recognition for the need for cooperation in health. This led to the establishment of the World Health Organization (WHO). As part of its constitution, the WHO (1948) defined health as:

> a state of complete physical, mental, and social wellbeing and not merely the absence of disease or infirmity

This marked a move away from the traditional definition of health which focused simply on the absence of disease. It emphasised a more holistic and wider approach, including physical health (the proper functioning of the body and the absence of physical ailments), mental wellbeing (emotional and psychological resilience, enabling individuals to cope with stress), and social wellbeing (quality of relationships and our interactions within society). This advancement of the definition of health to include wider perspectives has had a profound impact on health policies and practices around the world. It emphasised the importance of addressing social determinants of health, such as living conditions, education, and access to healthcare.

The WHO continues to promote this holistic view, advocating for health systems that support overall wellbeing. However, this definition has been critiqued for not accounting for those with long-term conditions, for whom (according to this definition) health can never be achieved, and that the complete state of wellbeing is unachievable.

From the 1960s, influenced by civil rights movements, disabled people began questioning societal assumptions about disability. They challenged the medical model, which viewed disability as an individual medical issue, and instead highlighted its limitations. By drawing attention to societal barriers, they exposed how these contributed to their exclusion and discrimination within society. Organisations like the *Union of the Physically Impaired Against Segregation* and *Liberation Network of People with Disabilities*, led by disabled individuals, advocated for significant changes (Inclusion London, 2015). This self-leadership was empowering and enabled a voice for those traditionally excluded from power. Their efforts led to the development of a new social model by disabled academic Mike Oliver (Oliver, 1983). The social model challenged the medical model by offering an alternative perspective, and had a significant positive impact in driving forward change and acknowledgement of other perspectives on disability, impairment, and health. Oliver (2004) progressed his work and outlined that the social model is based upon four key aspects:

1 Civil rights and equality advocating for equal rights and opportunities for disabled people as a basic human right
2 Shift from individual blame and need to 'fix' or 'cure' according to the medical model to instead highlighting how society excludes
3 Impairment (a physical, sensory, or cognitive condition such as being blind, deaf, having a learning difficulty, or living with a long-term condition) is distinguished from disability (the social consequences of impairment)
4 Barriers to inclusion within society which disable people (attitudinal, physical, and communication barriers).

The social model shifts the focus from what people 'can't do' to how society's organisation and attitudes create disabling barriers. In other words, it is not a physical impairment which is causing barriers for people with impairments, but the physical and social barriers that exist within society (Disability Rights UK, 2024). This new way of thinking challenges the medical model perspective that physical impairment is a personal tragedy or a condition needing cure or 'fixing'. This is shown in Figure 9.2.

Figure 9.2 shows that the social model views disability as the social consequences of having an impairment, such as the negative impact in relation to accessing work, transport, leisure, and domestic activities (Inclusion London 2015). The social model emphasises that individuals with impairments or health conditions are therefore negatively impacted by the barriers created by society, which exclude and discriminate against them. The social model highlights the importance of removing physical, organisational, and attitudinal barriers to ensure full participation and equality for people with impairments (Hogan, 2019; Inclusion London 2015).

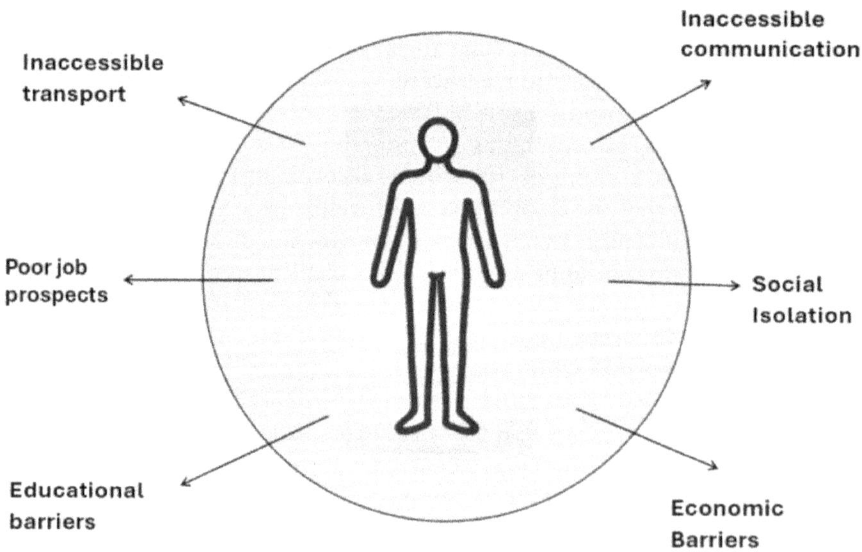

Figure 9.2 The social model of health.

The social model has evolved and expanded its scope over time, providing a framework for understanding and addressing the wider societal impacts on health, wellbeing, impairment and disability. Important factors within society which can negatively impact on a person's health outcomes such as education, employment, income, housing, healthcare access, transportation, social networks and social support are all included within the modern social model. Table 9.1 provides information about the categories of barriers identified by the social model and gives some suggested examples to demonstrate what these may look like in real life.

Table 9.1 Key barriers identified by the social model

Type of barrier/Description	*Examples*
Attitudinal Barriers: Negative social and cultural attitudes, prejudices and stereotypes that justify and perpetuate discrimination	Being overlooked for promotion based upon prejudice, poor attitudes of staff due to discrimination.
Physical Barriers: Inaccessible physical environments or inadequate facilities	Steps, narrow doorways, lack of accessible toilets, lack of essential equipment or the right facilities that facilitate engagement
Communication/Informational Barriers: Lack of accessible information and communication methods	Unsuitable information or communication such as important documents presented visually for someone who is visually impaired or verbally for someone who is deaf or in a language not understood by a person.
Organisational Barriers: Missing or inadequate policies, inadequate support services	No equality and diversity policy in place, no technology adaptations available to aid accessibility, poor career development opportunities.
Economic Barriers: Economic disparities, or social support, leading to financial instability	Limited access to well-paid jobs, little of no help with additional associated costs, no equipment available to support needs, e.g. hearing aids, hearing loops or no support with transport costs.
Educational Barriers: Inaccessible or unsuitable education and learning	Not being able to access education at all, or not accessing appropriate education. Inaccessible learning materials, curricula, facilities hindering learning and educational opportunities
Employment Barriers: Workplace environments or practices that exclude or disadvantage	Excluded from employment opportunities, job interviews, or promotions. Inflexible working hours, lack of reasonable adjustments.
Housing Barriers: Lack of suitable housing that meet needs, inaccessible accommodation	This includes physical inaccessibility, such as lack of elevators, housing policies that do not prioritise accessibility, or not being able to access appropriate accommodation.
Healthcare Access Barriers: Challenges in accessing appropriate care for health/medical needs	Inaccessible facilities, lack of trained healthcare providers, unable to access healthcare or equipment needed which can result in unmet health needs and poorer health outcomes.
Transportation Barriers: Limited or no availability of accessible public or private transport	Restricted access to essential transport services to aid engagement within a community, employment or educational opportunities.
Social Network and Support Barriers: Limited social networks that support an individual leading to social isolation	Friends or family support being limited due to physical distance, social isolation, lack of supportive networks that can provide emotional assistance, information, or practical help.

The barriers identified in Table 9.1 highlight the social model's focus on a more holistic and inclusive approach to health, considering both an individual's societal context and the barriers they face. By shifting the focus from individual physical limitations to societal structures, the social model advocates for the removal of barriers so individuals can fully participate in society and achieve a more inclusive, equitable and supportive community for all citizens.

Strengths of the social model

The social model of disability offers significant benefits, particularly in shifting the perspective of health from an individualistic view to a societal one, and the positive impact this can have at both individual and societal levels has been profound. As this model emphasises that disability is created by societal barriers, it can be a powerful tool for advocating for changes in the environment, attitudes and policies, and the strengthening of legislation to empower individuals with health concerns, impairments, or long-term conditions. For example, the history and development of the social model and the movements surrounding it were instrumental in paving the way for the *Disability Discrimination Act 1995* and the subsequent *Equality Act 2010*. A significant positive impact of social model is that it promotes equality and human rights by calling for adjustments in society to ensure equal access and equality of opportunity. It challenges discriminatory practices by highlighting that people with impairments or health conditions should have the same rights and opportunities as others, without being marginalised or excluded (Inclusion London, 2015).

Limitations of the social model

The social model, while groundbreaking in shifting the focus from individual impairments to disabling societal barriers, has faced significant critique. It is often considered too simplistic, as it portrays illness and impairment as entirely separate entities, neglecting the relationship between impairment and illness. This model does not account for the variety of ways barriers may be experienced, nor is it appropriate for all types of disability. For instance, it struggles to address the complexities of fluctuating impairments or health conditions, where an individual's lived experiences of a health condition or impairment may change over time, complicating the need for consistent adjustments. Additionally, the social model overlooks cultural factors and individual beliefs that influence perceptions and experiences of impairment, disability, and health conditions. For example, in some cultures mental health matters are considered taboo and are not acknowledged, leading to avoidance of seeking professional treatment or support due to concerns about family reputation and societal standing. It also assumes that adjusting the environmental barrier in society is feasible, which may not always possible due to practical, economic, or logistical constraints. Therefore, while the social model offers valuable insights, it may need to be integrated with other perspectives to fully understand and address the diverse experiences of disability (Owens, 2014).

Despite its limitations, the social model redefined impairment, disability and health conditions as a societal issue and it provides a framework for advocating systemic changes to achieve equality and inclusion in society. The social model can be used as a useful tool by health and social care students for identifying and removing barriers to support individuals. By highlighting and dismantling barriers, society can strive towards social justice, and provide individuals with greater independence, choice, and control.

The biopsychosocial (BPS) model of health

In 1977, George Engel proposed a new model for medicine, the 'biopsychosocial' model (Engel, 1977). The model sought to acknowledge the individual contribution of biological, psychological, and social issues to health presentations and interventions, hence the name 'biopsychosocial' (BPS) model. Engel developed the BPS model by highlighting the limitations of the medical model to psychiatry and sought to address these limitations.

Historically, biological factors were seen as the fundamental cause of mental disorders in psychiatry, and even when psychosocial elements were contributory factors they were viewed through a biological prism and the intervention implemented to help were based on a medical explanation (Guze, 1992). This meant that medical practitioners focused on assessment, diagnosis and treatment of mental/psychiatric disorders. This traditional medical approach tended to be paternalistic, and the medical model promoted a passive patient status which elevated the medical professional as expert in individuals' illness, as epitomised by the phrase 'doctor knows best'. However, in the 1970s and early 1980s, psychiatry was criticised for prioritising biology at the expense of psychosocial considerations.

Engel proposed the widening of the medical approach to address these limitations and developed the BPS model to provide a framework which acknowledges the importance of these other models (McKay *et al.*, 2012).

Since the 1970s, the BPS model has been accepted and widely applied as a means for understand health and disease in healthcare services. The BPS model has been described as the 'status quo of contemporary psychiatry' (Ghaemi, 2009; Lugg, 2021). Nevertheless, this model may have less influence depending on the area of healthcare involved, for example a surgeon may be less concerned with *how* the individual broke his leg than fixing it, giving higher status to the medical perspective. In summary, the BPS model is a holistic, person-centred, collaborative approach that values all the three levels, biological, psychological, and social in every healthcare task. Modern visual representations of the BPS emphasise this, as shown in Figure 9.3.

Figure 9.3 uses a Venn diagram to show how the BPS views biological (medical), psychological, and social (including environmental) factors as overlapping. This highlights that these domains are not isolated but are interconnected and interact to shape health and illness, as represented by the overlapping areas on the model. For example, a

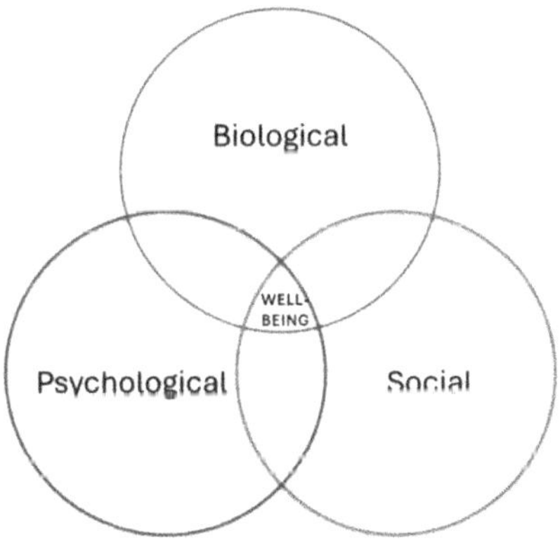

Figure 9.3 The BPS model.

biological condition like chronic pain may affect mood, which in turn, can impact social interactions. The overlapping areas demonstrate that health, illness, and behaviour must be understood through the interplay of all three factors. This holistic perspective rejects the simplistic approach of the medical model and highlights that in the real world there are complex interactions across all three elements. This means that effective care requires addressing each domain simultaneously, as changes in one can influence the others (e.g. psychological stress can lead to physiological changes such as increased blood pressure, which may be further affected by social pressures like work stress). Therefore, the BPS model reflects the fluid and dynamic nature of health and ill-health, recognising that changes in one domain can impact on the others.

Strengths of BPS model

The BPS model provides many strengths and benefits for practitioners to help them understand the underlying reasons behind health and illness by taking a more holistic approach. It encompasses a wide range of factors involved in health, connecting relevant aspects to build a bigger picture and recognising the interplay between these factors. This model aids in understanding health behaviours and is more aligned with modern health definitions that emphasise health and wellbeing beyond the mere absence of disease. By integrating these broader perspectives, the BPS model provides a more comprehensive understanding of health, addressing the complexities and nuances that influence an individual's overall wellbeing (Farre and Rapley, 2017). Understanding these additional dimensions from the BPS model helps healthcare professionals create more holistic and person-centred approaches, which in turn, can lead to more effective interventions and improved patient outcomes. Additionally, by considering the role of psychological and social factors in health, the BPS model encourages preventative measures, such as stress management and social support initiatives, which can reduce the risk of illness and promote and sustain overall wellbeing. In summary, the BPS model's integrative approach leads to a more nuanced understanding of health, enabling a person-centred approach to care and preventative strategies that collectively enhance outcomes for patients and service users.

Limitations of the BPS model

The impact of the BPS model in contemporary healthcare has been significant in terms of encouraging a shift from the medical model. However, it has been criticised in many key areas. It can be argued that medical practitioner's decision making is influenced by the concepts, ideas and understanding from which their knowledge and skills are based. This means that science and scientific methods have a significant influence on understanding and treatment of individuals, with a focus on disease. When applying the BPS model, it may be limited by the practitioner's knowledge, skills and issues, such as restrictions on the time spent with patients. Furthermore, the BPS model is often criticised for being too vague and generic, lacking specific guidance for application in professional practice, leading to inconsistent application among practitioners and potentially affecting the quality of care.

Additionally, the holistic nature of the BPS model necessitates thorough assessments, which can be time-consuming and inefficient in clinical settings where resources are limited. Understanding all the factors may take some time in engaging with the patient who also may not understand it. This can make it seem inefficient to use as a holistic approach. Bolton and Gillett (2019) point out that there are insufficient safeguards to protect against the dominance or under-representation of one of the three domains. Likewise, it does not provide clear directives on when or if certain aspects should be prioritised, creating ambiguity in determining appropriate interventions and potentially delaying treatment. Furthermore, its open-ended nature allows for varied interpretations, resulting in inconsistent implementation across different healthcare settings and potentially disparities in patient outcomes.

Borrell-Carrió *et al.* (2004) argues that complete reliance on the BPS model may never be possible, as the complexity of individuality means that it cannot be possible to know all the factors that contribute to any given health outcome. For example, individuals may be unreliable narrators, and omit some information, while exaggerating other areas. Additionally, the BPS model may struggle to remain relevant where an individual needs high level of direction and support and views the practitioner as the expert. Implementing the BPS model across diverse populations presents additional challenges, as cultural beliefs, socioeconomic factors, and access to healthcare resources can significantly impact its applicability and effectiveness. These limitations highlight the need for more precise frameworks to effectively integrate the BPS model into healthcare practice (Farre and Rapley, 2017).

Comparing the medical, social, and BPS models

Table 9.2 provides a comparative overview of the medical, social, and BPS models of health.

As Table 9.2 shows, each model offers a distinct perspective on health and illness, influencing approaches to diagnosis, treatment, and patient care. The medical model focuses primarily on biological factors, viewing health as the absence of disease and often relying on medical interventions. In contrast, the social model emphasises the impact of societal and environmental factors on health, advocating for changes in social structures

Table 9.2 Comparing features of the different models of health

	Medical model	*Social model*	*BPS model*
Definition of Health	Health is the absence of disease or illness.	Health is the ability to function well within an inclusive society.	'Health is a state of complete physical, mental, and social wellbeing' (WHO, 1948)
Focus	Biological factors: diagnosis and treatment of disease.	Social determinants: addressing societal barriers to health.	Holistic approach: integrating biological, psychological, and social aspects.
Approach to Illness/Disease	Identifies and treats the biological cause of disease.	Seeks to remove societal barriers and promote inclusion.	Considers the interplay of biological, psychological, and social factors.
Role of Healthcare	Provides medical interventions to cure or manage diseases.	Advocates for societal changes to improve health outcomes.	Employs a multidisciplinary approach, including medical treatment, therapy, and social support.
Intervention Strategies	Medical treatments, surgeries, and medications.	Policy changes, social support systems, and community inclusion.	Integrated care plans addressing medical, psychological, and social needs.

to improve wellbeing. The BPS model integrates biological, psychological, and social dimensions, promoting a holistic approach to understanding and managing health. By comparing these models, we can appreciate the strengths and limitations of each, leading to more comprehensive and effective healthcare practices. This comparison highlights the distinct perspectives and approaches each model offers in understanding and addressing health and illness.

Just as the models of health have evolved, how health is defined also evolves. For instance, in 1986 the WHO proposed an alternative defition of health as '*the extent to which an individual or group is able to realise aspirations and satisfy needs and to change or cope with the environment*' (WHO, 1986). This definition focuses on health being a resource needed for everyday life rather than an end goal. It also acknowledges the context within which we are situated and the need for adaptability and resilience for coping. Definitions of health are continuously adapting and evolving. Some involve adapting to life's challenges, fulfilling needs and achieving aspirations. Others focus on the connection between human wellbeing and environmental sustainability. Increasingly, there is recognition that human health and wellbeing is innately tied into our environment. The discourse on how best to define health will continue and evolve over time as our understanding increases and perspectives change.

Summary

Defining and understanding health, disease, and illness are essential for understanding the boundaries and scope of care. Models of health serve as useful tools for gaining insights into these complex topics, offering different lenses and perspectives that enhance comprehension. Despite the variety of models available, there is not a single approach which is considered universally 'best' within health and social care, as each has its own strengths and limitations. The medical model has dominated the UK healthcare system and the NHS for the past 75 years, significantly shaping current practice. This longstanding dominance underscores the model's influence, even as it highlights the need for incorporating diverse approaches to address the multifaceted and dynamic nature of health and care. Understanding these models is crucial for healthcare students, enabling them to navigate the healthcare systems and apply different frameworks effectively in their professional practice to gain deeper understanding from diverse perspectives to develop their person-centred approach to care.

References

Equality Act 2010, C.15. Available at https://www.legislation.gov.uk/ukpga/2010/15/contents (Accessed 2 February 2025).

Bolton, D. and Gillett, G. (2019) *The Biopsychosocial Model of Health and Disease: New Philosophical and Scientific Developments*. Palgrave Macmillan, Switzerland.

Borrell-Carrió, F., Suchman, A.L. and Epstein, R.M. (2004) 'The biopsychosocial model 25 years later: Principles, practice, and scientific inquiry', *Annals of Family Medicine*, 2(6), pp. 576–582.

Disability Discrimination Act (1995) C.50. Available at https://www.legislation.gov.uk/ukpga/1995/50/contents (Accessed 2 February 2025).

Disability Rights UK (2024) *Social model of disability language*. Available at https://www.disabilityrightsuk.org/social-model-disability-language (Accessed 13 June 2024).

Engel, G. (1977) 'The need for a new medical model: A challenge for biomedicine', *Science*, 196 (4286), pp. 129–136. https://doi.org/10.1126/science.847460

Farre, A. and Rapley, T. (2017) 'The new old (and old new) medical model: Four decades navigating the medical and psychosocial understandings of *health and illness*', *Healthcare (Basel)*, 5(4), p. 88.
Ghaemi, S.N. (2009) 'The rise and fall of the biopsychosocial model', *British Journal of Psychiatry*, 195(1), pp. 3–4.
Guze, S.B. (1992) *Why Psychiatry Is a Branch of Medicine*. New York: Oxford University Press.
Hogan, A.J. (2019) 'Social and medical models of disability and mental health: Evolution and renewal', *Medicine and Society*, 7(191), pp. E16–E18. https://doi.org/10.1503/cmaj.181008
Inclusion London (2015) *Factsheet: The social model of disability*. Available at https://www.inclusionlondon.org.uk/wp-content/uploads/2015/05/FactSheets_TheSocialModel.pdf (Accessed 13 June 2024).
Larsen, L.T. (2022) 'Not merely the absence of disease: A genealogy of the WHO's positive health definition', *History of the Human Sciences*, 35(1), pp. 111–131.
Lugg, W. (2021) 'The biopsychosocial history, controversy and Engel', *Australasia Psychiatry*, 30(1), pp. 55–59.
McKay, R., McDonald, R., Lie, D. and McGowan, H. (2012) 'Reclaiming the best of the biopsychosocial model of mental health care and "recovery" for older people through a "person-centred" approach', *Australasian Psychiatry*, 20(6), pp. 492–495.
Oliver, M. (1983) *Social Work with Disabled People*. Basingstoke: Macmillan.
Oliver, M. (2004) 'The social model in action: If I had a hammer', in Barnes C. and Mercer G. (eds.) *Implementing the Social Model of Disability: Theory and Research*. Leeds: The Disability Press, pp. 18–31.
Owens, J. (2014) 'Exploring the critiques of the social model of disability: The transformative possibility of Arendt's notion of power', *Sociology of Health and Illness*, 37(3), pp. 385–403.
Porter, R. (1997) *The Greatest Benefit to Mankind. A Medical History of Humanity from Antiquity to the Present*. London: HarperCollins.
Shah, P. and Mountain, D. (2007) 'The medical model is dead – Long live the medical model', *The British Journal of Psychiatry*, 191(5), pp. 375–377.
Wade, D.T. and Halligan, P.W. (2004) 'Do medical models of illness make for good healthcare systems?, *British Medical Journal*, 329(7479), p. 1398.
World Health Organization (WHO) (1948) *Constitution*. Available at https://www.who.int/about/governance/constitution (Accessed 1 February 2025).
World Health Organization (1986). *Ottawa Charter for Health Promotion*. First International Conference on Health Promotion, Ottawa, 21 November 1986. Available at https://apps.who.int/iris/handle/10665/349652 (Accessed 13 February 2025).
Zaks, Z. (2023) 'Changing the medical model of disability to the normalisation model of disability: Clarifying the past to create a new future direction', *Disability and Society*, 39(12), pp. 1–28.

10 The importance of anatomy and physiology for health and social care

Clive Sealey and Janet Osbaldiston

The aims of this chapter are to:

- **Define what anatomy and physiology are**
- **Explain the linkage between anatomy and physiology**
- **Analyse the importance of anatomy and physiology to improving health and social care**

Introduction

Anatomy and physiology describe the way that the human body is structured and the way that the human body functions. This includes basic human functions and processes, such as how we breathe, how we eat, how we walk and how we talk which enable us to live, love and learn. These functions and processes represent the essential core of health and social care, which is providing care that enables people to not only live, but to live well. It is important as a health and social care practitioner to understand these anatomy and physiology functions and processes in order to identify when they are healthy or when they are disrupted, as this can significantly impact on the health and wellbeing of an individual. For example, a disruption in the anatomy of the heart can lead to a heart attack, which can have a huge impact of the health and wellbeing of an individual. Similarly, a disruption in the physiology of the immune system can lead to instances of cancer and a number of long-term conditions, which again can have a huge impact on the health and wellbeing of an individual.

By understanding and monitoring the anatomy and physiology of the individual, it becomes possible to prevent, treat or manage such disruption, thereby improving the health and wellbeing of the individual. This highlights the importance of understanding the anatomy and physiology of the human body when healthy and unhealthy, as it is the essence of health and social care to improve the lives of individuals.

This chapter aims to outline how and why an understanding of anatomy and physiology makes this possible for you as a health and social care practitioner. The chapter starts with brief outlines of both anatomy and physiology, in terms of what they mean individually. It then outlines the importance of linking anatomy and physiology together. Finally, it explains three specific beneficial outcomes of understanding of anatomy and physiology for health and social care.

What are anatomy and physiology?

This section provides brief descriptions of anatomy and physiology, to enable a simple understanding of the terms. It highlights key features of each, as well as similarities and differences.

DOI: 10.4324/9781032619309-12

Anatomy

Anatomy is the concerned with studying and structure of the human body. This means studying how the body is made up and how it works. This includes the cells, tissues, organs and body systems, and how these are put together to make up the structure that we call the human body.

The human body is a very complex structure that is made up of lots of different components that work together as a whole system. A comparison could be made with the human body and a car, as a car has lots of different components that work together as a whole system to make the car work. For example, there is the engine, the brakes, the transmission, the clutch, the suspension and the cooling system. The car requires all of these components to work effectively and efficiently. Similarly, the human body has lots of different components that work together as a whole system to make it work. For example, there is the heart, the lungs, the eyes, the ears, the muscles and the brain to name a few. It is when these different components come together that we have what we term the human body. Anatomy is simply the study of what these different components of the human body are and how they are structured together to enable the human body to function as it does.

When studying anatomy, the starting point is what the components of the human body are. This is important as it enables us to identify the way that the human body is structured, which then enables us to progress to how these different components work together. Most of us can name and identify at least one body part, such as the brain, legs or arms. Just doing this enables us to make a distinction between the human body and a single-celled organism such as bacteria and algae, in that we can say that that the human body is not just one single entity but is made up of lots of different components. This is an important point to make as it means that at this point, the first thing we can say about human anatomy is that the human body is a collection of different parts. Anatomy is concerned with how these different parts work together to function as a whole human body.

The second thing that we can say about human anatomy at this point is that there are lots of body structures that are instantly visibly to the us, but many other body structures that are not. For example, we can see our hands, our feet and our skin, but we cannot see our heart, brain or stomach. Indeed, most of our anatomical features are hidden from us by our skin, or even further hidden by other means. When studying anatomy, we are not just interested in the visible part of our anatomy, we are also interested in the non-visible parts, as these are also important to us. While the human body functions as a single structure, it is actually also made of lots and lots of different smaller structures that are not visible to us. In anatomy, we can divide the components of the human body into four major structural categories: cells, tissues, organs and systems. This is shown in Table 10.1.

Table 10.1 Structures and description of the human body

Structures of the human body	*Description*
Cells	The smallest structure of the human body, the human body is made up of billions of cells
Tissues	A collection of similar cells that function together as a unit, e.g., muscle tissue, nervous tissue and connective tissue
Organs	A collection of tissues that combine to form a functional unit to perform a particular function, e.g., heart, lungs and kidney
Systems	A collection of organs that combine to together to perform a specific function, e.g., skeletal system, nervous system and reproductive system

Table 10.1 makes it clear that the anatomy of the human body is intricately linked together, with cells combining to make tissues, tissues combining to make organs and organs combining to make systems. This is an important starting point when trying to understand anatomy, as it indicates that understanding anatomy requires understanding the way that these structures are linked and connected together.

To summarise, anatomy is the study of structures of the human body, and the way that these structures are linked and connected together to make up the human body.

Physiology

Having identified the structures of the human body, the key focus of physiology is to identify how these structures work in a health body, and how they do not work when unhealthy. This links the structure of the body to the function of the body. For example, having identified the existence of a collection of organs which we call the nervous system through anatomy, the study of physiology is then focussed on identifying how the nervous system works both as an individual system and as part of the whole human body to ensure that all parts of the body communicate with each other. Physiology also focusses on how the human body responds and adapts to everyday life, and what happens when things go wrong leading to disease and illness.

As with anatomy, the starting point of physiology is how cells function, as these are the building blocks of the human body. However, unlike anatomy, the principal focus of physiology is not on the structure of the cells but how they work as part of the systems of the human body, such as the skeletal system, the nervous system and the reproductive system shown in Table 10.1. There are ten major systems of the body, as shown in Table 10.2. Studying how these ten major systems work and how these systems are integrated together to make the body function as a whole is the essential basis of physiology. When the human body is functioning normally, it requires these 10 major systems to work together in a series of complex and interlinked processes that react, overlap and anticipate what other parts of the body are doing. For example, in the act of eating, the teeth of the digestive system works to both mechanically break down and crush, as well as chemically breakdown through enzymes such as in our saliva, stomach juices and intestine to aid digestion of our food and eliminate waste, while at the same time the respiratory system works to keep us breathing, and after eating the endocrine system regulates the metabolism of the body to turn the food into energy that that the body can

Table 10.2 The ten major systems of the human body (refer to Waugh and Grant *et al.* (2023) for more detailed explanations)

System and description	*Function*
Skeletal system: bones, cartilages and tendons	Provides a strong frame to enable structure and support for the body when standing and moving and protects the soft organs of the body from damage. The bones contain bone marrow which generates red, white blood cells and platelets. Plus, bone marrow stores fat (energy reserve) and is a reservoir for calcium and other minerals.

(*Continued*)

Table 10.2 (Continued)

System and description	*Function*
Muscular system: muscle attached to skeleton, internal organs and the heart	Responsible for movement, posture, joint stability and heat production. Muscles also serve as a storage site for essential nutrient such as carbohydrates and amino acids.
Nervous system: brain, spinal cord and nerves	Regulates and communicates all physical and mental activity, including movement, digestion and memory. This involves voluntary and involuntary functions. It is the major control system of homeostasis in all body systems.
Endocrine system: glands that secrete hormones into the blood such as thyroid gland, testes and ovaries	Sends and controls chemical message called hormones that influence growth, development, reproduction and metabolic activities. The endocrine and nervous system communicate particularly closely to maintain homeostasis.
Cardiovascular system: heart, arteries, veins, capillaries and blood	Circulates and transports blood around the body carrying nutrients, oxygen and hormones, plus blood cells to and from the tissue cells. It also removes carbon dioxide and other waste products to organs for disposal.
Lymphatic system: lymph nodes, lymph vessels (thin tubes that carry lymph and white blood cells), bone marrow, spleen, thymus, tonsils and adenoids, and lymph tissue	Removes waste from the body's systems and also defends the body against infections and disease. Also helps regulate fluid balance in the body and absorption of fat from the digestive system.
Respiratory system: nose, mouth, throat, voice box, windpipe and lungs	Responsible for breathing by allowing the oxygen in the air to be taken into the body cells and organs and expels carbon dioxide in the air breathed out. This is called gaseous exchange. This system also helps regulate blood pH (acid/alkaline) levels.
Digestive system: the gastrointestinal tract, the liver, pancreas, and gallbladder.	Processes and breaks down food into nutrients/ molecules so that they can be absorbed by the body's cells. The main functions include, ingestion, propulsion (movement known as peristalsis), digestion both mechanical and chemical breakdown of food, absorption of nutrients, secretion of water and enzymes and elimination of waste products.
Urinary system: kidneys, renal pelvis, ureters, bladder and urethra.	Maintains the level of fluid in the body and eliminates waste from the body to regulate blood volume and blood pressure, control levels of electrolytes and metabolites, and regulate blood pH. Functions also include activation of vitamin D and control of red blood cell production.
Reproductive system: In women includes the ovaries, the fallopian tubes, the uterus, the cervix and the vagina. In men, it includes the prostate, the testes and the penis.	Responsible to enable sexual function and reproduction to ensure survival of the humans as a species.

Learning Box 10.1: Homeostasis

Homeostasis literally translates as 'one state', and means maintaining a stable internal balance. It refers to the ability of the body to maintain a stable internal balance during normal activities, and to return to a stable balance during non-normal activities, such as exercise, stress and ill health. For example, when the body experiences a cold environment, it responds by limiting the blood flow to the blood vessels to prevent heat loss and shivering to generate heat. Both of these are designed to return the body back to its stable internal balance, or homeostasis.

use. Physiology is concerned with the way that the body communicates with its different systems to ensure the effective integration of these processes.

Physiology is also concerned with how the body adapts to changes in the environment, and when we do or experience something that is out of the ordinary, to ensure that the body continues to function normally. This is called **homeostasis** (Learning Box 10.1) and refers to the way that the body maintains a steady state or tries to return to a normal state at all times. Physiology also analyses how the body adapts to the environment, stress and challenges that it encounters. For example, exercise challenges the body by requiring more energy than normal, and the systems of the body adapt in many ways to this, such as increased breathing by the respiratory system to increase the uptake of oxygen by the body, and increased blood flow from the circulatory system to increase the amount of oxygen to the cells and reduce the amount of carbon dioxide.

To summarise, physiology is the study of how the anatomical systems of the human body work together to ensure that the body continues to function normally even when changes in the environment, stress and other activities occur.

The important linkage between anatomy and physiology

So far, the chapter has divided anatomy and physiology into separate sections. This is because it is important to understand that they do study different aspects of the human body. However, it is important to understand that they are essentially linked together in order for the human body to function. They work together in varied and intricate ways to ensure the body works as smoothly as possible. Put simply, how the body is formed (its anatomy) largely determines what the body does (its physiology). For example, consider the fact that some species of monkeys and apes are able to hang from trees due to having what is called a prehensile tail. This enables them to grab and hold onto things, and means that they are able to live in trees safely. Humans do have a tail bone, but it does not function in the same way. It is largely redundant, and means that humans are not able to do the same things that monkeys and apes can. This shows how the anatomy of the body is linked to its physiology, in terms of its form affects its function. Similarly, the unique shape and length of the human hand (its anatomy) enables it to grab and hold things in intricate and delicate ways (its physiology) that the hand of other animals that are not so intricately shaped are unable to do.

Continually understanding and making this linkage between the anatomy and the physiology of the human body will improve your learning and understanding of both. It is harder to understand what something is if you do not understand what it does. To exemplify, try to describe a car without describing what it does. While it may be easy to describe the parts of the car, it becomes harder to do this without stating what they do. Similarly, imagine trying to describe the bones of the body without describing what they do. This should highlight that trying to understand what the parts of the body are (anatomy) without describing what they do (physiology) is not easy, and this should be borne in mind throughout your studies.

The benefits of understanding anatomy and physiology for health and social care

This section details how understanding anatomy and physiology specifically contributes to health and social care. There are three important ways in which this occurs, as detailed below.

Identify and understand the signs and symptoms of health and social care conditions

To be able to provide appropriate health and social care, the first thing that you need to be able to do as a health and social care practitioner is to correctly identify the condition that is occurring. This requires knowing the signs and symptoms of conditions and interpreting these signs and symptoms in relation to the way that the body should function. Sometimes, conditions are easy to identify as the sign and symptoms are clear. For example, an external broken limb can often be clear to identify as the break is evident. However, when that break is internal in the form of a fracture, it becomes harder to identify. This is where knowing the signs and symptoms becomes important, as it enables the correct identification of conditions. At this point, it is important to understand the **difference between signs and symptoms** (Learning Box 10.2), as sometimes the signs can match the symptoms, but other times the signs and symptoms do not match. For example, to go back to the example of a fractured limb, a stress fracture in the foot may have symptoms like a sprain, strain, or even plantar fasciitis, which is when pain occurs at the bottom of the foot, at or around the heel and arch of the foot. This can make it difficult to identify the condition just from the signs or just from the symptoms. Usually, it is the combination of the two that helps in most effectively identifying a condition.

The importance of anatomy and physiology to identifying conditions is perhaps most evident at times of emergency, where a quick understanding of the signs and symptoms can be crucial, or even lifesaving. Being able to do this quickly and immediately requires an understanding of basic concepts of anatomy and physiology. This applies to both health and social care workers, as this can help with the treatment of the condition until more specialised medical help is available.

> **Learning Box 10.2: The difference between signs and symptoms**
>
> People often think that signs and symptoms mean the same thing, but they do actually refer to different things. Symptoms are what a person feels, such as when a person has a cold, they may say that they have symptoms such as a sore throat, feel sweaty and have a runny nose. Signs are how the condition is observed by someone else. So while someone without a cold cannot feel a sore throat, feel sweaty or have a runny nose, they can observe a build-up of mucus in the throat, an increase in temperature and build-up of mucus in the nose. These are objective observations, which is what signs are, as opposed to subjective observations, which is what symptoms are.

It is important to note at this point that misdiagnosis of conditions does occur. For example, Walzl *et al.* (2019) observed a misdiagnosis rate of 4% for neurological diseases, with some diseases such as epilepsy having a misdiagnosis rate as high as 71%. Additionally, Miller and Levy (2015) identified a misdiagnosis rate of 15% for people with chronic obstructive pulmonary disease (COPD) in England and Wales. And Au-Yeung *et al.* (2019) observed that nearly 40% of autistic and over 50% of possible autistic individuals perceived that they had been misdiagnosed.

There can be many possible reasons for misdiagnosis. For example, Patel *et al.* (2024) observed that the misdiagnosis of COPD is largely a consequence of a lack of specialised knowledge of its signs from diagnostic equipment. Alternatively, Warrick *et al.* (2014) identified that a lack of knowledge of a disease (cognitive factors) was the most prevalent reason for diagnostic errors in children presenting with acute medical illness to a community hospital. Together, this suggests that a lack of anatomical or physiological knowledge can be a significant cause of misdiagnosis for a range of conditions.

It is also relevant here to note the effect that misdiagnosis can have on individuals. There can be a number of outcomes from this. Firstly, it can lead to the wrong treatment and care of the individual, Secondly, it can lead to no treatment at all if a condition has been missed. And thirdly, it can lead to a late diagnosis. All of these outcomes can either prolong the condition or make it worse. For the individual, this can lead to pain and suffering, financial issues such as loss of earnings, the need for prolonged care and a reduction in life expectancy. Misdiagnosis also has a financial cost to the health service, in terms of needing to provide more expensive treatment later on, needed to provide treatment for longer, and also financial compensation for misdiagnosis which between 2017 and 2021, cost the NHS £1.1 billion (Kelly, 2023). This is an expense that could be spent elsewhere on improving health and social care conditions and treatment.

Understand the short-term and long-term effects of health and social care conditions

Health and social care conditions can have both long-term (chronic) and short-term (acute) effects, which are important to identify and understand to provide the correct care and treatment. For example, stress is a condition which has short-term effects such as headaches, trouble sleeping and anger, and long-term effects such as increased blood pressure, increased risk of heart disease and increased risk of stroke (British Heart Foundation, 2024). Knowing these differences not only helps with a correct diagnosis of the condition, but also enables appropriate care and treatment to be provided depending on the condition. The relevant point here is that these short-term and long-term effects are often indicated by anatomical and physiological changes that help identification. For example, to go back to stress, a possible short-term anatomical change is tightness in the neck and jaw, and this can help with an identification of stress (Gallagher, 2024). Similarly, a possible short-term physiological effect of stress is an increase in the heart rate as the body prepares for possible 'fight and flight', which again can help with an identification of stress (Dhabhar, 2018). It is when these short-term anatomical and physiological conditions are combined that they provide a good indicator of the condition of stress that is being experienced, and this is the case for numerous other conditions.

For longer term conditions, there are also changes in anatomy and physiology which can help to understand the condition. For example, diabetes has long-term anatomical effects such as damage to large and small blood vessels, which can lead to significant physiological effects, such as high blood pressure, nerve damage and foot problems. Knowing these long-term effects can provide a good indicator of the extent to which the condition is affecting the individual as a way to decide relevant care and treatment.

An observation of a short-term or long-term condition can lead to a decision to monitor the condition in different ways, which, in turn, can confirm or reject the specific condition. For example, an anatomical observation of a broken rib can require that the condition is monitored either clinically or through an X-ray to ensure that it does not lead to more serious physiological conditions such as a collapsed lung or bleeding in the chest cavity. Even where the condition is not anatomically based, it can be still important to understand the short-term effect to ensure that the condition does not start to affect the body in other ways that are not expected. For example, a panic attack caused by anxiety can have an effect on the cardiovascular system in terms of leading to a significant increase in the heart rate. Identifying and understanding this as a short-term effect can lead to clinical observations to ensure that this does not continue over a longer period of time, or is not a sign of a more serious condition.

It is also important to understand that conditions can have effects on daily living that impact on the individual in short-term and long-term ways. For example, a short-term effect of diabetes can be a fatigue and a lack of energy, which can affect the ability of the individual to care for themselves and or do things that are important for daily living, such as washing, dressing and having social interaction with others. In the longer term, the effects of these can be loneliness, social isolation and neglect. Knowing the possibility of these short-term and long-term effects can make practitioners more aware of them when they occur, and accordingly put in place measures that limit their impact.

Enable planning, care and support for health and social care conditions

Understanding the anatomy and physiology of the human body and the conditions that can arise from them enables the better provision of planning, care and support for these conditions. Most conditions lead to changes in the anatomy, physiology or both of the body. The most obvious examples are the anatomy and physiology changes that occur during pregnancy. For example, anatomically the uterus expands, which puts pressure on the bladder and can lead to a need urinate more often than normal. Knowing this enables help and support to be put in place to limit these effects, such as exercises to increase pelvic floor muscles which will also potentially reduce the risk of long-term effects of urinary incontinence during and after pregnancy.

The identification and understanding of anatomical and physiological changes can also help to support the care of individuals. For example, when prescribing medication, it is important to understand what the effect of these can be on the anatomy and physiology of the body, in order to avoid harm or unnecessary suffering to the individual. Even when not prescribing medication but providing care for someone who is taking medication, it is important to understand how it is affecting the body in order to identify when medication may or may not be working, or having negative side effects. For example, there are a variety of types of medications for high blood pressure, all of which can cause varied and different side effects such as disturbed sleep, headaches, and constipation. However, these side effects are not the same for all individuals, meaning that while one individual may experience side effects from one particular type of medication, a different type of medication may not cause similar side effects. This means that a change of medication, or a change of dosage of the medication, can lead to the side effects become lessened or stopping. The key point here is that it is understanding the changes in anatomy and/or physiology, through the side effects that occur, which can lead to more effective treatment and care.

For some conditions, that nature of the anatomy and physiology changes are so evident that they enable care and support to be planned and designed well in advance. For example, dementia is a condition where there are significant anatomical changes, such as changes in the size of the brain, and physiological changes, such as changes to the nervous system. These changes can lead to social issues for the individual, such as memory loss or confusion. Knowing that these changes are likely to occur makes it possible to plan care and to provide care that limits the impact of these changes when they occur. For instance, the changes in memory linked to dementia has led to the development of 'Memory Cafes', as a way for people living with dementia, families, volunteers, and professionals to meet together to share information and experiences. These have been shown to 'contribute significantly to the psychosocial wellbeing of carers of those living with dementia and provide a positive outlet for carers to build social networks and become active in their community' (Protoolis *et al.*, 2022: 358).

Summary

The study of anatomy and physiology is the study of how the human body works, but its relevance to providing health and social care is often not evident or can seem not relevant. This chapter has hopefully made this provided an important understanding of this relevance. Anatomy and physiology bring to life what the body does and why it does it, which is important to understand when trying to enable individuals to not only live, but to live well, as the essential core of health and social care.

Anatomy is concerned with the form of the human body and how the human body structured as it is. Physiology is concerned with how the body functions as it does. However, they should be seen as intrinsically linked together, and learning them together as essential to understanding each. This is because the form of the human body affects the function, and vice versa, in the same way that the form of a machine affects its function.

For health and social care, the benefits of understanding anatomy and physiology vary from enabling the identification of signs and symptoms of conditions, understanding the short-term and long-term effects of conditions, and enabling planning care and support for conditions. All of these three beneficial outcomes can improve the treatment and care that you as a health and social care practitioner provide.

References

Au-Yeung, S.K. *et al.* (2019) 'Experience of mental health diagnosis and perceived misdiagnosis in autistic, possibly autistic and non-autistic adults', *Autism*, 23(6), pp. 1508–1518. Available at https://doi.org/10.1177/1362361318818167

British Heart Foundation (2024) Effects of stress on the body. Available at: https://www.bhf.org.uk/informationsupport/heart-matters-magazine/wellbeing/stress-and-the-body (Accessed 18 September 2025)

Dhabhar, F.S. (2018) 'The short-term stress response – Mother Nature's mechanism for enhancing protection and performance under conditions of threat, challenge, and opportunity', *Frontiers in Neuroendocrinology*, 49, pp. 175–192. Available at https://doi.org/10.1016/j.yfrne.2018.03.004

Gallagher, G. (2024) *Neck and jaw pain at the same time? Causes and treatment*, *Healthline*. Available at https://www.healthline.com/health/neck-and-jaw-pain (Accessed 17 June 2024).

Kelly, R. (2023) *What are the current medical misdiagnosis statistics?* Available at https://www.patientclaimline.com/article/medical-misdiagnosis-statistics/ (Accessed 11 June 2024).

Miller, M.R. and Levy, M.L. (2015) 'Chronic obstructive pulmonary disease: Missed diagnosis versus misdiagnosis', *BMJ*, 351, p. h3021. Available at https://doi.org/10.1136/bmj.h3021

Patel, K. *et al.* (2024) 'Exploring the causes of COPD misdiagnosis in primary care: A mixed methods study', *PLOS ONE*, 19(3), p. e0298432. Available at https://doi.org/10.1371/journal.pone.0298432

Protoolis, H.A. *et al.* (2022) 'More than memory: A qualitative analysis of carer-reported psychosocial benefits of memory cafés', *Health Promotion Journal of Australia*, 33(S1), pp. 358–366. Available at https://doi.org/10.1002/hpja.573

Walzl, D., Carson, A.J. and Stone, J. (2019) 'The misdiagnosis of functional disorders as other neurological conditions', *Journal of Neurology*, 266(8), pp. 2018–2026. Available at https://doi.org/10.1007/s00415-019-09356-3

Warrick, C. *et al.* (2014) 'Diagnostic error in children presenting with acute medical illness to a community hospital', *International Journal for Quality in Health Care: Journal of the International Society for Quality in Health Care*, 26(5), pp. 538–546. Available at https://doi.org/10.1093/intqhc/mzu066

Waugh, A. and Grant, A. (2023) *Ross & Wilson Anatomy and Physiology in Health and Illness*. 14th edn. London: Elsevier.

11 Safeguarding in health and social care

Progressive, proactive and preventative actions for practice

Clive Sealey

The aims of this chapter are to:

- **Outline legal definitions of safeguarding**
- **Differentiate between narrow and wide definitions of safeguarding**
- **Identify progressive, proactive and preventative actions for safeguarding practice**

Introduction

There have been many prominent cases and issues in the news which have raised the issue of safeguarding as a very important in society today. For example, the growth of social media has highlighted the need for safeguarding to deal with the harms that can occur from either its excessive use, such as in relation to online gaming, or exposure to harmful content, such as violence and graphic pornography. The primary concern here has been on the harm to children and young people, but safeguarding issues linked to social media can also occur for adults and older people, such as in relation to social media and gambling.

Safeguarding concerns can range from mild to severe to life-threatening. The high-profile death of Molly Russell in 2017 highlighted the life-threatening harm that can occur from social media, but there have been other cases that have also highlighted this, and also other types of safeguarding issues concerns that can occur. The death of ten-year-old Sara Sarif at the hands of her family in 2023 highlighted the safeguarding concerns that can occur to children in the family due to violence. The instances of grooming gangs in various towns and cities highlighted the safeguarding concerns that can occur to teenagers in communities due to sexual exploitation. The death of 57-year-old Errol Graham highlighted the safeguarding concerns that can occur to adults living in the community due to financial distress. And the death of 79-year-old Stanley Neill highlighted the safeguarding concerns that can occur for elderly people living in a care home due to neglect. These cases have emphasised that serious harm that can occur in the absence of appropriate safeguarding.

These cases also highlight other key features of safeguarding. The first is that safeguarding is relevant to all stages of life, as safeguarding issues in various forms can occur at any stage of life, whether during childhood, adolescence, adulthood or old age. Linked to this is that safeguarding is also important in relation to where we are, whether in the family, in the community, in society or in care. It is easy to think that safeguarding is not relevant to us when we are fit and healthy, but as these cases show, the reality is that our circumstances can change over time and very quickly, in which case our need for safeguarding becomes evident. For example, the cases of sexual exploitation of young people

DOI: 10.4324/9781032619309-13

described above occurred to young people that would not normally be thought of as vulnerable to abuse (Telford and Wrekin Council, 2016). This means that safeguarding is important at all stages of our life, whether we see ourselves as vulnerable or not. This means that safeguarding is everybody's business and safeguarding is everybody's responsibility.

This chapter focuses on outlining two key aspects of safeguarding, its meaning and key factors that can limit safeguarding issues and concerns. In terms of meaning, it outlines the difference between a narrow and a wide definition of safeguarding, the significance of this difference and how this is reflected in legislation. In terms of key factors that can limit safeguarding issues and concerns, it outlines nine factors which lead to progressive, proactive and preventative action on safeguarding. By the end of the chapter, you should have a clear understanding of what safeguarding is, and also a clear outline of action you can take in practice to progressively, proactively and preventatively limit safeguarding issues and concerns.

What is safeguarding?

If we look at some key definitions of safeguarding for both children and adults, it is noticeable that for both, there is usually a narrow emphasis on harm, abuse or neglect. For example, NSPCC (2025) states that 'A safeguarding issue or concern is anything that might impact on children and young people's safety and welfare, cause them harm, or put them at risk of harm'. Similar, in relation to adults, Age Concern (2023: 1) states that, 'Safeguarding means protecting people's right to live in safety, free from abuse and neglect'. This narrow emphasis is understandable when we consider that instances of harm and abuse have been the key to way that safeguarding issues have been made apparent to the general population, as emphasised in the examples above.

Safeguarding is required by law in health and social care organisations. For children and young people under 18 years old, the legal requirement originates in the *Children Act 1989*. For adults aged 18 and over, the legal requirement is in the *Care Act 2014*. These laws do not specifically define what safeguarding is, this is done in statutory guidance (see Chapter 6). These statutory guidance definitions are shown in Table 11.1.

These definitions have similarities that enable us to make two key points to define what safeguarding is. The first is the emphasis in the definitions on more than just responding to safeguarding issues or concern. In both definitions, safeguarding is specifically linked to improving the lives of all children and adults in a wide sense, such as in relation to the circumstances that children grow up and the wellbeing of adults. The assumption here is that the better the circumstances/wellbeing of an individual, the better they are able to protect themselves from safeguarding issues should they arise (Powell, 2016). For instance, consider the possible different response to a safeguarding issue of a child with strong social support systems to a child living in isolation without strong social support systems; or consider the possible different responses to a safeguarding issue of an adult in safe secure employment to an adult in temporary, unstable and insecure employment. This emphasises safeguarding not as a singular, one off act to deal with issues as they arise, but as an ongoing and enduring responsibility throughout the lives of all children and adults. For health and social care practitioners, this outlines safeguarding as a legal responsibility to focus on improving the circumstances of all children and adults at all times.

The second point to make about the legal definitions is that in contrast to the point made above, the legal definitions of safeguarding focus on issues wider than harm, abuse and neglect (the word harm does not even appear in the definitions). Instead, words like promote, protect and prevent are used in the definitions, which are words that highlight

Table 11.1 Legal definitions of safeguarding

Children and young people *Working together to safeguard children* (HM Government, 2023)	**Adult** *Care and Support statutory guidance* (Department of Health and Social Care, 2025)
• providing help and support to meet the needs of children as soon as problems emerge • protecting children from maltreatment, whether that is within or outside the home, including online • preventing impairment of children's mental and physical health or development • ensuring that children grow up in circumstances consistent with the provision of safe and effective care • promoting the upbringing of children with their birth parents, or otherwise their family network through a kinship care arrangement, whenever possible and where this is in the best interests of the children • taking action to enable all children to have the best outcomes in line with the outcomes set out in the Children's Social Care National Framework.	Safeguarding means protecting an adult's right to live in safety, free from abuse and neglect. It is about people and organisations working together to prevent and stop both the risks and experience of abuse or neglect, while at the same time making sure that the adult's wellbeing is promoted, including, where appropriate, having regard to their views, wishes, feelings and beliefs in deciding on any action. This must recognise that adults sometimes have complex interpersonal relationships and may be ambivalent, unclear or unrealistic about their personal circumstances.

that safeguarding requires taking actions before issues occur, not after they have occurred. This is an important point as often the focus in safeguarding is on what to do after harm, abuse or neglect has occurred, as is especially evident in the NSPCC definition above. However, the emphasis in the legal definitions on taking actions to promote, protect and prevent something occurring makes safeguarding primarily a *progressive* (meaning continuous), *proactive* (meaning planning well in advance) and *preventative* (meaning stopping something from happening) process, to stop things happening in the first place rather than a reactive process that acts after something that has happened. This is an important for health and social care practice as it places responsibility on practitioners to consider possible safeguarding concerns and issues that could occur and put measures in place to limit the possibility of these occurring.

From these two key points, we can more specifically define safeguarding broadly as *progressive actions to proactively improve the lives of all children, young people and adults, and which preventatively protect against issues and concerns occurring.* This definition highlights safeguarding as progressive, proactive and preventative action that improves lives.

Progressive, proactive and preventative safeguarding actions

Having identified progressive, proactive and preventative actions as important to safeguarding, the focus in this section is on detailing factors that enable this to occur. As shown in the adult definition of adult safeguarding in Table 11.1, the statutory guidance identifies 'promoting wellbeing' as a key requirement of safeguarding. This fits very well with the primary aim of health and social care as to promote the health

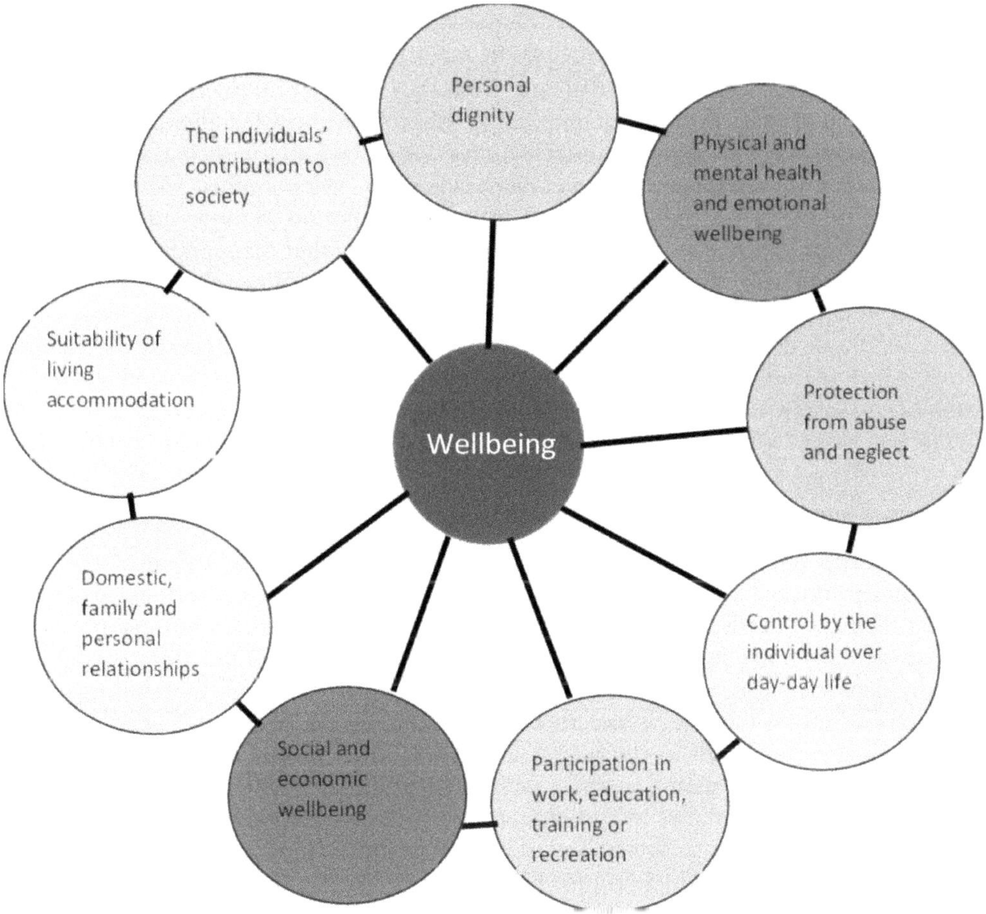
Personal dignity
Physical and mental health and emotional wellbeing
Protection from abuse and neglect
Control by the individual over day-day life
Participation in work, education, training or recreation
Social and economic wellbeing
Domestic, family and personal relationships
Suitability of living accommodation
The individuals' contribution to society
Wellbeing

Figure 11.1 Nine key wellbeing aspects.

Source: Adapted from Department of Health and Social Care (2019).

and wellbeing of individuals to enable them to participate in the activities of every-day life. The statutory guidance states nine key wellbeing aspects. These are shown in Figure 11.1.

In the statutory guidance, the aspects in Figure 11.1 are stated as expectations of how local authorities should approach and engage with people. In other words, they are not specific actions, but outline what a person could expect the local authority to try to do to ensure their wellbeing, not what they are obliged to do. For instance, there is no obligation to put in place action to ensure that a person participates in work, education, training or recreation, just an expectation that they will try to do this.

The aspects include things that are directly relevant to safeguarding, such as protection from abuse and neglect. It also includes aspects that you would not perhaps associate with safeguarding, such as the individual's contribution to society. These aspects are adapted below to show how acting upon them can take practice towards preventive, proactive and progressive safeguarding action.

Personal dignity

This refers to the way that we treat people. Its focus is on building relationships with children and adults who respect who they are, what they can do and the lives that they live. This means interactions that do not humiliate, embarrass or belittle individuals or groups, but treats them as equals and ensures respect for their views and wishes. For example, as a practitioner when interacting with a child, it is possible to ignore their views and wishes simply because they are a child in a way that you would not do so for an adult, and when talking to an adult, it is possible to speak to them in ways that maintain your status as a professional in an 'I am the professional and I know best' way. When this occurs, personal dignity is violated, which can lead to humiliation, degradation and dehumanisation (Peičius *et al.*, 2022), all of which can be relevant to safeguarding. For instance, in the example above, if a child thinks that they will be taken seriously, they would be more likely to raise issues of concern, which means that the issue can be progressed and prevented before it occurs or gets worse, which makes evident why personal dignity is important to safeguarding.

Physical and mental health and emotional wellbeing

Physical health refers to how the body works, mental health refers to how the mind works and emotional wellbeing refers to how people manage their emotions. To be able to meet their own needs, it is important for individuals to be healthy, not just physically but also mentally and emotionally. When one of these factors is not functioning well, then an individual may also not function well. For example, consider an Olympic athlete in peak physical fitness but who is experiencing a mental health illness. It is very likely that their physical performance in the field is affected by their mental health circumstances. This shows that each of these can affect each other, and that is why it is important to pay attention to all three equally. In specific relation to safeguarding, when either physical, mental, or emotional health is deprived, this increases the reliance that an individual has on other people for care, which in turn limits their ability to protect against and prevent safety concerns (WHO, 2024). An individual with good physical, mental and emotional health is more likely to accurately state what the problem is, which means that it can be progressively and/or preventatively dealt with before it becomes a bigger issue.

Protection from abuse and neglect

While abuse and neglect are similar, the difference between them is that abuse is primarily a harm that is caused by doing something to someone, such as hurting someone physically or using them, while neglect is primarily harm that is caused by not doing something to someone, such as not ensuring adequate care or not providing adequate food (Gonzalez *et al.*, 2025). As an example, where an adult physical hits a child, that would be abuse, but where an adult does not provide adequate clothes for a child that would be neglect. The most relevant point to take here is that, despite the difference, both abuse and neglect are key safeguarding concerns due as they both cause negative outcomes for children and adults.

There are 11 key types of abuse and neglect for safeguarding, and these are briefly detailed below.

1. Physical abuse

Physical abuse is an individual's body being injured or hurt due to, for example, assault, hitting, slapping or pushing. It can also be the wrong use of restrictive practices.

Examples include hitting, kicking, punching, biting, shaking, rough or inappropriate handling, misuse of medication and inappropriate use of restraint.

2. Domestic abuse

This is where abuse occurs where there is an intimate relationship between individuals, for example, a married couple or people recognised as being partners in a relationship. Examples include psychological, physical, sexual or financial harm within a domestic relationship.

3. Sexual abuse

Sexual abuse is when a person becomes involved in sexual relationships or activities that they do not want to be involved in. They may have said that they do not want to be involved, or they may be unable to give consent. Examples include sexual acts the person has not consented to, is pressurised into consenting to or does not have the capacity to consent to, contact sexual abuse such as touching inappropriately and rape, non-contact sexual abuse such as indecent exposure or forcing someone to watch acts, photographs and images, and grooming.

4. Psychological abuse

Psychological abuse is making a person feeling worthless, unloved or uncared for. Examples include shouting, swearing, name calling, insulting, humiliating, ridiculing, intimidating, threatening abandonment or institutional care, involuntary isolation or withdrawal from services, or controlling or coercive behaviour.

5. Emotional abuse

Emotional abuse is a consistent pattern of abusive words and bullying behaviours that wear down a person's self-esteem and undermine their mental health. Examples include name calling, shouting at a person even if someone has not done anything wrong, putting someone down, ignoring or leaving a person out of things, saying things that make a person feel bad about themselves and stopping someone from having friends.

6. Financial abuse

Financial abuse is the use of a person's money, assets or belongings without their permission. Examples include the misuse of funds, pressure or misappropriation of property, wills, bank accounts, welfare benefits, assets, cash, and investments, fraud, extortion, theft, deception, and threat of deprivation and assault or neglect to obtain money or other material gain.

7. Discriminatory abuse

Discriminatory abuse refers to an individual or group being treated unequally because of nine protected characteristics (age, race, gender reassignment, disability, sex, sexual orientation, religion or belief, marriage and civil partnership, and pregnancy and maternity) as set out in the *Equality Act 2010* (see Chapter 15). Examples include direct or indirect discrimination, harassment and hate crime (see Chapter 16).

8. Organisational abuse

Organisational abuse happens where services provided are focused on meeting the needs of the organisation and not on the needs of the individual. The focus is on working in ways because 'we always do it this way' or 'this is how we do it here'. As a consequence, the organisation's routines and practices are not responsive to or respectful to individuals' own needs. For example, a care home may insist on having a set early meal time for all individuals as this coincides with a change of shift, and not because it is beneficial to its residents. This may mean that in some instances, residents have to eat so early that they get hungry during the night.

9. Modern-day slavery

Modern slavery is where traffickers and slave masters use whatever means they have at their disposal to coerce, deceive and force individuals into a life of abuse, servitude and inhumane treatment. Examples include human trafficking, forced labour, domestic servitude, sexual exploitations such as escort work, prostitution and pornography, and debt bondage – being forced to work to pay off debts that realistically they never will be able to.

10. Neglect

Neglect is also known as the 'omission to act' or 'failure to act'. It is a failure to meet the basic needs of the individual, or to refuse to take care of their own basic needs. Examples include not providing, withholding or inadequate provision of necessities such as food, heating, medication and health care, not providing social stimulation, failure to give access to appropriate services such as health, social services, police or other, or not taking account of a person's educational, social, recreational, cultural or ethnic needs.

11. Self-neglect

Self-neglect refers to an extreme lack of self-care either as a consequence of being unable to such as due to a medical condition, or being unwilling to due to other issues such as addictions. Examples include lack of self-care to an extent that it threatens personal health and safety, neglecting to care for personal hygiene, health or surroundings, inability to avoid self-harm, failure to seek help or access services to meet health and social care needs, or inability or unwillingness to manage personal affairs.

From the list of 11 types of abuse and neglect above, we can make some key general points about abuse and neglect that are relevant when trying to safeguarding against them. These are that:

- Abuse and neglect can be perpetrated by anyone, including family, friends, intimate partners and colleagues
- Abuse and neglect can take place anywhere, including the home, at work, at leisure or just out and about
- Abuse and neglect often, but not always, occurs against an individual when they are in a position of less power or influence, for example in relation to age, gender, authority or status
- There is often more than one type of neglect or abuse occurring in any situation, meaning a need to be aware of the possibility that a specific sign of abuse or neglect should also be considering in relation to the possibility of other abuse or neglect occurring (Age Concern, 2023).
- Abuse and neglect can either be a **criminal offence or a civil offence** (Learning Box 6.1), meaning that they require action to be taken to both stop and punish the offender.

Protection from abuse and neglect is difficult because often they only become apparent once that have occurred. However, progressive action in the form of awareness of these can lead to proactive and preventive safeguarding responses on the part of individuals. Additionally, once abuse and neglect have been identified, it may be possible to take proactive action to prevent it from occurring again, such as practical help, care and support.

Control by the individual over day-to-day life

Having control over what we can do and how we can do it is important to us as individuals. Think about how important it is for you to be able to decide what to eat, what to wear, where to go and who we are friends with. When these are taken away from us, this negatively affects the way that we feel about ourselves. Maslow's (1943) theory of a '*Hierarchy of needs*' developed the concept of 'self-actualization' to describe the importance of having control over our lives. He argued that control, which he called 'self-actualization', led to morality, creativity, spontaneity, acceptance, purpose and meaning in our lives. These qualities enable us to feel happier and self-fulfilled, and therefore contribute fully to society (Sealey, 2015). In specific relation to safeguarding, this would enable individuals to take more responsibility for their own welfare and work out ways to meet this individually, instead of relying on other people to do this, which as we saw above in relation to physical and mental health and emotional wellbeing, can result in safeguarding issues.

Participation in work, education, training or recreation

Promoting participation is about getting people involved in doing things, rather than living in isolation or loneliness. Participation has several beneficial outcomes for individuals and communities. It can help people to have a sense of belonging, to make friends, identify sources of support, and improve their knowledge of issues (Thomas *et al.*, 2020). It can also help people overcome factors such as discrimination and prejudice (Turner, 2020), which are specially linked to safeguarding issues. For example, lack of participation by young people in education has been implicated in the issue of **county lines drug trade** (Learning Box 11.1), which has become a major issue in recent years in relation to safeguarding (The Children's Society, 2025). This is because such lack of participation works to isolate children away from their peers and family, which limits their ability to ask for and receive help when required. Providing these opportunities for participation increases their support systems which can help to prevent isolation and loneliness leading to other issues.

Learning Box 11.1: County lines drug trade

County lines drug trade is a term that refers to where drug criminals make friends with children and then exploit them by forcing them to carry out drug dealing. For example, they may start by being friendly to the young person by giving them gifts such as mobile phones to make them think that they are their friends. However, over time, they demand that the young person pays back the gift through doing task for them, which usually involves selling drugs. A refusal by the young person is often met by violence. The focus is on young people because they are less likely to be suspected of crime, and also the sentence for them is likely to be less if they are caught. Issues such as poverty have been identified as relevant to county lines occurring (Wroe, 2021).

Social and economic wellbeing

Closely linked to participation is social and economic wellbeing. Social wellbeing refers to how good your relationships are with people around you. Having good relationships is important for how we feel about ourselves, the things we want to do, and also when we need help (Jordan, 2023). Economic wellbeing refers to the financial security we have, and how we can use these to improve our lives, or use at times of need (Nozal, 2019). Both of these are important in providing stability and assurance in our lives, in terms of being able to call on these in times of need. The absence of either social or economic resources can lead to ill health, poverty, or isolation. For example, consider meeting friends on a weekly basis who ask you how you are and may notice if there is a deterioration in your health before you notice yourself. This is relevant to safeguarding as it can prevent issues becoming a more significant problem in the future, as is important to safeguarding.

Domestic, family and personal relationships

It is typically the case that our domestic, family and personal relationships are the most important to us, as these are the one that we refer and respond to the most often. For very young children especially, the family is especially important, as it is may be the only relationship that they know, and this influence can remain throughout life (Thomas *et al.*, 2017). For elder adults too, the family may also be very important. These relationships influence us in many various ways that sometimes we are not even aware of, and can have a huge influence on our lives. Positively, they can be sources of support, growth and development. Negatively, they can be areas of coercion, control and crisis. We can often become dependent on these relationships for many of our needs identified above, such as emotional, social and economic over long periods of time. This makes these relationships important in terms of providing resources to support us to develop and grow and also at times of need, to protect against safeguarding concerns.

Suitability of living accommodation

The suitability of our living accommodation is important for many reasons. Where we live positively provides us with shelter, warmth security and privacy. It also provides us with the space to be ourselves without having to worry about what others think. And it also allows us to express our creativity in terms of how we decorate the house. However, poor housing does not provide us with any of these, and additionally, housing that is damp, cramped and cold can have a serious detrimental effect on our health (Sealey, 2023). Having suitable accommodation progressively limits the possibility that such issues will occur. It is also important to acknowledge that where people live is where they tend to spend most of their lives, and so is where promoting and preventing safeguarding is likely to be highly effective.

The individuals' contribution to society

It is possible to contribute to society in many ways. This can be economically through work, communally through neighbourhood action, socially through volunteering, domestically through caring for family, and politically through sharing ideas. While the outcomes from these can be different in scope and effect, the key point is that they all have some effect, some of which may not be known for years later. For example, volunteering to run a sports team can not only have immediate benefits for individuals such as improving skills, but also long-term benefits, such as enabling them to work in a team environment. However, the evidence is that such action also has benefit to the contributor, in terms of improved life satisfaction, wellbeing and self-esteem (Department for Culture, Media and Sport and Department for Digital, Culture, Media and Sport, 2018). All of these are factors that improve the lives of individuals in significant ways, thereby progressively and preventatively limiting safeguarding issues.

To briefly summarise these nine key points, we can see that applying these nine aspects of wellbeing to safeguarding allows us to reinforce the point made above that safeguarding is not a narrow singular issue focused on harm, abuse and neglect. Instead, it highlights how safeguarding is only effective if the wider focus on progressive, proactive and preventative action that improves lives is the priority. For example, a focus on participation in work, education, training or recreation works progressively to limit the possibility of participating in issues that can be negative to safeguarding, such as county lines drugs trade. A focus on physical and mental health and emotional wellbeing works proactively to mean that individuals are more likely to make choices that are in their best interests and not influenced by others. And a focus on social and economic wellbeing works preventatively to limit issues related to poverty and discrimination occurring, which can lead to further safeguarding issues. Even if we do just narrowly focus on abuse and neglect, the importance of these other factors is evident. For example, a focus ensuring than an individual has control over day-to-day life is relevant to preventing abuse and neglect, in terms of its positive effect of limiting the reliance that an individual has on other people, which in turn increases their ability to protect against and prevent safety concerns.

The more extensive point to make about these aspects is that they should be seen as interconnected with each other, and not separate from each other. By this is meant that taking positive action in one factor has positive implications for the other factors. For example, ensuring personal dignity affects how an individual feels in terms of their mental and emotional wellbeing, which in turn makes it more likely that their physical and mental and emotional wellbeing are good, which in turn means that they are more likely to be able to protect themselves from abuse and neglect, which in turn means greater likelihood of control by the individual over their day-to-day life, which in turn means greater likelihood of participation in work, education training or recreation, which in turn means greater likelihood of social and economic wellbeing, which in turn means better likelihood of positive domestic, family and personal relationships, which in turn means better likelihood of suitability of living accommodation, which in turn means that the individual is better placed to contribute to society. The reverse of course is also true, as negative occurrence in one of these factors means a greater likelihood of negative occurrences in the other factors. So a key point here is that that all of these factors should be seen as equal, with no single factor being more important than the other (Department of Health and Social Care, 2025). This interconnective nature of safeguarding is highlighted in Figure 13.1 by the lines that connect them all together.

Summary

Safeguarding is everybody's business and safeguarding is everybody's responsibility. This is because safeguarding needs affect anyone at any time, whether young or old, rich or poor. The typically narrow focus on harm, abuse and neglect as the key focus of safeguarding is understandable in the context of current issues, but this does not reflect what is legally required. The legislation for both children and adults highlights the importance of promotion, protection and prevention of safeguarding issues, as well as improving the circumstances of individuals. This leads to a broader definition of safeguarding as *progressive actions to proactively improve the lives of all children, young people and adults, and which preventatively protect against issues and concerns occurring*. This definition highlights safeguarding as progressive, proactive and preventative action that improves lives.

To facilitate this, the chapter has adapted nine wellbeing aspects to show how acting upon them can take practice towards preventive, proactive and progressive safeguarding action. Applying these aspects reinforces the point that safeguarding is not a narrow singular issue focused on harm, abuse and neglect, but is only effective if the wider focus on progressive, proactive and preventative action that improves lives is the priority. Additionally, a further point to make about these aspects is that they should be seen as interconnected with each other, and not separate from each other. This means that to be effective, safeguarding action should always be on them collectively, and not as single entities.

References

Age Concern (2023) *Safeguarding* older *p*eople from *a*buse and *n*eglect. Factsheet 78. Available at https://www.ageuk.org.uk/siteassets/documents/factsheets/fs78_safeguarding_older_people_from_abuse_fcs.pdf (Accessed 25 March 2025).

Department for Culture, Media and Sport and Department for Digital Culture, Media and Sport (2018) *1. PEOPLE: Enabling a lifetime of contribution*. Available at https://www.gov.uk/government/publications/civil-society-strategy-building-a-future-that-works-for-everyone/1-people-enabling-a-lifetime-of-contribution (Accessed 24 March 2025).

Department of Health and Social Care (2019) *Strengths-based approach: Practice Framework and Practice Handbook*. Available at: https://assets.publishing.service.gov.uk/media/5c62ae87ed915d04446a5739/stengths-based-approach-practice-framework-and-handbook.pdf (Accessed: 18 September 2025).

Department of Health and Social Care (2025) *Care and support statutory guidance*. Available at https://www.gov.uk/government/publications/care-act-statutory-guidance/care-and-support-statutory-guidance (Accessed 20 March 2025).

Gonzalez, D., Bethencourt Mirabal, A. and McCall, J.D. (2025) 'Child abuse and neglect', in StatPearls. Treasure Island, FL: StatPearls Publishing. Available at http://www.ncbi.nlm.nih.gov/books/NBK459146/ (Accessed 20 March 2025).

HM Government (2023) *Working together to safeguard children*. Available at https://assets.publishing.service.gov.uk/media/669e7501ab418ab055592a7b/Working_together_to_safeguard_children_2023.pdf (Accessed 20 March 2025).

Jordan, M. (2023) 'The power of connection: Self-care strategies of social wellbeing', Journal of Interprofessional Education & Practice, 31, p. 100586. Available at https://doi.org/10.1016/j.xjep.2022.100586

Maslow, A.H. (1943) 'A theory of human motivation', Psychological Review, 50(4), pp. 370–396. Available at https://doi.org/10.1037/h0054346

Nozal, A. (2019) *The* Economy of Well-Being: Creating Opportunities for People's Well-Being and Economic Growth. OECD Statistics Working Papers. 2019/02. Available at https://doi.org/10.1787/498e9bc7-en

NSPCC (2025) *Safeguarding: Frequently asked questions*, *NSPCC learning*. Available at https://learning.nspcc.org.uk/research-resources/safeguarding-frequently-asked-questions (Accessed 25 March 2025).

Peičius, E. *et al.* (2022) 'Dignity violations and barriers to dignity assurance for terminally ill patients at the end of life: A cross-sectional Analysis', Medicina, 58(2), p. 294. Available at https://doi.org/10.3390/medicina58020294

Powell, C. (2016) Safeguarding and Child Protection for Nurses, Midwives and Health Visitors: A Practical Guide. 2nd edn. Maidenhead: Open University Press.

Sealey, C. (2015) Social Policy Simplified: Connecting Theory with People's Lives. London; New York, NY: Palgrave Macmillan. Available at http://find.shef.ac.uk/openurl/44SFD/44SFD_services_page?u.ignore_date_coverage=true&rft.mms_id=9983301999601441 (Accessed 19 July 2022).

Sealey, C. (2023) Applying Social Policy to Criminal Justice Practice: What Every Practitioner Should Know. Bristol: Policy Press. Available at https://doi.org/10.51952/9781447357490

Telford and Wrekin Council (2016) *Everyone's business scrutiny review of multi-agency working against child sexual exploitation*. Available at https://apps.telford.gov.uk/CouncilAndDemocracy/Meetings/Download/MTg0NDY%3D (Accessed 19 March 2024).

The Children's Society (2025) *What is county lines?* Available at https://www.childrenssociety.org.uk/what-we-do/our-work/child-criminal-exploitation-and-county-lines/what-is-county-lines (Accessed 25 March 2025).

Thomas, E.C. *et al.* (2020) 'An examination of the community participation interests of young adults with serious mental illnesses', The Journal of Behavioral Health Services & Research, 47(4), pp. 526–543. Available at https://doi.org/10.1007/s11414-019-09678-0

Thomas, P.A., Liu, H. and Umberson, D. (2017) 'Family relationships and well-being', Innovation in Aging, 1(3), p. igx025. Available at https://doi.org/10.1093/geroni/igx025

Turner, R.N. (2020) 'Reducing prejudice and discrimination', in Turner, R. N. (ed.) Oxford Research Encyclopaedia of Psychology. Oxford University Press. Available at https://doi.org/10.1093/acrefore/9780190236557.013.313

WHO (2024) *Abuse of older people*. Available at https://www.who.int/news-room/fact-sheets/detail/abuse-of-older-people (Accessed 24 March 2025).

Wroe, L.E. (2021) 'Young people and "county lines": A contextual and social account', Journal of Children's Services, 16(1), pp. 39–55. Available at https://doi.org/10.1108/JCS-10-2020-0063

12 Children and young people's mental health

Denisse Levermore

The aims of this chapter are to:

- Detail the current state of children/young people's mental health in the UK
- Analyse key factors that are currently impacting on children/young people's mental health
- Outline key factors that support good mental health for children/young people

Introduction

We are more aware of the importance of good mental health and the impact of poor mental health in relation to children and young people's development and lifelong health and wellbeing. We now understand that children and young people's mental health is not purely something to be thought about and understood by specialist services, but that there is a part to play for all practitioners in universal settings, in relation to building resilience, recognising difficulties, and supporting all children and young people to develop good mental health and wellbeing.

However, research has overwhelmingly supported the fact that over the past ten years, children and young people's mental health has worsened. For example, the number of children and young people struggling with mental health concerns has grown to one in five (NHS Digital, 2023) with the percentage reporting low happiness in relation to their mental health increasing in recent years (The Children's Society, 2022). The chapter outlines possible reasons for this occurring.

While data itself cannot inform us of the causes, there are a range of both national and international factors that cause children and young people to worry and that provide ongoing challenges to their mental health and wellbeing. These issues are wide-ranging and not all can be covered within this chapter. Those that are discussed here are the cost-of-living crisis, negative experiences using social media, the global COVID-19 pandemic impact on children and young people's mental health, abuse and neglect, the impact of racism, and poor parental mental health.

This chapter concludes by exploring and identifying key factors that can contribute to improving the mental health of children/young people. These factors can help to enable good mental health.

The current state of children/young peoples' mental health

The UK does not fare well in terms of overall life satisfaction of 15-year-olds in comparison to other European countries. Out of 27 European countries, the UK came last

DOI: 10.4324/9781032619309-14

Learning Box 12.1: Reflecting on and challenging statistics

Statistics in mental health and wellbeing help us to understand data, break findings down, and draw critical and meaningful responses, which can support a focus that enables purposeful change to practice and policy. However, when we review any health statistics, it is important that we are aware of how data is gained, who the source is, who collected the data, and what will happen with the data that has been gathered, to help to eliminate bias and the potential for relying on unreliable data/statistics. Since the COVID-19 pandemic, the UK public understand the need for good health data, but they want to be assured of confidentiality and reliability, with ongoing focus needed to build public trust in the use of their information (National Data Guardian, 2020). There is a need for caution in interpreting the data due to differences/difficulties in data collection (IT difficulties, infrastructure difference) that could lead to data gaps and limitations to interpretation (Child Outcomes Research Consortium, 2014).

on this scale, having the highest proportion of 15-year-olds reporting low life satisfaction (25.2%) in 2022 (OECD, 2023). Gender differences are also evident, with one in five boys (19.8%) and one in three girls reporting low life satisfaction at age 15 in the UK in 2022 (OECD, 2023).

It is important to note that reliable data on children and young peoples' mental health has only recently been collected and published regularly since 2014. Prior to this, the most up to date figures were from 2004 (UK Parliament, 2014) resulting in children/young people being let down and services working 'in a fog'. This emphasises **reflecting on and challenging statistics** (Learning Box 12.1) to support our knowledge of the current landscape of children/young people's mental health, to ensure appropriate support and services are available. However, there have been two important recently published reports which allow us to understand factors that are affecting children/young people's mental health. These are *The Good Childhood Report* and *The Mental Health of Children and Young People in England* survey.

The Good Childhood Report

The Children's Society produces an annual report titled *The Good Childhood Report* (The Children's Society, 2024) that explores how children/young people in the UK are feeling about their lives currently and in the future, including feelings about family, friends, school, appearance, their future and their safety in different contexts. The report states that out of nine areas of life that young people aged between 10 and 17 were asked to rate in terms of happiness, they were most happy with their family and least happy with school (The Children's Society, 2024). Happiness with family is a very important positive finding due to research that demonstrates positive relationships being key to children/young peoples' good mental health and wellbeing. However, the statistics in relation to children/young peoples' relationship with school are concerning, with school support for wellbeing and school absences being areas of concern (The Children's Society, 2024).

The context of *The Good Childhood Report* is important to consider when analysing the findings, as statistics presented in the 'Understanding Society' section are derived from data in 2021/22 when COVID-19 restrictions were in place. This meant that responses to the survey were reported as lower than previously (The Children's

Society, 2024). The authors state that it is difficult to assess whether these findings can be linked to the pandemic and so this requires further research to help us to understand the importance of context in relation to statistics and children/young peoples' mental health.

The Mental Health of Children and Young People in England survey

The *Mental Health of Children and Young People in England* survey (NHS Digital, 2023) provides an analysis of the mental health of children/young people during the COVID-19 pandemic, offering valuable context to children/young people's lives during the pandemic and beyond. Statistics from these reports and other research in relation to children/young people's mental health highlight specific issues that currently impact on children and young peoples' mental health, such as COVID-19, social media, abuse and neglect and racism.

According to the survey, one in five children/young people aged between 8 and 25 had a probable mental disorder. This compares with previous statistics from 2004 (Office for National Statistics (ONS), 2004), which showed that the ratio of children/young people aged 5–16 years having a probable mental disorder was one in ten. This indicates that the number of young people with a probable mental disorder has doubled over the last 20 years. The breakdown between these ages demonstrates that young people aged between 17 and 19 years are the most likely to struggle with a mental health difficulty (23%).

Factors affecting children/young people's mental health and wellbeing

Poverty

The *Good Childhood Report* (The Children's Society, 2024) is also clear on the impact that financial strain for families is having on children and young people, as shown in Figure 12.1.

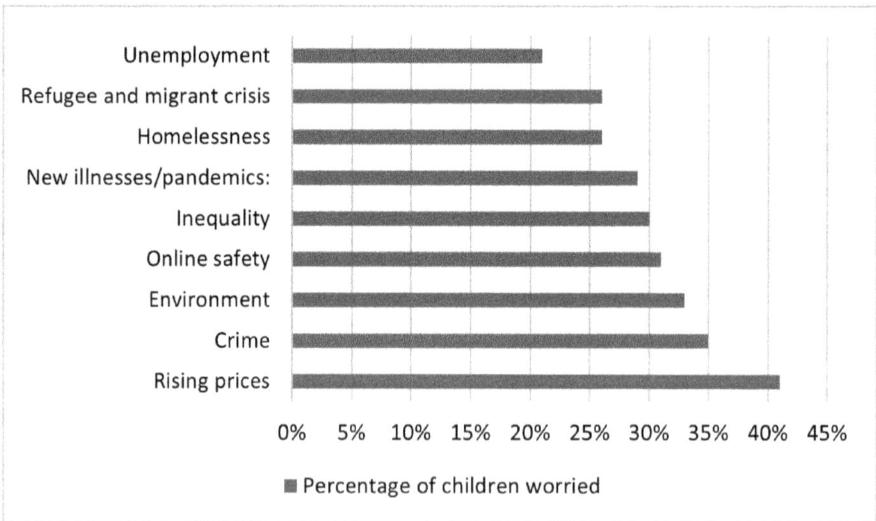

Figure 12.1 Children's and young people's worries about societal issues.

Source: The Children's Society (2024).

Figure 12.1 demonstrates that out of nine other societal issues, 41% or two in five children were 'very' or 'quite worried' about rising prices. The Children's Society (2024) findings also show that 17% (one in six children) reported low life satisfaction when their family is under financial strain, and 9% (under one in ten children) when their family is not under financial strain. This reinforces Morrison Gutman *et al.'s* (2015) observation that by age 11, children from the lowest 20% income households are four times more likely to experience significant mental health challenges compared to those from the top 20% wealthiest households.

For children/young people, the effect of poverty accrues throughout childhood, intensifying mental health problems over time (Treanor and Troncoso, 2023), which in turn negatively impact on family dynamics and relationships. There is widespread recognition and research demonstrating the impact of poverty on children/young people, and financial strain being associated with lower wellbeing (Adjei *et al.*, 2024; The Children's Society, 2022). A report by the Centre for Mental Health, the Children and Young People's Mental Health Coalition, and Save the Children UK highlights the impact of poverty on children's mental health and calls for UK government action on mental health and education policies (Rainer *et al.*, 2024).

Children growing up in poverty face numerous disadvantages that can accumulate throughout their lives. These disadvantages can lead to inequalities in health, cognitive development, psychosocial development, and educational attainment (Graham and Maughan, 2025). Adjei *et al.* (2024) states that for one in ten children, parental health is also affected by stress related to family poverty. Poverty has lifelong impacts due to the stress that it causes to vulnerable, developing brains and bodies, with chronic stress able to significantly alter brain development. The amygdala, responsible for processing emotional reactions in the brain, may exhibit prolonged heightened activity, causing an exaggerated response to everyday stressors. Elevated levels of stress hormones (cortisol) within the brain can impede the development of the hippocampus, essential for memory and cognitive processing, thereby hindering effective learning (McEwen, 2011). Moreover, chronic stress can induce changes in the prefrontal cortex (white matter) and other brain regions, leading to emotional dysregulation, hypervigilance, and impaired executive function, these being critical for rational thinking and decision-making (Blair and Raver, 2016).

Research often looks at future outcomes of child poverty, but it is important to understand the impact on children *during* their childhood. Children living in poverty, especially older young people, often miss out on social, leisure, and celebratory activities. They might feel excluded and stigmatised because they cannot keep up with trends which in turn, can affect their friendships and self-esteem, with low self-esteem being a risk factor for mental illness, suicide or poor academic achievement (Doi *et al.*, 2019). There are educational barriers as poverty limits children's ability to fully benefit from learning opportunities. The UK ranks third among the wealthy countries in the OECD for having the highest levels of inequality in access to basic educational resources, based on income (UNICEF, 2010) with parents facing challenges in covering extra school costs. A higher perceived income inequality, as compared to friends, has also been found to have an association with poor adolescent mental health, with young people who saw themselves as belonging to families equal in wealth having better mental health outcomes (Piera Pi-Sunyer *et al.*, 2023).

It is important to emphasise that while many children growing up in poverty face significant challenges, not all will have poor mental health outcomes as adults

(Adjei *et al.*, 2024) and protective factors like strong family relationships and peer inclusion can help mitigate negative impacts (Kintrea *et al.*, 2011).

COVID-19

The outbreak of the COVID-19 pandemic and subsequent lockdowns affected children's mental health, causing negative impacts globally. Ng and Ng (2022) observed that children from low-income families were especially affected. The pandemic worsened their financial situation, leading to stress and poor parenting practices, which harmed children's mental health, with crowded living conditions adding to this. Other findings suggest being an only child was a risk factor, due to larger families mitigating some of the negative effects of social isolation (Ng and Ng, 2022).

Bronfenbrenner's (1979) ecological systems theory (Figure 12.2) supports an explanation of the pandemic's impact on children's mental health. This theory describes how children develop through interactions within different systems, from close (family – microsystem) to broad (societal influences – macro-system), and shape an individual's development, from immediate environments like family to broader societal influences like culture.

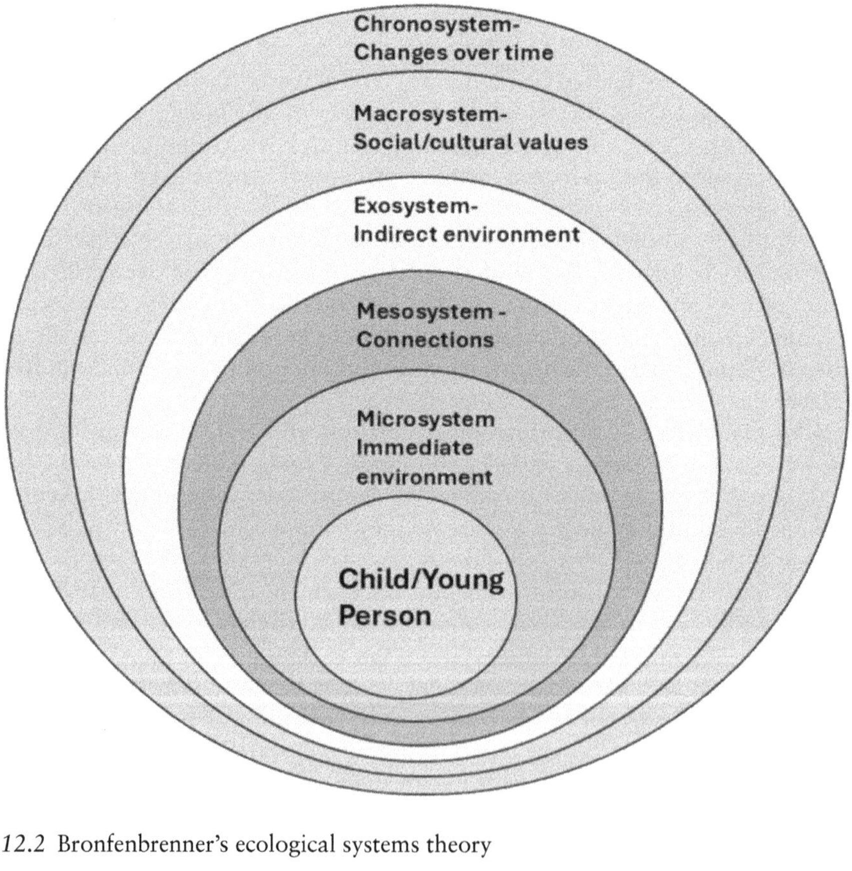

Figure 12.2 Bronfenbrenner's ecological systems theory

Source: Author's own diagram.

The pandemic disrupted these systems, increasing stress and mental health issues for both children and parents (Ng and Ng, 2022). School closures and reduced support from teachers affected children's mental health, as feeling connected to school helps buffer against negative outcomes (Hertz *et al.*, 2022). Parents working from home experienced stress that impacted their children indirectly, as the economic impact of the pandemic also worsened parents' mental health, which in turn, affected children. The two-way relationship between parents and children in the microsystem helps to understand how both parents and children are affected in a reciprocal manner (Ng and Ng, 2022).

Many young people have been affected by the pandemic in different ways. People with a stable home life and financial security found spending more time at home during lockdown easier and more enjoyable, with 22% reporting that their mental health had improved (NHS Digital, 2021). In contrast, those from disadvantaged backgrounds, who may rely on school meals and resources or have strained family relationships, faced greater challenges. Also, for children with negative school experiences, such as bullying or high academic pressure, the lockdowns likely brought relief rather than anxiety (KCL, 2022). Resilience was a factor that supported young people to be able to cope with the overwhelmingly negative effects of the pandemic. Panchal *et al.* (2023) found that 93% of children could cope with lockdown measures and adapt, and that family relationships improved for most children.

Supporting children and young people's mental health recovery post pandemic is a public health priority, requiring actions at multiple levels to recover from the negative effects of the pandemic. According to Ng and Ng (2022), ensuring adequate support for parents' mental health is essential in mitigating parental stress, anxiety, and depression. This recognition underscores the importance of providing sufficient support to parents as a fundamental aspect of effectively supporting children's wellbeing.

Social media

The rapid transformation of social media from a simple networking site to a comprehensive tool has brought about many advantages. Nevertheless, it has also presented considerable challenges to children and young people's mental health. Liu *et al.* (2024) investigated how social media affects children aged 6-13 years mental health. Results showed both positive and negative impacts, influenced by factors, such as age, gender, social support, and parental involvement. In relation to young people, research has demonstrated mixed results regarding the relationship between social media use and adolescent mental health (Keles *et al.*, 2020). Some studies indicate that increased social media use is associated with depression, anxiety, and psychological distress, while other studies suggest that social media can enhance social support, strengthen connections, and reduce feelings of social isolation and loneliness (Best *et al.*, 2014; Keles *et al.*, 2020; Orben *et al.*, 2020). Plackett *et al.* (2024) conducted a longitudinal study (an analysis of changes over time) and found minimal evidence suggesting that increased social media usage is linked to future mental health issues in UK adolescents. Self-esteem was found to be a significant mediator, meaning that social media might affect young people's mental health partly because it impacts their self-esteem, however, it is clear that more research is needed to understand this relationship (Plackett *et al.*, 2024).

These findings indicate that mental health interventions focusing on factors, such as self-esteem and its relationship with social media could be more effective than those that solely focus on social media use (Plackett *et al.*, 2024). The need to balance social media use, while underscoring the importance of strong family and school support systems to lessen any adverse effects is emphasised. Liu *et al.* (2024) suggests practical parent training programmes and school-based curricula, to encourage collaboration between parents and educators, and to foster healthy social media habits.

Abuse and neglect

Childhood maltreatment, encompassing physical, sexual, and emotional abuse, as well as neglect, represents a worldwide public health and human rights crisis. It affects over one-third of children under the age of 18 (World Health Organization, 2017). Many studies have shown that experiencing abuse or neglect during childhood can lead to serious and lasting health effects, greatly increasing the risk of developing mental and physical health problems later in life. Individuals who suffered childhood abuse were over twice as likely to develop severe mental health conditions (psychoses, schizophrenia, and bipolar disorder) or to need medication, compared to those without a history of maltreatment (Chandan *et al.*, 2019). Additionally, they were at double the risk of developing mental illnesses, including depression and anxiety (Chandon *et al.*, 2019). It is well known that adverse childhood experiences (ACEs), such as abuse and neglect, are negatively associated with numerous physical, social, emotional, and behavioural difficulties in adulthood (Felitti *et al.*, 1998).

ACEs are extremely stressful events where a child either suffers direct harm or lives in a detrimental environment. Within the original research (Felitti *et al.*, 1998), participants were asked if they had experienced any of seven different adversities as a child, these responses culminated in an ACE score. The higher the score, the greater the relationship with poor mental and physical health outcomes in adult life. These experiences can include physical, sexual, or emotional abuse, neglect, or living in a household with issues, such as parental mental health problems, domestic violence, or substance misuse. ACEs significantly increase the risk of children experiencing poorer mental and physical health, difficulties in forming friendships, and academic underachievement. It is important to note that while ACEs increase vulnerability, they do not always lead to negative outcomes, as the impact varies for each child. Some may experience trauma that affects their development, learning, health, and behaviour, whereas others, supported by protective factors like a safe environment and personal resilience, might not be as affected. In relation to children and young people, up to two thirds of the population experience at least one ACE before the age of 18, and one quarter experience four or more ACEs (Hughes *et al.*, 2017). However, it is important to acknowledge that there are limitations of ACEs screening in this way. For instance, an ACEs score alone does not effectively distinguish between individuals who will develop health problems later in life and those who will not. Many individuals with a high ACEs score may not experience poor health outcomes, while most health issues in the population are often seen in those with a low ACE score, due to other factors (Baldwin *et al.*, 2021). Therefore, there is a need for caution and curiosity in relation to using ACEs scores alone as a predictor for future health problems. Increasing public awareness of ACEs within a Trauma-Informed approach and ensuring that we look beyond to the broader structural cases of ACEs (such as poverty) are key considerations when developing policy and interventions to support children/young people (Lacey and Minnis, 2019).

Maltreated children may be more likely to develop mental health difficulties due to abuse and neglect, alternatively this could be due to other genetic and environmental factors (Baldwin *et al.*, 2023). These factors include family history of mental illness, higher genetic risk scores for psychiatric disorders, socioeconomic disadvantage, bullying and victimisation. Co-occurring risks have been overlooked in previous research; holistic interventions that address both the experiences of abuse (e.g. trauma-focused CBT) and the wider mental health risk factors should be considered to help minimise the risk of psychopathology (Baldwin *et al.*, 2023).

Racism

Racism is a structured system of oppression that constructs race by classifying and ranking social groups. It devalues, disempowers, and unequally distributes desirable societal opportunities and resources to groups deemed inferior (Bonilla-Silva, 1997; Williams and Whitfield, 2004). While racism has progressively been recognised as a significant determinant of poor mental health, most research predominantly examines its effects on adults. There is an even more pronounced dearth of studies addressing the impact of racism on the mental health of children and adolescents, particularly in relation to younger children, leading to a substantial gap in the evidence base necessary for informing policy and practice within the UK (Ghezae *et al.*, 2025).

Simela *et al.* (2024) outline the vicarious nature of racism in the context of parent-child relationships with both parents and young people reporting symptoms like fear, worry, and sadness in children, related to depression and anxiety. These symptoms were not only driven solely by parents' experiences of racism, but also by children's own direct and indirect experiences with racism outside the family, demonstrating how parent's experiences of racism can impact on children and vice versa (Simela *et al.*, 2024). This highlights a need to consider a family approach to understanding the pervasive nature of racism experienced by all within the family in order to fully recognise its impacts on the child's mental health and wellbeing.

Parental mental health

Starting a family is a big milestone and the transition to parenthood can be difficult for both men and women, leading to or worsening mental health problems (Challacombe *et al.*, 2022). Around 68% of women and 57% of men with mental health difficulties are parents and many parents manage their condition, thereby reducing its impact on their children with the right support (Mental Health Foundation, 2025). Poor mental health in mothers and fathers is linked to poor outcomes in children. The effect on children depends on the severity and type of the parent's mental health condition, as well as the child's age and development stage. It is important to note that it remains unclear if the link between parental mental health and childhood outcomes is due to direct cause or genetic factors (Larsson, 2023). However, it is recognised that parental mental health difficulties can affect the family environment (Challacombe *et al.*, 2022).

A combination of mental health of both primary and secondary caregivers, along with family poverty, can significantly impact on children/young people's mental health, with both factors combining to create severe negative effects. Adjei *et al.* (2024) estimate that 22–40% of adolescent mental health problems can be attributed to having persistent mental health problems in both caregivers, combined with household poverty. In the UK, there are few policy efforts designed to address both poverty and mental health, although there are numerous separate reports and studies outlined to address parental mental health problems and poverty (Elliott, 2016). Adjei *et al.* (2024) suggest a need to think holistically about the clustering of childhood adversity, rather than focus on single issues, as this could have a dramatic impact on mental health outcomes for adolescents in the UK.

What is good mental health for children and young people?

Consideration of good mental health for children and young people starts in the womb. Advances in neuroscience and infant mental health inform us that pregnancy, childbirth and the first year of life are critical times of brain and relationship changes and the time when interventions can make a positive difference to an infant and mother's mental health and wellbeing (Whitters, 2023). Positive infant mental health can be defined as the developing capacity of the infant to:

- form close and secure relationships,
- experience, manage, and express a full range of emotions,
- explore the environment,
- learn, all in the context of family, community, and culture (Zeanah and Zeanah, 2019).

The Parent-Infant Foundation (2024) outlines that the first 1,001 days of an infants life (which equates to just under 3 years) is very important to their social/emotional wellbeing and development within this time, and so also very important to their mental health. During this time, sensitive, responsive parenting is crucial to developing good mental health, with severe and persistant difficulties in early relationships and emotional development potentially having pervasive and lifelong impacts. This means that the relationship with the infant's primary carer is the key to future relational capacities, and it is this relationship that provides the infant with the medium with which they learn to regulate their emotions, behaviours, and actions. Therefore, it can be proposed that it is this relationship that supports and promotes good infant mental health and wellbeing above others. Stress factors that impact on this relationship, whether external or internal, will, in turn, increase the potential for poor infant mental health.

These early experiences shape the architecture of the developing brain and lay the foundations for good mental health. The brain is particularly sensitive during the period 0–3 years and 11–24 years with 'windows of opportunity' for learning and developing at their optimum within these periods (Dahl *et al.*, 2018; Schneider *et al.*, 2022). Moreover, changes to brain plasticity within adolescence also increases vulnerability, thereby potentially increasing the risk of mental ill health (Fuhrmann *et al.*, 2015).

Neuroscience advances support our knowledge of brain development and how this affects our mental health, strengthening awareness of our expectations in relation to emotional health and what supports good mental health, and this will be impacted by context. In consideration of children and young people's good mental health, this is reflected in their ability to form, maintain, and repair relationships, to maintain high levels of resilience so that they can cope with change and uncertainty, to reach developmental milestones and be able to manage and express both positive and negative emotions, including being able to self-regulate.

Important factors for good mental health for children and young people

Several key factors contribute to fostering and maintaining mental health, including supportive relationships with family, peers and other adults, a safe and stable living environment, access to quality education, and opportunities to reach developmental milestones throughout childhood. Additionally, promoting emotional intelligence, resilience, and coping skills can equip young individuals to navigate life's challenges effectively. These elements, when combined, create a nurturing environment that supports the mental and emotional growth of children and adolescents. Within the following section some of these factors are explored in more detail.

The role of supportive relationships in promoting mental health

The availability of supportive relationships during childhood is an important determinant of positive mental health (Butler *et al.*, 2022). A 2024 study by the OECD highlights that parental emotional support is a crucial determinant of children's wellbeing and academic success. The study found that greater parental emotional support is associated with higher test scores and better subjective wellbeing (OECD, 2024).

Other relationships in a child's life are also important to consider here. For example, supportive relationships between students and teachers positively influence a child/young person's ability to problem solve, build social skills, positively influences school engagement and achievement, fostering a sense of purpose and increasing their autonomy, all of these being both promotive and protective of good mental health (Butler *et al.*, 2022). Moreover, Bellis *et al.* (2017) state that high levels of support from any trusted adult in childhood, regardless of the relationship, reduces the risk of low mental wellbeing in adulthood by 50%.

Peers also contribute to a child/young person's resilience. Moreira *et al.* (2021) highlight the significant role of positive peer relationships in enhancing children's subjective wellbeing and resilience. Additionally, Butler *et al.* (2022) recognise the protective and promotive role of peers in relation to positive mental health, suggesting children/young people with low peer support being over six times more likely to experience low mental wellbeing. Therefore, as we can see, positive relationships within a child/young person's life matter, as they support good mental health and wellbeing, with it taking one trusted adult to make a difference, with peers also being of huge importance.

The importance of resilience to good mental health

Resilience is strongly associated with mental health in children and young people and is best defined as a multisystemic dynamic process of successful adaptation in the context of risk or threat (Mesman *et al.*, 2021).

As a simple way to understand what resilience means, visualise a seesaw with the child/young person in the middle. On one side of the seesaw are protective experiences and coping skills, such as supportive relationships, safety, good health, financial security, and on the other side are negative factors, such as poverty, mental illness, violence, and poor/difficult education. Resilience is present when a child/young person's health and development leans towards the positive, protective factors, even with lots of negative, adversity factors stacked on the other side. Resilience is a combination of protective factors but as we know from above, the single most common protective factor is a stable supportive relationship with one trusted adult. Other protective factors include self-efficacy and perceived control, opportunities to strengthen adaptive skills and self-regulation, and mobilising sources of faith, hope, and cultural traditions (Harvard Centre of the Developing Child, 2024).

However, some people argue that resilience is a Western construct and thereby insensitive to cultural factors (Dhar and Dixit, 2022), and that resilience places responsibility on the individual, positioning the child/young person/family as the locus of change. This means that those in power take no responsibility for the child's circumstances, despite having power to change external factors that impact on mental health (Fisher and Jones, 2023). As resilience is often positioned as a cure all elixir for children/young people's mental health, we need to be mindful of these arguments against resilience, especially where children/young people and families are managing mental health in such dire circumstances that surviving is the aim, meaning that in such circumstances, resilience becomes a meaningless slogan.

The importance of developmental milestones

Emotional development and self-regulation are critical components of a child's wellbeing and social adjustment to support their development into adulthood (Aghaziarati and Nejatifar, 2023). We have become increasingly aware of the importance of developmental milestones as supportive of good mental health.

Developmental milestones are stages of development that a child is expected to reach at certain times in their lives, e.g., smiling, crawling, and walking. They help professionals and parents track infant/child/young person's physical, emotional, social and language development, and help identify any potential delays or problems. Each child develops at different rates and in their own way but failure to reach a milestone enables further investigation as to why and to give support early if required. Developmental milestones and growth are recorded within a Personal Child Health Record (often referred to as the 'red book') within the UK and this is monitored by health professionals, such as Health Visitor, Midwife, and GP. Percentile charts within the red book based on average growth and recorded by gender/age are used to plot the child's growth.

Adolescent emotional developmental milestones are characterised by increased self-awareness, formation of identity and experiencing a wide range of emotions. Young people will be exploring personal values, establishing, and negotiating peer and romantic relationships while endeavouring to regulate intense emotions and navigate convoluted social dynamics, as part of more complex social/emotional development at this life stage.

When negative emotions (usually sadness, fear, anger) are more intensely experienced/expressed, or are exceedingly long, they fail to become adaptive and become maladaptive (Beauchaine *et al.*, 2007). This is known as 'emotional dysregulation'. Emotional dysregulation has been identified as a significant factor contributing to poor mental health for children/young people, including depression and anxiety (Young *et al.*, 2019). Trauma and ACEs contribute to the likelihood of emotional dysregulation, with a variety of mental health and neuro-developmental disorders also associated with emotional dysregulation, such as conduct disorder, attention deficit hyperactivity disorder (ADHD), autism, self-harm, and suicidality (Copeland *et al.*, 2014).

Summary

The most recent data shows that children/young people's mental health is in a poor state. There are several contemporary challenges significantly impacting children/young people's mental health, including poverty, the ongoing effect of COVID-19, social media, abuse/neglect, racism, and parental mental health. These can often lead to increased anxiety, reduced access to mental health resources, and difficulties meeting basic needs, all of which influence children and young people's emotional wellbeing.

Developing good mental health in children and young people is essential for their emotional, social, and cognitive development. It enables them to manage emotions, build relationships, and cope with challenges effectively. There are a number of ways in which this can be done. Building resilience is crucial in this context. Resilience, fostered through positive relationships with family, peers, and trusted adults, equips children to navigate adversity. Supportive relationships provide stability, encouragement, and a sense of belonging, all of which are vital for mental wellbeing, especially in challenging times. Strengthening these connections alongside systemic interventions offers a comprehensive approach to addressing the complex mental health needs of children and young people.

References

Adjei, K. *et al.* (2024) 'Impact of parental mental health and poverty on the health of the next generation: A multi-trajectory analysis using the UK millennium cohort study', *Journal of Adolescent Health*, 74 (1), pp. 60–70. Available at https://doi.org/10.1016/j.jadohealth.2023.07.029

Aghaziarati, A. and Nejatifar, S. (2023) 'Emotional development and regulation in children: A review of recent advances', *KMAN Counseling and Psychology Nexus*, 1 (1), pp. 118–125. Available at https://doi.org/10.61838/kman.psynexus.1.1.14

Baldwin, J. *et al.* (2023) 'Childhood maltreatment and mental health problems: A systematic review and meta-analysis of quasi-experimental studies', *American Journal of Psychiatry*, 180 (2), pp. 117–126. Available at https://psychiatryonline.org/doi/full/10.1176/appi.ajp.20220174

Baldwin, J.R. *et al.* (2021) 'Population vs individual prediction of poor health, results of adverse childhood experiences screening', *JAMA Paediatric*, 175 (4), pp. 385–393. Available at https://doi.org/10.1001/jamapediatrics.2020.5602

Beauchaine, T. *et al.* (2007) 'Polyvagal theory and developmental psychopathology: Emotional dysregulation and conduct problems from preschool to adolescence', *Biological Psychology*, 74 (2), pp. 174–184. Available at https://pmc.ncbi.nlm.nih.gov/articles/PMC1801075/

Bellis, M. *et al.* (2017) 'Does continuous trusted adult support in childhood impart life-course resilience against retrospective childhood experiences: A retrospective study on adult health-harming behaviours and mental well-being', *BMC Psychiatry*, 17, pp. 1–12. Available at https://bmcpsychiatry.biomedcentral.com/articles/10.1186/s12888-017-1260-z

Best, P. *et al.* (2014) 'Online communication, social media and adolescent wellbeing: A systematic narrative review', *Children and Youth Services Review*, 41, pp. 27–36. Available at https://www.sciencedirect.com/science/article/abs/pii/S0190740914000693

Blair, C. and Raver, C.C. (2016) Poverty, stress, and brain development: New directions for prevention and intervention. *Academic Pediatrics*, 16. Available at https://doi.org/10.1016/j.acap.2016.01.010

Bonilla-Silva, E. (1997) 'Rethinking racism: Toward a structural interpretation', *American Sociological Review*, 361, pp. 465–480. Available at https://www.sciencedirect.com/science/article/pii/S0277953624007780

Bronfenbrenner, U. (1979) *The Ecology of Human Development: Experiments by Nature and Design*. Harvard: Harvard University Press.

Butler, N. *et al.* (2022) 'The contributing role of family, school, and peer supportive relationships in protecting the mental wellbeing of children and adolescents', *School Mental Health*, 14 (3), pp. 776–788. Available at https://www.ncbi.nlm.nih.gov/pmc/articles/PMC8818094/#CR58

Challacombe, F. *et al.* (2022) 'Paternal perinatal stress is associated with children's emotional problems at 2 years', *The Journal of Child Psychology and Psychiatry*, 64 (2). Available at https://acamh.onlinelibrary.wiley.com/doi/10.1111/jcpp.13695

Chandan, J. *et al.* (2019) 'The burden of mental ill health associated with childhood maltreatment in the UK, using the health improvement network database: A population-based retrospective cohort study', *The Lancet Psychiatry*, 6 (11), pp. 926–934. Available at https://doi.org/10.1016/S2215-0366(19)30369-4

Child Outcomes Research Consortium (CORC) (2014) Written evidence submitted by *Child Outcomes Research Consortium (CORC)* (CMH0141). Available at https://committees.parliament.uk/writtenevidence/49614/pdf/

Copeland, W. *et al.* (2014) 'Adult diagnostic and functional outcomes of DSM-5 disruptive mood dysregulation disorder', *American Journal of Psychiatry*, 171 (6), pp. 668–674. Available at https://doi.org/10.1176/appi.ajp.2014.13091213

Dahl, R. *et al.* (2018) 'Importance of investing in adolescence from a developmental science perspective', *Nature*, 554, pp. 441–450. Available at https://doi.org/10.1038/nature25770

Dhar, A. and Dixit, S. (2022) 'Making of a crisis: The political and clinical implications of psychology's globalization', *Journal of Theoretical and Philosophical Psychology*, 42 (2), pp. 108–130. Available at https://psycnet.apa.org/doiLanding?doi=10.1037%2Fteo0000187

Doi, S. *et al.* (2019) 'Pathway of the association between child poverty and low self-esteem: Results from a population-based study of adolescents in Japan', *Frontiers in Psychology*, 10. Available at https://pmc.ncbi.nlm.nih.gov/articles/PMC6511812/

Elliott, I. (2016) *Poverty and mental health: A review to inform the Joseph Rowntree Foundation's anti-poverty strategy*. Available from https://www.mentalhealth.org.uk/sites/default/files/2022-08/poverty-and-mental-health-report.pdf

Felitti, V.J. *et al.* (1998) 'Relationship of childhood abuse and household dysfunction to many of the leading causes of death in adults. The adverse childhood experiences (ACE) study', *American Journal of Preventive Medicine*, 14 (4), pp. 245–258. Available at https://doi.org/10.1016/S0749-3797(98)00017-8

Fisher, J. and Jones, E. (2023) 'The problem with resilience', *International Journal of Mental Health Nursing*, 33 (1), pp. 1–4. Available at https://onlinelibrary.wiley.com/doi/10.1111/inm.13220

Fuhrmann, D. *et al.* (2015) 'Adolescence as a sensitive period of brain development', *Trends in Cognitive Sciences*, 19 (10), pp. 558–566. Available at https://doi.org/10.1016/j.tics.2015.07.008

Ghezae, F.T. *et al.* (2025) 'The association between experiences of racism and mental health on children and young people in the UK: Rapid scoping review', *BJPsych Open*, 11 (1). Available at https://www.cambridge.org/core/journals/bjpsych-open/article/association-between-experiences-of-racism-and-mental-health-on-children-and-young-people-in-the-uk-rapid-scoping-review/E3A4F958A2A5C74AADDDB285196CAB44

Graham, P. and Maughan, B. (2025) 'Child mental health problems and poverty', *BJPsych Bulletin*, pp. 1–3. Available at https://doi.org/10.1192/bjb.2024.111

Harvard Centre of the Developing Child, (2024) *A guide to resilience*. Available at https://developingchild.harvard.edu/resource-guides/guide-resilience/

Hertz, M.F. *et al.* (2022) 'Adolescent mental health, connectedness, and mode of school instruction during COVID-19', *Journal of Adolescent Health*, 70 (1), pp. 57–63. Available at https://doi.org/10.1016/j.jadohealth.2021.10.021

Hughes, K. *et al.* (2017) 'The effect of multiple adverse childhood experiences on health: A systematic review and meta-analysis', *Lancet Public Health*, pp. 356–366. Available at https://doi.org/10.1016/S2468-2667(17)30118-4

KCL (Kings College London) (2022) *How has Covid-19 impacted children and young people?* Available at https://www.kcl.ac.uk/an-isolated-generation-the-impact-of-covid-19-on-children-and-young-people

Keles, B. *et al.* (2020) 'A systematic review: The influence of social media on depression, anxiety and psychological distress in adolescents', *International Journal of Adolescence and Youth*, 25 (1), pp. 79–93. Available at https://doi.org/10.1080/02673843.2019.1590851

Kintrea, K. *et al.* (2011) *The Influence of Parents, Places and Poverty on Educational Attitudes and Aspirations*. York, Joseph Rowntree Foundation. Available at https://pascalobservatory.org/sites/default/files/young-people-education-attitudes-summary.pdf

Lacey, R. and Minnis, H. (2019) 'Practitioner review: Twenty years of research with adverse childhood experience scores – Advantages, disadvantages and applications to practice', *The Journal of Child Psychology and Psychiatry*, 61 (2), pp. 116–130. Available at https://acamh.onlinelibrary.wiley.com/doi/10.1111/jcpp.13135

Larsson, H. (2023) 'Children of parents with depression or anxiety: Long-term follow-up, causality and resilience', *JCPP Advances*, 3 (4). https://pubmed.ncbi.nlm.nih.gov/38054050/https://pubmed.ncbi.nlm.nih.gov/38054050/

Liu, T. *et al.* (2024) 'The impact of social media on children's mental health: A systematic scoping review', *Healthcare (Basel)*. Available at https://pmc.ncbi.nlm.nih.gov/articles/PMC11641642/

McEwen, B.S. (2011) *Effects of stress on the developing brain. Cerebrum.* Available at https://pmc.ncbi.nlm.nih.gov/articles/PMC3574783/#:~:text=McEwen's%20laboratory%20discovered%20adrenal%20steroid,differences%20in%20these%20brain%20regions.

Mental Health Foundation (2025) *Family and parenting: statistics.* Available at https://www.mentalhealth.org.uk/explore-mental-health/statistics/family-parenting-statistics

Mesman, E. *et al.* (2021) 'Resilience and mental health in children and adolescents: An update of the recent literature and future directions', *Current Opinion in Psychiatry*, 34 (6), pp. 586–592. Available at https://www.ncbi.nlm.nih.gov/pmc/articles/PMC8500371/

Moreira, A. *et al.* (2021) 'Children's subjective well-being, peer relationships and resilience: An integrative literature review', *Child Indicators Research*, 14, pp. 1723–1742. Available at https://doi.org/10.1007/s12187-021-09843-y

Morrison Gutman, L. *et al.* (2015) *Children of the new century: Mental health findings from the Millennium Cohort Study.* Available at https://www.researchgate.net/publication/308083993_Children_of_the_new_century_mental_health_findings_from_the_Millennium_Cohort_Study

National Data Guardian (2020) *Polling indicates growing public understanding about importance of using health and care data.* Available at https://www.gov.uk/government/news/polling-indicates-growing-public-understanding-about-importance-of-using-health-and-care-data

Ng, C.S.M. and Ng, S.S.L. (2022) 'Impact of the COVID-19 pandemic on children's mental health: A systematic review', *Front Psychiatry*, 13. Available at https://pmc.ncbi.nlm.nih.gov/articles/PMC9622998/

NHS Digital (2021) *Mental health of children and young people in England, 2021 - wave 2 follow up to the 2017 survey.* Available at https://digital.nhs.uk/data-and-information/publications/statistical/mental-health-of-children-and-young-people-in-england/2021-follow-up-to-the-2017-survey

NHS Digital (2023) *Mental health of children and young people in England, 2023 - wave 4 follow up to the 2017 survey.* Available at https://digital.nhs.uk/data-and-information/publications/statistical/mental-health-of-children-and-young-people-in-england/2023-wave-4-follow-up#

OECD. (2023) *PISA 2022 Results (Volume I): The State of Learning and Equity in Education.* Available at: https://www.oecd.org/en/publications/2023/12/pisa-2022-results-volume-i_76772a36/full-report/the-state-of-learning-and-equity-in-education-in-2022_e65c570e.html

OECD (2024) Parental emotional support and adolescent well-being: A cross-national examination of socio-economic and gender gaps based on PISA 2018 surveys, OECD Papers on Well-Being and Inequalities. Available at https://doi.org/10.1787/2b7a2ac6-en

Office for National Statistics (ONS) (2004) *Mental health of children and young people in Great Britain, 2004.* Available at https://sp.ukdataservice.ac.uk/doc/5269/mrdoc/pdf/5269technicalreport.pdf

Orben, A. *et al.* (2020) 'The effects of social deprivation on adolescent development and mental health', *The Lancet Child & Adolescent Health*, 4 (8), pp. 634–640. Available at https://doi.org/10.1016/S2352-4642(20)30186-3

Panchal, U. *et al.* (2023) 'The impact of COVID-19 lockdown on child and adolescent mental health: Systematic review', *European Child & Adolescent Psychiatry*, 32, pp. 1151–1177. Available at https://doi.org/10.1007/s00787-021-01856-w

Parent-Infant Foundation (2024) *What is infant mental health? Why does it matter?* Available at https://parentinfantfoundation.org.uk/1001d-resource/what-is-infant-mental-health/

Piera Pi-Sunyer, B. *et al.* (2023) 'The relationship between perceived income inequality, adverse mental health and interpersonal difficulties in UK adolescents', *Journal of Child Psychology and Psychiatry*, 32, pp. 417–425. Available at https://doi.org/10.1111/jcpp.13719

Plackett, R. *et al.* (2024) 'The longitudinal impact of social media use on UK adolescents' mental health: Longitudinal observational study', *Journal of Medical Internet Research*, 25, e43213. Available at https://doi.org/10.2196/43213

Rainer, C. *et al.* (2024) *A dual crisis. The hidden link between poverty and children's mental health.* Available at https://cypmhc.org.uk/wp-content/uploads/2024/07/CentreforMH_ADual-Crisis.final_.pdf

Schneider, N. *et al.* (2022) 'Connecting inside out: Development of the social brain in infants', *Child Development*, 93 (2), pp. 359–371. Available at https://srcd.onlinelibrary.wiley.com/doi/full/10.1111/cdev.13649

Simela, C. *et al.* (2024) Intergenerational consequences of racism in the United Kingdom: a qualitative investigation into parents' exposure to racism and offspring mental health and well-being, pp. 181–191. Available at https://acamh.onlinelibrary.wiley.com/doi/10.1111/camh.12695

The Children's Society (2022) *The Good Childhood Report*. Available at https://www.childrenssociety.org.uk/information/professionals/resources/good-childhood-report-2023

The Children's Society (2024) *The Good Childhood Report*. Available at https://www.childrenssociety.org.uk/sites/default/files/2024-08/Good%20Childhood%20Report-Main-Report.pdf

Treanor, M. and Troncoso, P. (2023) 'The indivisibility of parental and child mental health and why poverty matters', *Journal of Adolescent Health*, 73 (3), pp. 470–477. Available at https://www.jahonline.org/article/S1054-139X(23)00210-0/fulltext

UK Parliament (2014) *Children's and adolescents' mental health and CAMHS - Health Committee*. Available at https://publications.parliament.uk/pa/cm201415/cmselect/cmhealth/342/34205.htm

UNICEF (2010) *The Children Left Behind: A League Table of Inequality in Child Wellbeing in the World's Rich Countries*. Florence: Innocenti Research Centre. Available at https://www.unicef.org.uk/publications/report-card-13-fairness-for-children/

Whitters, H. (2023) *A Study into Infant Mental Health*. Oxon: Routledge.

Williams, D. and Whitfield, K. (2004) 'Racism and health'. in *Closing the Gap: Improving the Health of Minority Elders in the New Millennium*. The Gerontological Society of America. Available at https://pmc.ncbi.nlm.nih.gov/articles/PMC3863357/

World Health Organization (2017) *Violence info – Child maltreatment*. Available at http://apps.who.int/violence-info/child-maltreatment/

Young, K.S. *et al.* (2019) 'Positive and negative emotion regulation in adolescence: Links to anxiety and depression', *Brain Sciences*, 9 (4). Available at https://doi.org/10.3390/brainsci9040076

Zeanah, C. and Zeanah, P. (2019) *Infant Mental Health: The Clinical Science of Early Experience*. 4th Edition, pp. 5–24. New York: Guildford Press.

13 The rights of children and young people within health and social care settings

Kirsty Fraser

The key aims of this chapter are:

- **To provide an understanding of the importance of rights for children and young people**
- **To highlight the importance of the UNCRC to children's and young people's rights**
- **To identify the practical application of children and young people's rights within health and social care settings**

Introduction

Children's rights are fundamental in ensuring that children and young people receive appropriate care and protection within the UK's health and social care systems. These rights are enshrined in various legal frameworks, including the United Nations Convention on the Rights of the Child (UNCRC), which the UK ratified in 1991. Article 24 of the UNCRC states that children have the right to the highest attainable standard of health. This includes access to necessary medical services, nutritious food, clean water, and a safe environment. Ensuring these rights are met helps promote the overall health and well-being of children (OHCHR, 2025).

This chapter provides an overview of children's and young people's rights within health and social care settings. It emphasises the importance of understanding and upholding these rights to ensure the well-being and protection of children and young people. The chapter is particularly relevant for professionals who will be working with children and young people. It also holds significance for those working with adults, as the principles of rights and protections are universally applicable. This chapter assumes we exist and operate within a society and culture that acknowledges the existence of rights, often shaping our everyday lives, understanding that not all societies and cultures are the same, and attitudes towards rights can vary.

What is a right?

Before we think specifically about children's rights, it can be helpful to think about rights more generally. A right can be defined as a moral or legal entitlement to have or obtain something or to act in a certain way. Rights are fundamental to the functioning of a fair society, ensuring that individuals have the freedom to pursue their interests and protect their well-being. They are based on fundamental principles, such as dignity, justice, respect, and fairness, in order to safeguard individuals regardless of their identity, location, or lifestyle. They can be classified into various categories, such as human rights, civil rights, and legal rights.

DOI: 10.4324/9781032619309-15

Another way of thinking about rights in general is the difference between liberty rights and welfare rights. In simplistic terms, liberty rights protect the right to act freely, such as freedom of religion, freedom of speech, freedom to play, freedom to rest, and the guarantee of a fair, unbiased trial. Welfare rights are often classed as 'positive rights', and they exist in many parts of the world as legal rights (Griffin, 2000). Examples of welfare rights are a right to food, shelter, education, a right to be safe, healthcare and transgender bathrooms. Some of our human rights mean that we need to do something to practise our rights actively. For other rights, there are systems in place that ensures laws, policies, and services exist that mean our rights should automatically be met.

There are two main types of rights, passive rights and assertive rights (Castaños-Cervantes, 2024).

Passive rights

Passive rights are those that individuals benefit from without needing to take specific actions. These rights require the state or other entities to refrain from interfering with the individual's freedoms. Examples include:

- **Right to Privacy:** Being free from unwarranted surveillance or intrusion.
- **Right to be Free from Torture:** Protection from torture or inhumane treatment.
- **Right to Non-Discrimination:** Being treated equally regardless of race, gender, religion, etc.

Assertive rights

Assertive rights are those that individuals actively claim or exercise. These rights require action by the individual or the state to uphold them. Examples include:

- **Freedom of Speech:** The ability to share one's thoughts and ideas, whether talking to friends, writing stories, or drawing pictures.
- **Right to Vote:** The right to have a say in choosing leaders, such as picking class representatives or voting in school elections.
- **Right to Education:** Going to school to learn new things, make friends, and discover your favourite subjects.

Children and young people may require support from an adult to help them access their assertive rights. There are several reasons for this. For example, children may not fully understand their rights or how to exercise them. Additionally, some children and young people may feel shy or unsure about speaking up.

The difference between passive rights and assertive rights is that passive rights involve protection from interference or harm, while assertive rights involve active participation or claiming rights. Both types of rights are crucial for ensuring that individuals are free to act in certain ways, protected from harm within society, and treated with equality, respect, and dignity.

What are children's rights?

Children's rights are rights specifically tailored to the needs and vulnerabilities of individuals under 18. Children's rights are important because they make the point that children must be treated with equality, respect, and dignity, not because they are 'the future' or the 'adults of tomorrow', but because they are human beings today. Children should enjoy the same human rights as everybody else – from the right to freedom of expression to privacy. This means all rights should apply equally to children and adults.

However, the reality is that in various decision-making processes, adults, particularly those in positions of leadership or power, may overlook the applicability of rights to children and young people due to the power disparity between adults and children, or not seeing situations from a child or young person's perspective (Alshammari *et al.*, 2025). This is further compounded by the limitations often experienced by children and young people, such as relying on adults for survival, not being able to express their views, or the inability to participate in the electoral process. Also, it is often the case that we view rights and processes from an adult perspective rather than that of a child or young person. This is called 'adultism' (Flasher, 1978). We can use this term to describe and explain children's disadvantaged position in society and their positioning within an adult-centric world (LeFrançois, 2013; Watts and Flanagan, 2007).

The heightened vulnerability of children (Viterbo and Ioffe, 2024) is evidenced by their dependency on adults for care and protection, making it imperative for societal structures to ensure robust safeguarding measures are in place (Children's Commissioner for England, 2019). This is particularly crucial in contexts where children may face additional risks, such as those living in poverty or with disabilities, who are disproportionately affected by harm and abuse (Chambers *et al*, 2021).

The United Nations Convention on the Rights of the Child (UNCRC)

Children's rights are enshrined in various international and national legal frameworks, most notably the United Nations Convention on the Rights of the Child (UNCRC, 1989). The UNCRC is a 54-article document that outlines the rights of every child from civil, political, social, economic, and cultural perspectives. It is structured around four core principles:

- non-discrimination,
- the best interests of the child,
- the right to life, survival, and development,
- child's participation.

(Fairhall and Woods, 2021).

It is the most widely ratified human rights treaty in the world, and all United Nations members except the United States incorporate it into their own legislation, the UK bringing it into force in 1992. The UNCRC was established in response to injustices reported during the International Year of the Child in 1979, including poor healthcare, limited educational opportunities, high infant mortality rates, and children suffering from abuse and exploitation. The UNCRC was created to establish standards for the treatment of children and has an emphasis on children and young people's participation. As a treaty, the UNCRC acknowledges children and young people as valuable members of the community (OHCR, 2024). The convention set out minimum standards protecting the rights of all children without discrimination.

To date, the UNCRC has improved the lives of millions of children and young people, prompting countries worldwide to make necessary changes to laws, policies and services that have made significant improvements in various aspects of their lives, including in the UK. For instance, the *Children Act 1989* and the *Children and Families Act 2014* incorporate principles from the UNCRC, ensuring that children's rights are considered in legal proceedings and policymaking. In a more practical application of the UNCRC, the United Nations Children's Fund (UNICEF) launched the *Rights Respecting Schools* initiative in 2004, which aims to embed children's rights into the ethos and culture of UK based schools. Since its creation, approximately 5,000 schools across the UK have participated, with more than 2,000 schools reporting awards (UNICEF, n.d.). Participating schools reported significant improvements in students' respect for themselves and others, engagement with learning, and educational attainment, contributing to a positive school environment, and many schools also experienced a reduction in bullying incidents and exclusions (Quennerstedt, 2022).

There are many examples globally of the positive changes that have happened in response to the UNCRC. For example, in Kenya, the implementation of the UNCRC has contributed to a rise in primary school enrolment rates from 62% in 1990 to 95% in 2018 (UNICEF, 2025). This improvement is attributed to policies aligning with the UNCRC's principles, such as abolishing school fees and introducing free primary education. The UNCRC has also had a profound impact on children's health. *Article 24* of the Convention highlights the right to the highest attainable standard of health. In Bangladesh, the UNCRC has influenced national health policies, significantly reducing child mortality rates. Between 1990 and 2015, the under-five mortality rate in Bangladesh decreased from 144 to 38 deaths per 1,000 live births (World Bank, 2016). This achievement is linked to improved healthcare services, vaccination programmes, and nutrition initiatives that align with the UNCRC's guidelines (World Bank, 2016).

Protection from violence is another critical area where the UNCRC has made a difference. *Article 19* of the Convention mandates the protection of children from all forms of physical or mental violence. In Sweden, the UNCRC has been pivotal in shaping child protection laws, leading to the prohibition of corporal punishment in all settings, including the home (Global Initiative to End All Corporal Punishment of Children, 2020). As a result, Sweden has seen a decline in child abuse cases and an increase in public awareness about children's rights.

However, there are still countries where children do not fully enjoy their rights. (Stoecklin *et al.*, 2023). In the UK, despite children's rights being incorporated into the UNCRC and other policy documents and legislation, such as the *Human Rights Act 1998*, *Equality Act 2010*, and *Data Protection Act 2018*, disparities remain in how they are applied. The harsh reality is that, in terms of health and well-being, children born in the UK are often worse off than those born in other comparably wealthy countries. This is especially true if the child is experiencing socio-economic hardships (Royal College of Paediatrics and Child Health 2020).

Children's Rights can be divided into three broad groups.

- **Participation rights:** These relate to children's rights to participate in and be involved in things, including decisions that affect them.
- **Protection** rights concern keeping children safe and ensuring their well-being.
- **Provision rights:** These rights are associated with ensuring children have the necessary things.

Participation rights

Participation rights are fundamental to recognising children and young people as active agents in their own lives. This means children are not just passive recipients of adult decisions but individuals capable of forming opinions, making choices, and taking actions that impact their surroundings. At the core of participation rights is the principle that children should have the opportunity to express their views on matters affecting them and should be taken seriously according to their age and maturity. This principle is enshrined in *Article 12* of the UNCRC, which mandates that children's perspectives must be considered in decision-making processes (McCafferty and Mercado Garcia, 2024). Research highlights that enabling children to participate in decisions about their education, healthcare, and community involvement supports their sense of autonomy and self-worth (Lansdown, 2019). This principle involves listening to children and creating environments where their voices can influence decisions.

Participation rights extend to various parts of children and young people's lives. Children should be encouraged to take part in community activities, cultural events, and political processes where appropriate. This involvement helps them develop resilience, a sense of belonging, and responsibility towards their community and society (Davidov *et al.*, 2015). These rights include expressing views freely, being heard in judicial and administrative proceedings, and accessing information relevant to their well-being (Lundy *et al.*, 2020). Implementing these rights can enable children and young people to engage meaningfully in family, cultural, social, and political life, contributing to their development as informed and engaged citizens.

Children and young people should be given platforms to voice their opinions on curriculum development, school policies, and classroom management in educational settings. A study by Lundy *et al.* (2024) emphasises that when children are given opportunities to contribute to their learning environments, they demonstrate increased motivation and academic engagement. Similarly, in healthcare, children have the right to be informed about their medical conditions and treatment options, allowing them to participate in decisions concerning their health (Coyne *et al.*, 2016). Providing age-appropriate information ensures that children are not excluded from crucial discussions about their well-being.

Participation in family life is also essential. Research suggests that when children are involved in family decision-making, such as choices about their living arrangements or education, they develop a stronger sense of responsibility and self-efficacy (Fattore *et al.*, 2017). This involvement prepares them for active citizenship in adulthood, reinforcing democratic values and critical thinking skills from an early age.

A crucial component of participation rights is access to information, which enables children to make informed decisions about various aspects of their lives. *Article 13* of the UNCRC affirms that children have the right to seek, receive, and share information, supporting their ability to engage meaningfully in society (UNICEF, 2023). The availability of child-friendly and accessible information is essential in ensuring that children can exercise this right effectively. For instance, in healthcare settings, providing children with clear and understandable explanations of medical conditions can empower them to take an active role in their treatment and care (Coyne *et al.*, 2016). Similarly, in education, access to information about school governance and policies allows students to advocate for improvements in their learning environments (Lundy *et al.*, 2024). Participation rights go beyond individual decision-making to collective social, cultural, and political engagement. Encouraging children and young people to participate in community initiatives, youth groups, and cultural activities can foster a sense of belonging and civic responsibility (Davidov *et al.*, 2015). Research indicates that when children and young people are given platforms to contribute to their communities, they develop resilience and a proactive attitude towards social change (Percy-Smith and Thomas, 2023).

Protection rights

Protection rights are designed to safeguard children from all forms of harm, abuse, neglect, and exploitation. These rights include protection from physical and mental violence, protection from sexual exploitation and abuse, and protection from child labour. Additionally, protection rights ensure that children are not subjected to torture or other cruel, inhuman, or degrading treatment or punishment. These rights are fundamental to ensuring that children grow up in a safe and nurturing environment, free from fear and harm.

They also encompass the right to special protection and assistance for children who are in vulnerable situations, such as those affected by armed conflict, refugees, or those with disabilities. Children and young people have the right to be protected from harm due to their inherent vulnerability and developmental needs, which are recognised under international and national frameworks, such as the UNCRC, the *Children Act 2004*, and the *Children and Social Work Act 2017*. These frameworks mandate that children must be safeguarded from abuse, neglect, and exploitation, acknowledging that their physical and psychological immaturity makes them more susceptible to harm compared to adults (Wilkinson and Bowyer, 2017). For instance, research indicates that exposure to violence and neglect during childhood can lead to long-term detrimental effects on mental health, academic performance, and social relationships (Equality and Human Rights Commission, 2022) (see Chapter 12). Additionally, children are more likely to be victims of online exploitation and bullying, which can severely impact their well-being and development (Chambers *et al.*, 2021).

Provision rights

Provision rights focus on ensuring children have access to the necessary resources and services for their development and well-being. The UNCRC states that every child has the right to a standard of living adequate for their physical, mental, spiritual, moral, and social development (UNICEF, n.d.). Ensuring the fulfilment of provision rights is fundamental in promoting equity and reducing disparities among children from different socio-economic backgrounds. One of the core aspects of provision rights is the right to adequate food, clothing, and housing. *Article 27* of the UNCRC states that governments must provide material assistance and support programmes to help families secure these necessities (Convention on the Rights of the Child, 1989). Access to nutritious food is essential for children and young people's physical and cognitive development, with malnutrition linked to long-term health issues, including stunted growth and learning difficulties (World Health Organization, 2024). Similarly, safe and secure housing is vital for children's well-being, as unstable living conditions can negatively impact their mental health and educational attainment (Sharma, 2020). In the UK, the *Education Act 1996* establishes the duty of local authorities to ensure that children receive an appropriate education, whether in school or otherwise. However, socio-economic factors continue to create disparities in educational access and outcomes, with children from disadvantaged backgrounds more likely to experience barriers such as inadequate resources and digital exclusion (Children's Commissioner for England, 2019).

In the UK, the National Health Service (NHS) provides free healthcare to children, ensuring access to medical treatment regardless of financial status. However, disparities exist in health outcomes, particularly in relation to mental health services, which have seen increased demand with limited availability of timely support (NHS Digital, 2023). The importance of early intervention in children's mental health has been widely recognised, with research highlighting that access to appropriate support can significantly improve long-term well-being (Department of Health and Social Care, 2024). Provision rights also include social welfare support, which plays a vital role in assisting children and families, particularly those experiencing poverty. Financial assistance schemes, such as Universal Credit, provide crucial support for low-income families, helping to meet basic needs (Department for Work and Pensions, 2022). Childcare services and early years education programmes, such as the UK's free early education entitlement, contribute to children's cognitive and social development while supporting parents' ability to work (Education Policy Institute, 2016).

Another fundamental aspect of provision rights is the right to play and recreational activities, as recognised in *Article 31* of the UNCRC. Play is essential for children's cognitive, social, and emotional development, contributing to creativity, problem-solving skills, and overall well-being (Gleave and Cole-Hamilton, 2012). In the UK, organisations, such as Play England advocate for safe and accessible play spaces, highlighting the importance of outdoor play in promoting physical health and social interaction (Play England, 2025). However, children in low-income communities often face barriers to accessing quality play facilities, which make inequalities in developmental opportunities worse.

The importance of a child rights approach in health and social care

A child-rights-based approach means respecting the children or young person's views, opinions, strengths and potential. It emphasises the importance of involving children in situations as experts on their own lives in decision-making and implementation. They have a right to be consulted listened to and to have their views and feelings validated hear their views. This means as people working within health and social care settings, we can ensure that our practice takes a rights-based approach. A child's rights approach may be adopted by individuals, such as healthcare professionals, teachers, and youth workers, or by services and organisations, such as schools, healthcare settings, and local authority services. A rights-based, child-centred approach recognises the individuality of each child, meaning that no child is the same, and no childhood experience is the same. Therefore, we should not treat all children the same. Each child has their own story and experiences, so there is no one-size-fits-all solution. Children are the experts in their own lives. It's essential to enable their participation, build their self-esteem, and provide opportunities to build self-efficacy. This will better prepare young people for a rights-based society.

A child rights approach is based on four key principles of:

- participation and inclusion
- non-discrimination
- equality and equity
- empowerment

Participation and inclusion

All children and young people have the right to express their opinions in matters that concern them, and to have their views respected and included. To be active members of their family, community, and society as a whole, children and young people require support and chances to participate. They need access to information that is accessible to them, a platform to share their thoughts and emotions, and opportunities to ask questions. Children's participation can be explained further using Hart's (1992) ladder of participation, as shown in Figure 13.1. Hart's ladder of participation outlines eight levels of children's involvement in decision-making processes. This starts at the bottom with manipulation, in which adults make decisions with little regard for the child or young person, to child-initiated with shared decisions from adults, in which the child or young person makes decisions that affect their lives and is supported by the adult.

The examples in Figure 13.1 illustrate how children's participation can range from minimal involvement to full health and social care services partnership. Participation in decision-making processes can significantly enhance children's self-esteem, health, and overall well-being. When children are given opportunities to express their views and have them respected, they develop a sense of agency and self-worth. Meaningful participation helps children see themselves as valuable contributors to their communities, which boosts their self-esteem (McCafferty and Mercado Garcia, 2025). Positive self-esteem is closely linked to children's well-being, confidence, and social competence. The health benefits of participation are also well-documented, such as engaging children in decisions about their healthcare, which can lead to better health outcomes (Keshky and Samak, 2017). When children and young people feel heard and involved, they are more likely to adhere to medical advice and engage in healthy behaviours. This is supported by research indicating that participatory approaches in healthcare settings can improve children's mental and physical health (McCafferty and Mercado Garcia, 2024). Participation is crucial for the overall well-being of children and young people as it fosters a sense of belonging and inclusion, which are essential components of well-being. Percy-Smith's (2023) *A Handbook of Children's Participation* highlights that involving children in community and school activities can lead to improved social skills, reduced feelings of isolation, and greater life satisfaction (Percy-Smith, 2023).

Non-discrimination

Non-discrimination is crucial in health and social care settings for children and young people as it ensures equal access to services, promoting an inclusive environment where every child and young person feels valued. This principle is outlined in *Article 2* of the UNCRC and protected by the *Equality Act 2010*. It aims to help mitigate the negative impacts of discrimination, such as limited access to essential services and chronic stress, which can lead to long-term health issues (United Nations Children's Fund, 2022). By promoting a non-discriminatory environment, health and social care providers can support children's psychological and emotional development, helping them develop a positive self-image and resilience. Providers have a legal and ethical obligation to uphold non-discrimination, as mandated by the *Human Rights Act 1998*. Embedding these practices leads to better health outcomes and a more supportive environment for all children and young people (Priest *et al.*, 2021).

Child-Initiated, Shared Decisions with Adults	Children initiate projects and invite adults to join in decision-making. Example: Young people create a peer support group for chronic illness and collaborate with healthcare professionals to provide accurate information and resources.
Child-Initiated and Directed	Children initiate and direct their own projects. Example: A group of teenagers start a mental health awareness campaign in their school, organising events and resources independently.
Adult-Initiated, Shared Decisions with Children	Adults initiate projects, but decision-making is shared with children. Example: A community health program is developed by adults, but children help decide the activities and outreach methods.
Consulted and Informed:	Adults design and run projects, but children are consulted and their opinions are considered. Example: A hospital surveys children about their experiences and uses the feedback to improve paediatric care services.
Assigned but Informed:	Children are assigned specific roles and understand the purpose of their involvement. Example: Children are asked to distribute health pamphlets and are informed about the pamphlet's content and importance.
Tokenism	Children appear to be given a voice, but in reality, have little or no choice about how they participate. Example: A health service invites a few children to a meeting to discuss new services, but their input is not genuinely considered in the final decisions.
Decoration	Children take part in activities but have no real influence. Example: Children are invited to a health fair to perform a dance, but they have no input on the event's planning or content.
Manipulation	Children are used to support projects without understanding the issues. Example: A health campaign uses children in promotional materials without explaining the campaign's purpose to them.

Figure 13.1 Hart's ladder of participation applied to children and young people.

Equality and equity

Equality and equity are essential in health and social care settings for children and young people, ensuring that all individuals receive the care and support they need regardless of their background or circumstances. Equality involves providing everyone with the same level of care and access to services, promoting fairness and justice. However, equity recognises that different individuals have different needs and adapts services accordingly to achieve the same health outcomes. This is particularly important for children and young people, who are vulnerable to health inequalities due to their developmental stages and dependence on adults. Ensuring equality and equity helps address their unique developmental needs, provides access to necessary services, reduces health disparities, and promotes social inclusion. By implementing these principles, health and social care services can support the healthy development of children and young people, leading to better health outcomes and a more inclusive society (Institute of Health Equity, 2024)

Empowerment

Empowerment is about providing opportunities for individuals to participate in community decision-making, which can enhance their lives and the welfare of their communities. Where empowerment occurs, decision-makers recognise children and young people as valuable contributors, actively seeking their input on community issues. This inclusive approach encourages widespread participation and helps shape civic agendas that genuinely reflect the concerns and voices of younger generations.

In the context of health and social care, empowerment involves enabling children and young people to have greater control over decisions affecting their lives. This participatory approach ensures their voices are heard and valued, leading to more inclusive and effective care planning and delivery. Empowered children and young people are more likely to engage actively in their care, resulting in better health outcomes and overall well-being (Abraczinskas and Zarrett, 2020) Research has shown that empowerment is a critical factor in resilience among children and young people, especially those with emotional and behavioural difficulties. Empowerment helps young people achieve successful outcomes across academic, social, and behavioural areas of their lives, particularly during major transitions (Huscroft-D'Angelo *et al.*, 2017).

Applying the UNCRC to health and social care practice

The UNCRC can be used in practice in various ways when working with children and young people to improve their lives.

Access to health and social care

Article 24 of the UNCRC states that children and young people have the right to the highest attainable standard of health, including access to healthcare services without discrimination. This means that young people have the right to get information about their health in private, without a parent or guardian's knowledge. While as a child it might have been in their best interests for a parent or guardian to make decisions about their health, young people should be able to choose which services they need. Children under the age of 16 can consent to their own treatment if they are believed to have enough intelligence, competence and understanding to appreciate what's involved in their treatment fully. There are frameworks in place to make sure young people do have the capacity to understand the decisions that they are making. Two primary examples used frequently by professionals are the **Fraser guidelines and Gillick competence** (Learning Box 13.1). Both Fraser guidelines and Gillick competence originated from a legal case from the 1980s, which looked at whether doctors should be able to give contraceptive advice or treatment to young people under 16 years old without parental consent.

Adults in power may overlook children's rights due to a lack of perspective or understanding of their specific needs. Children, who are naturally more vulnerable and reliant on adults, have the right to protection from harm, which sometimes is not fully realised.

To uphold these rights in health and social care, policies should explicitly prioritise children's rights, ensuring equal access to services and creating child-friendly environments. Services must be tailored to the unique needs of children and young people providing age-appropriate care and involving them in decision-making processes. Furthermore, professionals working with children should receive training on child rights principles to effectively advocate for and uphold these rights. Regular monitoring and evaluation of

Learning Box 13.1: Fraser Guidelines and Gillick Competence

Fraser Guidelines and Gillick Competence are critical concepts in medical law, particularly when dealing with the consent of minors under 16 years old.

Fraser Guidelines

The Fraser Guidelines were established following a legal case in the 1980s and are specifically used to assess whether a child under 16 can receive contraceptive advice and treatment without parental consent. The guidelines include the following criteria

1 The child understands the advice provided.
2 The child cannot be persuaded to inform their parents.
3 The child is likely to continue having sexual intercourse with or without contraceptive treatment.
4 The child's physical or mental health may suffer without the treatment.
5 The treatment is in the child's best interest.

Gillick Competence

Gillick Competence, also stemming from the same legal case, is a broader concept used to determine whether a child under 16 has the maturity to make their own medical decisions. A child is considered Gillick competent if they have sufficient understanding and intelligence to fully comprehend the proposed medical treatment and its implications.

These guidelines and competence assessments are essential for healthcare professionals to balance respecting a child's autonomy with ensuring their safety and well-being (Griffith, 2016; NSPCC, 2024).

practices is essential for ensuring compliance with child rights, alongside independent advocacy for those struggling to be involved in their healthcare. Creating welcoming and age-appropriate healthcare environments, complete with supportive staff and resources, is vital for empowering young patients and alleviating anxiety.

Accountability

Accountability in this context means that individuals and institutions responsible for protecting children's rights are answerable for their actions. This involves various forms of accountability, including legal, political, administrative, and social accountability (Gibbons and Bell, 2015). Legal accountability ensures that there are laws and regulations in place to protect children's rights and that these laws are enforced.

Political accountability involves holding elected officials responsible for their commitments to children's rights. Administrative accountability refers to the internal mechanisms within organisations that ensure policies and procedures are followed. Social accountability, however, involves the active participation of children, young people, and the community in monitoring and evaluating the performance of those responsible for protecting children's rights (Gibbons, 2015).

Transparency

Transparency is closely linked to accountability. It involves making information about policies, procedures, and outcomes readily available and accessible to the public and accessible to children and young people. Transparency helps to build trust and ensures that actions taken by those in power can be scrutinised. In the context of children's rights, transparency means that children, young people, and their advocates have access to information about their rights and the mechanisms in place to protect those rights (Alshammari *et al.*, 2025). This access to information can enable children and young people to hold those in power accountable.

For example, transparency in health and social care can be achieved by publishing reports on service performance, making information about complaints procedures readily available, and ensuring that children and young people are informed about their rights and how to exercise them. When children and young people know their rights and the mechanisms available to protect them, they are better equipped to hold service providers accountable (Alshammari *et al.*, 2025).

Children's commissioner

In the United Kingdom, each of the four nations of England, Scotland, Wales, and Northern Ireland employ a Children's Commissioner to advocate for children's rights and ensure their voices are heard in matters affecting them (Children's Commissioner for England, 2025). These Commissioners play a crucial role in promoting and protecting children's rights as outlined in the UNCRC. They work to ensure that children's rights are respected and upheld in all areas of society, including education, health, and social services.

One of the key responsibilities of Children's Commissioners is to ensure that children's perspectives are considered in policymaking and legislative processes. They conduct consultations with children and young people to gather their views and represent these views to government bodies and other organisations. Additionally, Children's Commissioners play an important role in raising awareness about children's rights among the public, professionals, and policymakers. They provide information and resources to help people understand and respect children's rights, and they work to educate children about their own rights. Commissioners monitor the implementation of children's rights and report on the progress and challenges in this area. They publish annual reports and other documents to highlight issues affecting children and to recommend actions for improvement. In some cases, Children's Commissioners have the authority to conduct independent investigations into issues affecting children, such as cases of abuse or neglect, and make recommendations for changes to policies and practices to protect children and young people better.

Summary

This chapter has provided a brief overview of the rights of children and young people within health and social care settings. Key points covered include the definition and importance of children's rights, the legal frameworks that protect these rights, and the practical application of these principles in everyday practice. The chapter has emphasised the significance of the UNCRC as a foundational document that guides the global protection and promotion of children's rights. Reflecting on the significance of the UNCRC, it is clear that understanding and implementing its principles is crucial for health and social care students and professionals. The UNCRC sets the standard for children's rights and provides a framework for ensuring that these rights are respected and upheld in all aspects of care.

A call to action for promoting and protecting children's rights in health and social care practice is essential. Professionals must actively advocate for children's and young people's rights, ensuring their voices are heard and their needs are met. This involves creating children and young people friendly environments, providing age-appropriate care, and involving children and young people in decision-making processes. Incorporating child rights principles into health and social care policies and practices is essential for promoting children's well-being, development, and protection. By prioritising children's rights in policy formulation, service provision, training, and monitoring, stakeholders can create environments that uphold the principles of dignity, equality, and respect for every child. This approach contributes to a healthier and more inclusive society, where every child has the opportunity to thrive.

References

Abraczinskas, M. and Zarrett, N. (2020) 'Youth participatory action research for health equity: Increasing youth empowerment and decreasing physical activity access inequities in under-resourced programs and schools', *American Journal of Community Psycho*, 66(3–4), pp. 232–243.

Alshammari, S.M. *et al.* (2025) 'Healthcare professionals' understanding of children's rights: A systematic review of the empirical evidence-base', *Systematic Reviews*, 14(1), pp. 9–17.

Castaños-Cervantes, S. and Atristain-Suárez, C. (2024) *Assertiveness in the Context of Human Rights, Ethics, and Classical Virtues*. Cham: *Springer*.

Chambers, D., Cantrell, A. and Booth, A. (2021) 'Recognition of risk and prevention in safeguarding of children and young people: a mapping review and component analysis of service development interventions aimed at health and social care professionals, *BMC Health Services Research*, 21(1), pp. 1–11.

Children Act 2004, c. 31. Available at https://www.legislation.gov.uk/ukpga/2004/31/contents (Accessed 11 March 2025).

Children and Social Work Act 2017, c. 16. Available at https://www.legislation.gov.uk/ukpga/2017/16/contents (Accessed 11 March 2025).
Children's Commissioner for England (2019) *Childhood vulnerability in England 2019*. Available at https://www.childrenscommissioner.gov.uk/resource/childhood-vulnerability-in-england-2019/#:~:text=We%20estimate%20that%202.3%20million,therefore%20not%20getting%20any%20support (Accessed 11 March 2025).
Children's Commissioner for England (2025) *Our priorities*. Available at https://www.childrens-commissioner.gov.uk/our-priorities/ (Accessed 11 March 2025).
Convention on the Rights of the Child (1989) Treaty no. 27531. United Nations Treaty Series, 1577, pp. 3-178. Available at: https://treaties.un.org/doc/Treaties/1990/09/19900902%2003-14%20AM/Ch_IV_11p.pdf (Accessed: 21 September 2025).
Coyne, I., Hallström, I. and Söderbäck, M. (2016) 'Reframing the focus from a family-centred to a child-centred care approach for children's healthcare', *Journal of Child Health Care*, 22(1), pp. 36–46. Available at https://doi.org/10.1177/1367493518795341 (Accessed 11 March 2025).
Davidov, M. *et al.* (2015) 'The influential child: How children affect their environment and influence their own risk and resilience', *Development and Psychopathology*, 27(4 Pt 1), pp. 947–951.
Department for Work and Pensions (2022) *The Universal Credit (Local Welfare Provision Disregard) (Amendment) Regulations 2022: Explanatory Memorandum. London: Department for Work and Pensions*. Available at: https://www.legislation.gov.uk/uksi/2022/448/pdfs/uksiem_20220448_en.pdf (Accessed: 21 September 2025).
Department for Work and Pensions (2025) *Universal credit statistics*. Available at https:// www.gov.uk/government/collections/universal-credit-statistics (Accessed 11 March 2025).
Department of Health and Social Care (2024) *Improving the mental health of babies, children and young people: A framework of modifiable factors*. Available at https://www.gov.uk/government/publications/improving-the-mental-health-of-babies-children-and-young-people/improving-the-mental-health-of-babies-children-and-young-people-a-framework-of-modifiable-factors (Accessed 11 March 2025).
Education Policy Institute (2016) *Widening the gap? The impact of the 30-hour entitlement on early years education and childcare*. Available at https://epi.org.uk/publications-and-research/widening-gap-impact-30-hour-entitlement-early-years-education-childcare/ (Accessed 11 March 2025).
Equality Act 2010, c. 15. Available at https://www.legislation.gov.uk/ukpga/2010/15/contents (Accessed 11 March 2025).
Equality and Human Rights Commission (2022) *Children's rights in Great Britain*. Available at https://www.equalityhumanrights.com/sites/default/files/11706_ehrc_executive_summary_report_english_accessi_1.2.pdf (Accessed 10 March 2025).
Fairhall, N. and Woods, K. (2021) 'Children's views on children's rights: A systematic literature review', *The International Journal of Children's Rights*, 29(4), pp. 835–871.
Fattore, T., Mason, J. and Watson, E. (2017) *Children's Understanding of Well-Being: Towards a Child Standpoint*. Dordrecht: Springer.
Flasher, J. (1978) 'Adultism', *Adolescence*, 13(51), pp. 517–523.
Gibbons, E.D. and Bell, W. (2015) Accountability for children's rights: With special attention to social accountability and it's potential to achieve results and equity for children. UNICEF Working Paper, Human Rights Unit, Programme Division. Available at: https://content.sph.harvard.edu/wwwhsph/sites/2464/2017/12/Accountability-for-Childrens-Rights-UNICEF.pdf (Accessed: 21 September 2025).
Gleave, J. and Cole-Hamilton, I. (2012) *A World without Play: A Literature Review*. London: Play England.
Global Initiative to End All Corporal Punishment of Children (2020) *Corporal punishment of children in Sweden*. Available at https://www.endcorporalpunishment.org/wp-content/uploads/country-reports/Sweden.pdf (Accessed 11 March 2025).
Griffin, J. (2000) 'Welfare Rights', *The journal of ethics*, 4(1/2), pp. 27–43.
Griffith, R. (2016) 'What is Gillick competence?', *Human Vaccines and Immunotherapeutics*, 12(1), pp. 244–247. https://doi.org/10.1080/21645515.2015.1091548
Hart, R.A. (1992) *Children's participation. From tokenism to citizenship*. Available at https://www.unicef-irc.org/publications/pdf/childrens_participation.pdf (Accessed 1 May 2024).
Human Rights Act 1998, c. 42. Available at: https://www.legislation.gov.uk/ukpga/1998/42/contents (Accessed: 27 February 2025).

Huscroft-D'Angelo, J., Trout, A.L., Lambert, M.C. and Thompson, R. (2017) 'Reliability and validity of the youth empowerment scale–mental health in youth departing residential care and reintegrating into school and community settings', *Journal of Emotion*, 40(4), pp. 547–570.

Institute of Health Equity (2024) *Children and young people health equity collaborative.* [online] Available at https://www.instituteofhealthequity.org/resources-reports/children-and-young-people-health-equity-collaborative (Accessed 11 March 2025).

Keshky, M.S. and Samak, Y.A. (2017) 'The development of self esteem in children: Systematic review and meta-analysis', *International Journal of Psychology and Behavior Analysis.* https://doi.org/10.15344/2455-3867/2017/128

Lansdown, G. (2019) *A toolkit for monitoring and evaluating children's participation.* Save the Children UK. Available at https://resourcecentre.savethechildren.net/pdf/me_toolkit_booklet_5.pdf (Accessed 11 March 2025).

LeFrançois, B.A. (2013) 'Queering child and adolescent mental health services', *Children and Society*, 27(1), pp. 1–12.

Lundy, L., Murray, C., Smith, K. and Ward, C. (2024) 'Young children's right to be heard on the quality of their education: Addressing potential misunderstandings in the context of early childhood education', *British Educational Research Journal* [Preprint]. https://pure.qub.ac.uk/en/publications/young-childrens-right-to-be-heard-on-the-quality-of-their-educati

Lundy, L., Kilkelly, U., Forde, L. and Kelleher, D. (2020) *The Right of Children to Participate in Public Decision-Making Processes.* London: Save the Children. Available at https://resourcecentre.savethechildren.net/library/right-children-participate-public-decision-making-processes

McCafferty, P. and Mercado Garcia, E. (2024) 'Children's participation in child welfare: A systematic review of systematic reviews', *The British Journal of Social Work*, 54(3), pp. 1092–1108.

McCafferty, P. and Mercado García, E. (2025) 'Children's participation in social work research', *The British Journal of Social Work.* https://doi.org/10.1093/bjsw/bcaf017.

NHS Digital (2023) *Mental health of children and young people in England: 2023 Wave 4 Follow Up.* Available at https://digital.nhs.uk/data-and-information/publications/statistical/mental-health-of-children-and-young-people-in-england/2023-wave-4-follow-up (Accessed 11 March 2025).

NSPCC (2024) *Children and the law.* [online] Available at https://learning.nspcc.org.uk/child-protection-system/children-the-law (Accessed 11 March 2025).

OHCHR (2025) *'Children and Health'*, OHCHR. Available at https://www.ohchr.org/en/children/children-and-health (Accessed 24 February 2025).

Percy-Smith, B., Thomas, N.P., O'Kane, C. & Twum-Danso Imoh A. (eds.) (2023). *A Handbook of Children and Young People's Participation: Conversations for Transformational Change.* 2nd ed. London: Routledge. https://doi.org/10.4324/9781003367758

Percy-Smith, B. and Thomas, N. (2023) *A Handbook of Children and Young People's Participation: Perspectives from Theory and Practice.* 2nd edn. London: Routledge.

Play England (2025) *The importance of play.* Available at https://www.playengland.org.uk (Accessed 11 March 2025).

Priest, N., Guo, J., Doery, K., Perry, R., Thurber, K., Jones, R., Gibaju, L. and Skelton, F. (2021) 'Racism, racial discrimination and child and youth health: A rapid evidence synthesis'. Victorian Health Promotion Foundation, Melbourne.

Quennerstedt, A. (2022) 'UNICEF'S *rights respecting schools award* as children's human rights education', *Human Rights Education Review*, 5(3), pp. 1–23. https://doi-org.apollo.worc.ac.uk/10.7577/hrer.4761

Royal College of Paediatrics and Child Health (2020) *State of Child Health 2020: England.* [online] Available at https://stateofchildhealth.rcpch.ac.uk/wp-content/uploads/sites/2/2020/03/SOCH-ENGLAND-02.03.20.pdf (Accessed 11 March 2025).

Sharma, R. (2020) *Briefing: The Impact of Homelessness and Bad Housing on Children's Education.* Shelter: Available at https://england.shelter.org.uk/professional_resources/policy_and_research/policy_library/briefing_the_impact_of_homelessness_and_bad_housing_on_childrens_education (Accessed 11 March 2025).

Stoecklin, D., Rizzini, I., Mizen, P., Johnson, V. and Cardozo Sarli, A. (2023) 'Children in street situations and their rights', in *The Palgrave Handbook of Global Social Problems*. Cham: Palgrave Macmillan. https://doi-org.apollo.worc.ac.uk/10.1007/978-3-030-68127-2_27-1

UNICEF (2023) *Convention on the rights of the child: Text*. Available at https://www.unicef.org/child-rights-convention/convention-text (Accessed 11 March 2025).

UNICEF (2025) *Education*. [online] Available at https://www.unicef.org/kenya/education (Accessed 11 March 2025).

UNICEF UK (n.d.) *The right to participation for rights respecting schools*. Available at https://www.unicef.org.uk/rights-respecting-schools/the-right-to-participation/ (Accessed 10 March 2025).

Viterbo, H. and Ioffe, Y. (2024) 'No refuge from childhood: How child protection harms refugees', *European Journal of International Law*, 35(3), pp. 647–677.

Watts, R.J. and Flanagan, C. (2007) 'Pushing the envelope on youth civic engagement: A developmental and liberation psychology perspective', *Journal of Community Psychology*, 35(6), pp. 779–792.

Wilkinson, J. and Bowyer, S. (2017) *The Impacts of Abuse and Neglect on Children; and Comparison of Different Placement Options: Evidence Review*. Dartington: Research in Practice. Available at https://www.researchinpractice.org.uk/children/publications/2017/march/the-impacts-of-abuse-and-neglect-on-children-and-comparison-of-different-placement-options-evidence-review-open-access/ (Accessed 11 March 2025).

World Bank (2016) *Bangladesh health, nutrition, and population: Improving capacity to meet growing needs*. [online] Available at https://www.worldbank.org/en/results/2016/10/07/bangladesh-health-nutrition-population-improving-capacity-meet-growing-needs

World Health Organization (2024) *World health statistics 2024: Monitoring health for the SDGs, Sustainable Development Goals. Geneva: World Health Organization*. Available at: https://iris.who.int/bitstream/handle/10665/376869/9789240094703-eng.pdf (Accessed: 21 September 2025).

14 Disability

Perspectives, experiences and implications for health and social care practice

Daniel Howarth

The aims of this chapter are to:

- **Explore different perspectives on disability**
- **Explain and analyse experiences of disability using Thompson's Personal, Cultural and Structural (PCS) analysis model**
- **Identify implications for health and social care practice from using the PCS analysis model**

Introduction

This chapter focuses on disability, which is a very wide-ranging and complex topic. It is not a clinical or medical chapter, nor is it based on what it is like to live with a disability as I do not have that experience. There are several brilliant books, documentaries and other sources that can give windows into this perspective (see, for example, Sealey *et al.*, 2022). This chapter is focused on you as a current or future health and social care professional who works alongside service users with a disability. It aims to help you consider academic and cultural ideas around disability and explore, or begin to explore, your own ideas, values and beliefs around disability. The chapter explores some factors and possible examples of discriminatory ideas that likely cause oppression for people with a disability, which as a care professional you should try to be aware of as we hopefully work towards anti-oppressive practice (Karim, 2023) (see Chapter 15). To facilitate this, the chapter is largely structured around the theoretical model of Thompson's PCS analysis which looks at aspects of discrimination across Personal, Cultural and Structural levels (Thompson, 2021: 28). This is important as exploring and understanding these can be central to helping you provide the best care (Cuthbert and Quallington, 2017).

Ultimately, this chapter is not about the PCS model itself but it is about you and your health and social care practice. However, the PCS model should be a framework or a 'lens' (see Chapter 8) for you to take into your practice, so that you are aware of aspects across all of the three levels that affect your service users, such as your own thoughts and beliefs, their thoughts and beliefs, as well as legislation and societal attitudes. It is worth noting here that the title of the Thompson book where he outlines the PCS model is 'Anti-Discriminatory Practice', and this is really the clue to the purpose of Thompson's PCS model (Thompson, 2021).

The chapter is based on teaching I do in various ethics and values modules across the courses I support, and it takes this approach to the topic. I have studied various disability and learning disability courses at university and worked in social care for several years, especially working with children and young people with learning disabilities.

DOI: 10.4324/9781032619309-16

In this chapter, there are points that might be new or different or uncomfortable, so do be aware of yourself and practice self-care, and also be aware that this chapter asks more questions than it answers.

Definition of terms

To start the chapter, write a short definition of about a sentence for these terms:

- Disability
- Learning/Intellectual Disability
- Physical Disability
- Hidden/Non-Visible Disability
- Learning Difficulty

Now some of these, if not all of them, may have felt quite simple to define for most people; however, the more these are looked at and considered, the more potential complexity and nuance may emerge. We explore some of these terms later in the chapter, so hold on to your definitions.

Thompsons PCS analysis model

The main theory that supports this chapter is the PCS analysis model developed by Neil Thompson. The PCS model is a way of considering the different factors and levels around discrimination and inequality that can cause oppression. It contains three levels, **Personal/Psychological**, **Cultural** and **Structural**, hence PCS, represented as circles within circles. There are many slightly different diagrams of this model and Thompson outlines that the three levels are 'closely interlinked and constantly interact with one another' (Thompson, 2021: 35). Figure 14.1 shows a version of the model.

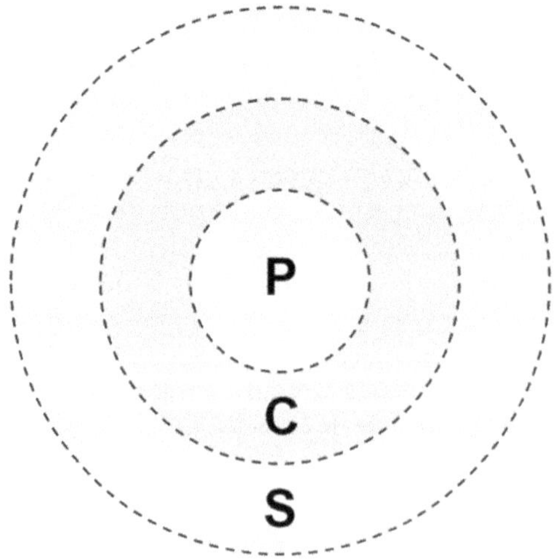

Figure 14.1 The PCS model.

Source: Adapted from Thompson (2021).

The three levels of the PCS model are explained below:

- P is the **Personal** or **Psychological** level. It is the individual level that reflects a persons, or your own, 'thoughts, feelings, attitudes and actions' (Thompson, 2021: 35). This includes how your personal biases and prejudices could lead to discriminatory practices in relation to disability. For example, someone may view people with physical disabilities differently from people with non-physical disabilities, and accordingly treat them differently.
- C is the **Cultural** level. It is the 'shared ways of seeing, thinking and doing ... about what is right and what is normal' (Thompson, 2021: 36), and how the shared beliefs that we have as a society about disability affect the outcomes for disabled groups and individuals. For example, until recently, there was a lot of stigma in society associated with having a disability, it is only recently that this stigma has decreased. This historic and current stigma has important negative implications for disabled people.
- S is the **Structural.** It is the 'wider level of social forces' in which oppression and discrimination is woven into society, 'the sociopolitical dimension' (Thompson, 2021: 36). This refers to how institutions, laws and policies shape and are shaped by the cultural beliefs that exists in society, which enables discrimination and oppression to occur. For example, the low number of disabled people working occurs from the cultural stigma that exists, and laws and policies can reinforce this discrimination in the workforce against people with a disability.

The difference between these three levels can be exemplified if we use the PCS model to consider how people experience disability.

Using the PCS model to explain and analyse experiences of disability

Using the PCS model, we can explain and analyse how disability is experienced and known by a disabled service user on a daily basis. This helps us to consider personal perspectives on disability, cultural perspectives on disability, and structural perspectives on disability.

Personal perspectives on disability

We started the chapter by asking you to define some terms connected to disability. Now you have these definitions, let us take it a step further with an initial exploration of yourself and your own personal experiences, awareness and understanding of disability. Below are a few questions about disability for you to consider:

- Do you have a disability?
- Do you have a family member or close friend with a disability?
- Do you work with people with a disability?
- What disabilities can you name?

In answering these questions, consider whether it was simple to say yes or no to each, or whether it was more complicated than that.

There are also more difficult and deeper questions to consider at this **Personal** level, for example:

- What do you think and feel when you hear the word disability?
- Someone is physically disabled and appears to be struggling, do you help?

- Are you cautious or wary around people with a learning disability?
- What opinions or news stories have you heard about people with mental health diagnoses?

It is likely that none of these questions has a simple yes or no answer, and it may also be the case that you are surprised or disappointed by some of your answers. There may also be a difference between the answer in your head and the answer you would tell someone else. If this is the case, this is an example of how critical personal reflection works and that if it is done honestly and genuinely, it can often feel difficult to fully explore, especially in areas where there may already be a level of discomfort for whatever reason. But this does not mean that you should avoid it, although equally be careful of yourself and seek support as and when necessary. For more on the importance of self-reflection to health and social care, see Chapter 17.

Ideas are constantly refined over time and this leads to changes in preferred terminology over time. This is why this chapter is not readily offering you definitions, as these are written at a fixed point in time and it may well be that even in a couple of years preferred terms and definitions change. A somewhat recent example of this for me was around the difference between the terms 'autistic person' and 'person with autism'.

In my previous professional settings and in my teaching, I would have expected and did indeed use the term 'person with autism' as I had received multiple trainings and guidance that made clear that this was the correct term to use. This was the **Culturally** correct way to express this because it literally puts the person first, so you prioritise the person not the diagnosis (Botha *et al.*, 2023; Vivanti, 2020).

Some of you may recognise this person-first language concept and this chapter still broadly follows this approach generally using phrases like people with a disability rather than disabled person. However, my perspective has changed following participation in the **Oliver McGowan training** (Learning Box 14.1). This training discusses 'identity-first language' and argues that autism is not something someone carries around with them or that can just be dropped, but that it is an integral part of them, so 'autistic person' is preferred.

Learning Box 14.1: Oliver McGowan Training and LeDeR

Oliver McGowan's 'avoidable death' in 2016 'shone a light' on the need for better training for healthcare staff on learning disability and autism. This is because people with a learning disability and autistic people often have poorer health and greater barriers to accessing care, which leads to a higher percentage of 'avoidable deaths' than the general population. After campaigning, a part of the *Health and Care Act 2022* introduced the requirement that Care Quality Council (CQC) regulated service providers must ensure their staff receive learning disability and autism training appropriate to their role. The Oliver McGowan Mandatory Training on Learning Disability and Autism is the standardised training that has been developed for this purpose and is the government's preferred and recommended training for health and social care staff (NHS England, 2024).

Since 2017, these issues around 'avoidable deaths' have been tracked by the 'Learning from lives and deaths – people with a learning disability and autistic people' or LeDeR service improvement programme to hopefully change services and improve health (King's College London, 2023; NHS England, no date).

How widespread across all of health and social care this approach will become is unclear. For example, within dementia it is still seen as best to have person-first language, so person with dementia, as well as other specific best practices for talking about dementia that are perhaps **Cultural** to this condition, like avoiding the term 'sufferer' (Alzheimer's Society, 2018). This is just one example of changing terms and definitions just within the world of autism. There are others such as the dropping of Asperger's syndrome as a specific diagnosis (National Autistic Society, 2023), the emergence of the term 'allistic' as a word for people without autism (Cambridge Dictionary, 2024) and even in some online areas the creation and attempt at usage of the term 'Neurospicy' as a more fun and positive spin on the term Neurodiversity.

So all definitions and terms are subject to change, but even the changes in terms is not always agreed upon (Keating *et al.*, 2022; Zajic and Gudknecht, 2024). **Personally** different people may prefer different terms or have different definitions and it is important to respect people as individuals (Bury *et al.*, 2023). You may have a **Personal** response and preference for these or other terms, but it is important to consider when you are a professional whether your preference matters, or whether you should just use whatever language your service users prefer. The advice from the Autistic Society is to use what you are asked to use (National Autistic Society, no date) but this can or may be difficult, especially if they prefer a term you struggle with. Language can be powerful and therefore create powerful feelings and responses, and if you are new to the term allistic and are allistic, or not on the autistic spectrum, it may feel strange to you **Personally** to have this new label attached to you. Or if you are neurodivergent, the term 'neurospicy' attached to you may also create feelings.

Cultural perspectives on disability

As stated in the Introduction, the levels of PCS are interconnected and from my personal experience, it sometimes feels that the **Cultural** level is the hardest to get to grips with. Thompson makes various points about how to recognise and understand culture in terms of the PCS analysis model, perhaps most clearly by linking it to what people consider normal 'values and patterns of thought and behaviour, an assumed consensus about what is right and what is normal' (Thompson, 2021: 35). 'Normal' itself as a specific word when used in relation to disability can be loaded with assumptions, creating complex feelings and responses itself (Shyman, 2016). You can, for example, see the changing cultural perceptions of what is ok or normal with the increasing number of warnings at the start of older TV shows and movies saying they contain language or jokes that may be now considered offensive.

Ultimately when talking about **Culture**, it is important to understand that each person has their own culture and each person's culture comes through their own unique experiences and surroundings. This is both in small more direct ways, for example, who your family is, all the way up to much wider elements like which country you grew up in. This has similarities to other theories like the Bronfenbrenner Systems model (Hayes *et al.*, 2023), which argues that you are shaped by who is around you and how you grew up.

Arguably, the two main **Cultural** lenses or academic frameworks in terms of considering disability are the *medical model of disability* and the *social model of disability* (Byrnes and Muller 2017: 2–3). Both of these are core ideas and concepts when working in health and social care in relation to disability and both are subject to much writing and debate and are open to challenge and/or development. The medical model and the social model are such significant mainstream theories that they, along with the Biopsychosocial model, are discussed in more detail in Chapter 9. We provide here a brief look at them before moving on to perhaps less widely used academic theories or cultural lenses of disability. When looking at the medical and social model here, consider Thompson's point about **Cultural** understandings and how they might link to an idea about what is 'normal'.

Medical model of disability

The medical model is the traditional model of disability that as the name suggests is largely based on and arguably perhaps still a foundation of medical or clinical approaches to disability. In simplified terms, this model sees that there is some sort of 'problem' or 'impairment' within the person that needs fixing. As a straightforward example, this means that a person is disabled by a broken leg and the break needs fixing so the person is no longer disabled. This seems fairly clear and straightforward, and these are some of the advantages of the medical model perspective. However, it perhaps gets more complicated when considering long-term or lifelong conditions, or when there is no 'cure' for the condition (Shyman, 2016). This quickly moves into more contentious areas that shift from fixing an impairment to fixing a person, and perhaps trying to fit people into a narrow definition of what is 'normal'. This approach runs quickly into other theories/cultural responses, particularly *Ableism* and the *Personal Tragedy Model*, both of which are outlined below.

Social model of disability

The social model came through from the development of the Disability Rights Movement or Disabled Peoples Movement. The core idea here is that it is the barriers in society that disable people not their conditions or impairments. So, if a person is in a wheelchair this is not what is disabling them, it is the fact that the building they need to access does not have a ramp, which means that they cannot access the building. The 'problem' is in society not in the person.

As with the medical model discussion, this is a fairly simple example to start with, but unpicking and exploring these ideas further links quickly to more complex and interesting examples and ideas. The social model was and still is very popular for organisations and charities that work with people with disabilities. Many of them make some reference to believing in and following the ideas of the social model, but that does not mean it is perfect and unchallengeable. Some key challenges are explored more in Chapter 9, but some aspects to consider are that it would be impossible to design a society that does not cause some disablement to some people, and that there is likely no person that has no impairment (Shakespeare, 2006, 2017). For example, needing reading glasses would not generally be seen as a disability, but is an aid that is required to overcome an impairment to allow the person to fully participate.

If the medical model and the social model are the two main theoretical/academic theories for general study and consideration of disability in its broadest sense, then perhaps in a similar way the two main lenses for considering the discrimination experienced by people with disabilities are ableism and disablism.

Ableism and disablism

These two terms have somewhat open definitions and can be a little confusing to understand and separate as there is some overlap in their meanings. They are also newer and much less mainstream than other '-isms' that define the similar ideas for other characteristics, for example, racism or sexism. Sense (2022) provide definitions of both as:

> In general, ableism can be used to describe the way society and people tend to favour non-disabled people. Disablism can be used to describe more direct, conscious acts of discrimination or abuse against disabled people.

Using Sense's definition here as a starter, let us begin to explore these as concepts. Ableism is the broad way that society is generally shaped towards a preference or assumption of 'normality' in a way that excludes people with a disability (Gappmayer, 2021). This links back to the previous section on the medical model and the idea of needing to 'cure' or 'fix' people with a disability. The key point is that even if you believe those ideas come from a genuine, kind and positive place, sometimes or even potentially the very basis of this idea is that a person with a disability is somehow less than someone without a disability.

Disablism has clear links to discrimination, which tends to occur when one group of people does not consider another group of people as equal, in this case disabled people. The discrimination may be conscious, i.e. actively carried out, such as where a person with a disability is not employed because of their disability, or unconscious, such as where a disabled person is given a limited role because of an assumption that their disability limits what they can do.

As you begin to work in health and social care, especially if you work with people with lifelong conditions or disabilities, try to remember these ideas and consider what language and experiences you are using and seeing in your workplace and what that might feel like for your service users.

'Personal Tragedy Model' and 'Inspiration Porn'

The Personal Tragedy Model has a base or links to the medical model, and is the term used for things that frame disabilities or being disabled as a tragedy, or portrays disability as an enemy, which frames disability as 'abnormal'. This is the viewpoint that says disability should be avoided at all costs as it robs enjoyment of life and makes people a burden on society (Swain and French, 2008). You can see this specifically from how disability is often described in the news, to how governments and politicians sometimes talk about disability. This viewpoint, the PCS model suggests, then trickles down to individuals, including those you are or will work with.

The term 'Inspiration porn' is perhaps less academic/mainstream than the other ideas and models identified. The term was originally coined by Stella Young (Kelly, 2023; Young, 2012) and it is when disabled people are viewed as objects for the benefit of a non-disabled viewer. It is perhaps most commonly seen online when an image is created of a visibly disabled person performing a physical activity accompanied by a caption to inspire the non-disabled viewer, such as someone with a prosthetic leg running or similar with text about excuses or attitude. The key question here is what purpose does that image serve and who is it designed for? Essentially this idea argues these images and other similar pieces of media objectify a disabled person for the benefit of a non-disabled audience with the purpose of making them think that at least their life is not as bad as a disabled person (Grue, 2016). As an exercise, go and watch Stella Young's TED talk from 2014 (Young, 2014) called *'I'm not your inspiration, thank you very much'* to get an understanding of this idea and how it relates to the other models in this chapter and ultimately hopefully back to yourself and your work in care.

Structural perspectives on disability

Finally, the **Structural** level is the largest/broadest level of the PCS model, as represented by the outside layer of the circle. This represents the 'sociopolitical dimension of interlocking patterns of power and influence' (Thompson, 2021: 36). In some ways, the easiest element of the **Structural** level to consider for a chapter like this is national or governmental legislation. These are usually rules that set out what is allowed or not allowed across a whole society either nationally, with things like the *Equality Act 2010* or the *Human Rights Act 1998* or even internationally such as the *United Nations Convention on the Rights of Persons with Disabilities*. This section focuses primarily on the *Equality Act 2010,* because it links most relevantly to the PCS analysis model and the overall theme of this chapter. You can read more about other relevant legislation in Chapter 6.

Equality Act 2010

The *Equality Act 2010* is the main disability legislation in the UK in terms of discrimination. In the previous sections, we see that the way that we personally and culturally define disability says a lot about our personal and cultural perspective on disability. It is also the case that the way that we define disability in legislation says a lot about how we structure disability as a society. There was early legislation such as the *Idiots Act 1886* and the *Mental Deficiency Act 1913*, which described disabled people as 'feeble-minded' and 'moral defectives'. More recent legislation has been the *Chronically Sick and Disabled Persons Act 1970*, the *Disabled Persons Act 1986*, the *Equality Act 2010* and the *Care Act 2014*. Just looking at the names of these Acts over time, it is interesting to consider how they reflect how our perspectives on disability have changed over time.

The *Equality Act 2010* defines disability as 'a physical or mental impairment and the impairment has a substantial and long-term adverse effect on his or her ability to carry out normal day-to-day activities' (Office for Disability Issues, 2011). What is perhaps most interesting to consider from this legislation and its guidance in terms of the **Structural** level of the PCS model is that there are specific conditions listed as being excluded from the definition of disability and certain conditions which are stated as specifically included within the definition of disability. For example, the Act states that a person who has cancer, HIV infection or multiple sclerosis (MS) is a disabled person (Office for Disability Issues, 2011). Research has shown that there is still within health and social care discrimination around disabilities, including about different conditions and the significant impact this can have on access to care and final outcomes, despite legislation like the *Equality Act 2010* (Ames *et al.*, 2024; Silva *et al.*, 2024).

However, the list of excluded conditions include 'tendency to set fires', 'tendency to steal', 'voyeurism', 'seasonal allergic rhinitis (e.g. hayfever)' and perhaps most interestingly 'addiction to, or dependency on, alcohol, nicotine, or any other substance (other than in consequence of the substance being medically prescribed)' (Office for Disability Issues, 2011). This is particularly interesting as it essentially has an exclusion within the exclusion, so if you are addicted to alcohol or drugs that is not a disability, but if you become addicted because it was prescribed to you, then it is considered a disability in terms of the *Equality Act 2010*. This leads to some interesting questions around what we as a society think and believe about disability and addiction. This is explored by Flacks (2012), who discusses what this means about how we think about those that receive or require legislative protection from discrimination. Looking at categories, including 'dependents' and 'deviants', and how the distinction between these labels is whether people have 'chosen' their condition. This raises a number of questions such as:

- Do people choose to become addicts?
- Should they be considered as disabled?
- Would your answer to these questions change if you had a disability or an addiction?

These also have implications for practice around ideas of choice or blame, such as if you are asked to care for someone who has become disabled through an addiction, for example, to alcohol or tobacco, and they continue to drink alcohol or smoke. Consider as well perhaps the likely experiences of those with multiple disabilities or rare diagnoses trying to access care services, seeking the support and input of professionals who have not heard of their condition. Or indeed, if as a professional your definition of disability or carer is not the same as your service users, as people may well have a disability but may not consider themselves disabled or want to be labelled that way. Consider what the consequences are if you label and treat that service user as 'disabled'.

The international symbol of access

Figure 14.2 shows the main single image used to represent disabilities. It is used almost exclusively internationally in any public place or setting, denoting where there is disabled parking or disabled toilets or for a range of other reasons and is perhaps as **Structural** as an image can be. Now we have identified what this image is take a moment to consider it, and what if anything you think about this image. You should also consider what you think it says about society's view of disabled people. Usually when I ask this question

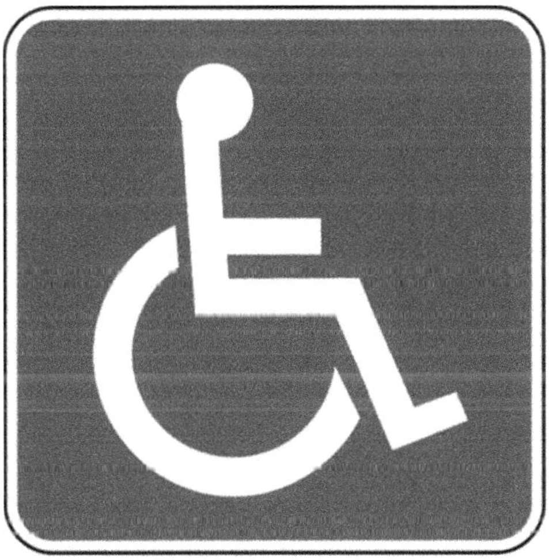

Figure 14.2 The international symbol of access.

Source: U.S. Department of Transportation (2003).

to a classroom of students, there is kind of a stilted silence as either they have not really understood what I am asking, or they just have no opinions on it – usually because they have not considered this before. If this is you, do not worry, this is normal!

The first and perhaps easiest point to understand here is that the image is of a person in a wheelchair. The most recent government figures, taken from the Family Resources Survey, put the total number of people with a disability in the UK in 2022/2023 at 16.1 million people, or about 24% of the total population (Department for Work and Pensions, 2024). Figures specifically for wheelchair use are harder to find and tend to give broad ranges, such as a 2022 report from Motability and The Wheelchair Alliance which estimated that in 2018/2019 there were between 688,000 and 860,000 wheelchair users (Motability and The Wheelchair Alliance, 2022). So we could estimate roughly using these figures that only 1 in 20 disabled people in the UK uses a wheelchair, which should lead us to reflect on why basically the only symbol used of a disabled person is that of a person in a wheelchair? A possible answer to this is that, across all levels of the PCS model, there is still a tendency to think of disability firstly, or only, as physical disability. Think back to your answers to those starter questions, perhaps when you initially think of disability it is of someone in a wheelchair. What might that mean for you when you come to work in health and social care with people perhaps with a hidden or invisible disability? This is perhaps why increasingly we are seeing the use of additional signs or stickers saying things like 'not all disabilities are visible' on disabled toilets or parking spaces and the recent uptake in use of the 'Hidden Disabilities Sunflower' (Hidden Disabilities Sunflower, 2024).

In terms of the symbol, the difficulty really comes when considering what would you swap the image for to be more inclusive whilst still being so clear. This is also perhaps where we consider the image a little more deeply, beyond just suggesting that the only disabilities are physical disabilities to consider: What does the symbol suggest about how we view people with a disability?

The Accessible Icon Project

This is where The Accessible Icon Project comes in, as shown in Figure 14.3. This is an 'ongoing work of design activism' (The Accessible Icon Project, no date), which offers a tweaked version of the symbol. Consider now the difference between Figures 14.2 and 14.3.

The main difference is that the person in Figure 14.3 is actively and independently pushing themselves forward. In contrast, looking back to Figure 14.2, does it now suddenly seem like the person is very passive, requiring help (Museum of Modern Art, 2024). Use these two images to consider yourself and your approach to people with a disability, especially as a health and social care worker, such as what are your default assumptions when working with someone in a wheelchair?

Implications for practice from using the PCS model

Thompson states that 'good practice is anti-discriminatory practice' (Thompson, 2021:9) and calls on us to 'eradicate discrimination and oppression from our own practice and challenge them in the practice of others and the institutional structures in which we operate' (Thompson, 2021: 51). And so, if we are to provide effective care for people with disabilities and those around them, we need to honestly face the reality of the experiences

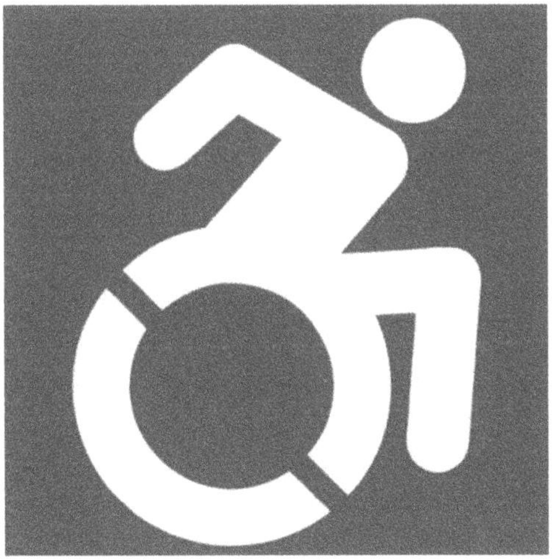

Figure 14.3 The Accessible Icon.

of ourselves and disabled people in our society both generally and then within our care services. The hope is that you take the points from this chapter and the questions we have considered across the PCS levels into your practice. This means being aware of your personal beliefs in connection to disability, and concepts like ableism and disablism. Carrying these concepts and the PCS analysis model forward in your practice will hopefully help you create and accomplish work that strives to be anti-discriminatory and anti-oppressive. This is discussed more in Chapter 15.

Summary

Overall, this chapter has begun to explore some concepts around disability primarily through the lens of Thompson's PCS analysis model that those starting, or continuing to, work with people with a disability in a health and social care setting should consider. The PCS model is a way of considering topics, in particular discrimination, through Personal, Cultural and Structural layers. Initially, we explored the Personal level, examining what you consider in terms of disabilities and people with disabilities and explored some points on the person-to-person experience such as terminology and language. At the Cultural level we explored some theories and approaches to studying and working with disability, including the medical model alongside the social model and ableism connected to disablism. We then explored some Structural level topics around legislation, in particular the *Equality Act 2010* and how it defines and applies disability. Ultimately, hopefully this chapter has provided information and questions to make you consider yourself and your thoughts and experiences in connection to disability, so that when you are working in health and social care you are aware of yourself and switched on, ready to work with people.

References

Alzheimer's Society (2018) *Positive language*. Available at https://www.alzheimers.org.uk/sites/default/files/2018-09/Positive%20language%20guide_0.pdf (Accessed 10 June 2024).

Ames, S. *et al.* (2024) 'Impact of disability-based discrimination in healthcare on parents of children with medical complexity', *Developmental Medicine and Child Neurology*, 66, pp. 1226–1233. Available at https://doi.org/10.1111/dmcn.15870

Botha, M., Hanlon, J. and Williams, G. (2023) 'Does language matter? Identity-first versus person-first language use in autism research: A response to Vivanti', *Journal of Autism and Developmental Disorders*, 53, pp. 870–878. Available at https://doi.org/10.1007/s10803-020-04858-w

Bury, S. *et al.* (2023) 'Understanding language preference: Autism knowledge, experience of stigma and autism identity', *Autism*, 27(6), pp. 1568–1600. Available at https://doi.org/10.1177/13623613221142383

Byrnes, J. and Muller, J. (eds.) (2017) *Bioarchaeology of Impairment and Disability: Theoretical, Ethnohistorical, and Methodological Perspectives*. Switzerland: Springer International Publishing AG.

Cambridge Dictionary (2024) 'Allistic'. Available at https://dictionary.cambridge.org/dictionary/english/allistic (Accessed 10 June 2024).

Cuthbert, S. and Quallington, J. (2017) *Values and Ethics for Care Practice*. Banbury: Lantern Publishing Limited.

Department for Work and Pensions (2024) *National statistics Family Resources Survey: financial year 2022 to 2023*. Available at https://www.gov.uk/government/statistics/family-resources-survey-financial-year-2022-to-2023/family-resources-survey-financial-year-2022-to-2023#disability-1 (Accessed 26 April 2024).

Equality Act 2010, c. 15. Available at: https://www.legislation.gov.uk/ukpga/2010/15/contents (Accessed: 6 December 2024).

Flacks, S. (2012) 'Deviant disabilities: The exclusion of drug and alcohol addiction from the Equality Act 2010', *Social & Legal Studies*, 21(3), pp. 395–412. Available at https://doi.org/10.1177/0964663912437991

Gappmayer, G. (2021) 'Disentangling disablism and ableism: The social norm of being able and its influence on social interactions with people with intellectual disabilities', *Journal of Occupational Science*, 28(1), pp. 102–113. Available at https://doi.org/10.1080/14427591.2020.1814394

Grue, J. (2016) 'The problem with inspiration porn: A tentative definition and a provisional critique', *Disability & Society*, 31(6), pp. 838–849. Available at https://doi.org/10.1080/09687599.2016.1205473

Hayes, N., O'Toole, L. and Halpenny, A. (2023) *Introducing Bronfenbrenner*. 2nd edn. Oxon: Routledge.

Hidden Disabilities Sunflower (2024) *What is the hidden disabilities sunflower?* Available at https://hdsunflower.com/uk/ (Accessed 11 June 2024).

Karim, S. (2023) 'Power-informed practice in social work', *Journal of Social Work*, 23(6), pp. 1062–1079. Available at https://doi.org/10.1177/14680173231180307

Keating, C. *et al.* (2022) 'Autism-related language preferences of English-speaking individuals across the globe: A mixed methods investigation', *Autism Research*, 16, pp. 406–428. Available at https://doi.org/10.1002/aur.2864

Kelly, N. (2023) 'Why is inspiration porn entrenched in our attitudes towards disability?', *Disability Rights UK,* 17 November. Available at https://www.disabilityrightsuk.org/news/why-inspiration-porn-entrenched-our-attitudes-towards-disability-ned-kelly (Accessed 10 January 2025).

King's College London (2023) *Learning from lives and deaths - people with a learning disability and autistic people (LeDeR)*. Available at https://www.kcl.ac.uk/research/leder (Accessed 11 June 2024).

Motability and The Wheelchair Alliance (2022) *An economic assessment of wheelchair provision in England*. Available at https://www.motabilityfoundation.org.uk/media/zsjnh4un/wheelchair-economic-study-final.pdf (Accessed 26 April 2024).

Museum of Modern Art (2024) *Accessible icon*. Available at https://www.moma.org/collection/works/174871 (Accessed 26 April 2024).

National Autistic Society (no date) *How to talk and write about autism*. Available at https://dy55nndrxke1w.cloudfront.net/file/24/xT2FqU_xTh5_JA5xTMYZxb.dfV0x/NAS_How%20to%20talk%20and%20write%20about%20autism.pdf (Accessed 26 April 2024).

National Autistic Society (2023) *Asperger syndrome (Asperger's)*. Available at https://www.autism.org.uk/advice-and-guidance/what-is-autism/the-history-of-autism/asperger-syndrome (Accessed 26 April 2024).

NHS England (no date) *Learning from lives and deaths – People with a learning disability and autistic people (LeDeR)*. Available at https://www.england.nhs.uk/learning-disabilities/improving-health/learning-from-lives-and-deaths/ (Accessed 11 June 2024).

NHS England (2024) *The Oliver McGowan mandatory training on learning disability and autism*. Available at https://www.hee.nhs.uk/our-work/learning-disability/current-projects/oliver-mcgowan-mandatory-training-learning-disability-autism (Accessed 11 June 2024).

Office for Disability Issues (2011) *Equality Act 2010 Guidance: Guidance on matters to be taken into account in determining questions relating to the definition of disability*. Available at https://assets.publishing.service.gov.uk/media/5a80dcc8ed915d74e6230df4/Equality_Act_2010-disability_definition.pdf (Accessed 26 April 2024).

Sealey, C., Fillingham, J. and Unwin, P. (eds.) (2022) *Social Policy, Service Users and Carers: Lived Experiences and Perspectives*. Cham: Springer International Publishing.

Sense (2022) *Ableism and disablism*. Available at https://www.sense.org.uk/information-and-advice/life-with-complex-disabilities/ableism-and-disablism/ (Accessed 26 April 2024).

Shakespeare, T. (2006) *Disability Rights and Wrongs*. Oxon: Routledge.

Shakespeare, T. (2017) 'The social model of Disability', in L. Davis (ed.) *The Disability Studies Reader*. 5th edn. New York: Routledge, pp. 145–152.

Shyman, E. (2016) 'The reinforcement of ableism: Normality, the medical model of disability, and humanism in applied behavior analysis and ASD', *Intellectual and Development Disabilities*, 54(5), pp. 366–376. Available at https://doi.org/10.1352/1934-9556-54.5.366

Silva *et al.* (2024) 'Discrimination and access to healthcare for people with disabilities: An integrative literature review', *Aquichan*, 24(3), pp. 1–16. Available at https://doi.org/10.5294/aqui.2024.24.3.4

Swain, J. and French, S. (2008) 'The tragedy view of impairment and disability', in Swain, J. and French, S. (eds.) *Disability on Equal Terms*. London: SAGE, pp. 7–20.

The Accessible Icon Project (no date) *The Accessible Icon Project*. Available at https://accessibleicon.org/ (Accessed 26 April 2024).

Thompson, N. (2021) *Anti-Discriminatory Practice*. 7th edn. London: RED GLOBE PRESS.

US Department of Transportation (2003) Manual on Uniform Traffic Control Devices for Streets and Highways. Available at: https://mutcd.fhwa.dot.gov/pdfs/2003r1r2/mutcd2003r1r2complet.pdf (Accessed 5 November 2025)

Vivanti, G. (2020) 'Ask the editor: What is the most appropriate way to talk about individuals with a diagnosis of autism?, *Journal of Autism and Developmental Disorders*, 50, pp. 691–693. Available at https://doi.org/10.1007/s10803-019-04280-x

Young, S. (2012) 'We're not here for your inspiration', *ABC News*, 3 July. Available at https://www.abc.net.au/news/2012-07-03/young-inspiration-porn/4107006 (Accessed 10 January 2025).

Young, S. (2014) *I'm not your inspiration, thank you very much*. April 2014. Available at https://www.ted.com/talks/stella_young_i_m_not_your_inspiration_thank_you_very_much?subtitle=en (Accessed 29 August 2024).

Zajic, M. and Gudknecht, J. (2024) 'Person- and identity-first language in autism research: A systematic analysis of abstracts from 11 autism journals', *Autism*, 00(0), pp. 1–17. Available at https://doi.org/10.1177/13623613241241202

15 Anti-discriminatory and anti-oppressive ACTion for health and social care

Clive Sealey

The aims of this chapter are to:

- **Define anti-discriminatory and anti-oppressive practice**
- **Outline relevant anti-discriminatory and anti-oppressive practice legislation**
- **Explain the benefits of anti-discriminatory and anti-oppressive practice to health and social care, and propose ACTion as a strategy to promote anti-discriminatory and anti-oppressive practice**

Introduction

The focus of this chapter is on discrimination and oppression, and specifically on encouraging practice that is not discriminatory and not oppressive. Discrimination and oppression are words that have strong negative meanings attached to them, and yet it is likely that you have come across these in your lives, either directly or indirectly. For example, the recent Post-Office Horizon IT Scandal, in which many employees were wrongly convicted of fraud by their employers and sent to prison, displays how the imbalance of power between employees and employers has led to oppressive practices. Similarly, the emergence of the Black Lives Matter movement followed the death of George Floyd, which occurred directly as a consequence of an imbalance of power that led to discriminatory practice. Both of these examples show how discriminatory and oppressive practices can lead to significant negative outcomes for individuals.

The examples above also highlight that discrimination and oppression most often occur when there is a negative balance, or imbalance, of power between individuals. A key point to note here is that within health and social care practice, this imbalance of power exists as an everyday norm. This is because the nature of health and social care practice is working with people who have care and support needs at a time when they are at their most vulnerable. For example, consider the imbalance of power that exists between a health and social care practitioner when providing care for someone living with dementia, someone suffering from a chronic illness or a young person requiring mental health support. In all of these examples, the balance of power is most likely with the health and social care practitioner providing care, and not the service user requiring care. This existence of an imbalance of power in its self need not be a problem, it only becomes a problem when it is acted upon, either directly or indirectly in the form of discriminatory and oppressive practice.

It is relevant to note here that discrimination and oppression in care are everyday occurrences. For instance, Mateo and Williams (2020: S5) state that in the UK, '63% of respondents experienced, and 56% witnessed, discrimination during their health professions

DOI: 10.4324/9781032619309-17

training. Sources of discrimination vary and include patients and patients' families, physicians, nurses, staff, and other trainees'. These high instances of discrimination and oppression make tackling them relevant and urgent. This makes it evident as to why it is important for you as a practitioner to be aware of this possibility, as it is only from such awareness that you are able to actively provide care that is anti-discriminatory and anti-oppressive in nature.

This chapter details the importance of anti-discriminatory practice (ADP) and anti-oppressive practice (AOP) for health and social care. The chapter firstly defines what ADP and AOP are, and links them to relevant legislation. The chapter then briefly details relevant ADP and AOP legislation. It then explains why and how ADP and AOP can impact on the quality of health and social care that you provide. The chapter concludes by proposing ACTion as a strategy that you can use to provide and promote ADP and AOP.

Defining anti-discriminatory and anti-oppressive practice

In trying to define what we mean by ADP and AOP, we first have to consider what we mean by discrimination and oppression. The prefix anti- means not, so defining what they are first of all helps us to consider what they are not.

Discrimination and anti-discriminatory practice

Discrimination at its most basic level is where we identify that a difference exists between two or more things. Discrimination is something that we do on an everyday basis. For example, when we choose a particular pen to use, when we prefer a certain type of food over another and where we choose one university over another to study are all examples of where we have discriminated. This type of discrimination is not a problem. Where it becomes a problem is when we use this difference as the basis to treat an individual worse than another individual (Raineri and Calcaterra, 2018), for example, based on their physical, health or social circumstances/characteristics. Table 15.1 shows a list of circumstances/characteristics that can define people and what they mean.

Table 15.1 Descriptions of circumstances and characteristics that define people

Circumstances/ Characteristics	*Description*
Age	how old a person is at a particular time, e.g., 47, 12, 65
Race	The physical characteristics that people share, e.g., skin colour, hair texture and facial features
Ethnicity	The social and or cultural characterises that people share, e.g., language, religion and beliefs
Sex	The biological differences between individuals, e.g., XX female and XY chromosomes, different sex organs and body size differences
Gender	The socially constructed differences between the sexes, e.g., male, female and trans
Social class	The economic circumstances of a person, e.g., working class, middle class and upper class
Sexuality	The sexual orientation that a person has, e.g., heterosexual, homosexual and bisexual
Ability	The physical or mental capabilities that a person has, e.g., differences in speed, thought, or mental health
Looks	The physical appearance that a person has, e.g., physical appearance, facial appearance and colour hair

Table 15.1 is not meant to provide an exhaustive list of all categories that can define people. It does show, however, that there is a lot of ways in which people can differ from each other, and it is certain that you fit into one of these categories. Actually, it is likely that you fit into all of these categories somewhere. So you can be categorised based on your age, race, ethnicity, gender, sex, social class, ability and looks. This in itself is not problematic, and can be a way to define who we are.

Where it does become problematic is when these categorises are used as a basis to treat people differently in a way that negatively affects their health and well-being. In this context, this is what we mean as discrimination, which refers to 'the unequal treatment of similar individuals placed in the same situation but who differ by one or several characteristics, such as race, ethnicity, gender, (dis)ability, sexual orientation, or other categorical statuses' (Fibbi *et al.*, 2021: 13). Examples of where discriminatory practice has occurred in health and social care are of older people having experience of a poor service because of their age (Jackson *et al.*, 2019), poorer maternity care for some women based on their race and ethnicity (Silverio *et al.*, 2023) and LGBTQ+ (Lesbian, Gay, Bisexual, Transgender, Questioning/Queer, Plus) individuals experiencing some form of unequal treatment from healthcare staff simply as a consequence of being LQBTQ+ (Bachman and Gooch, 2018).

In contrast to the discriminatory practices above, we can define ADP as practice that works 'to ensure that everyone is treated fairly and equally, and has access to the same opportunities' (Lane, 2017: 37). This highlights that the focus of ADP is on ensuring that the categories outlined in Table 15.1 do not affect the care that is provided. This requires having an awareness of the existence of these categories and the effect that they can have on individuals trying to access care, so that their potential to cause discrimination is reduced or eliminated to the extent that the care provided is equal regardless of circumstances or characteristics (Thompson, 2020).

Oppression and anti-oppressive practice

Oppression works in a similar way to discrimination in that it relies on the differences to operate. Taylor (2016: 520) provides a definition of oppression as occurring when 'one social group is subordinated while another is privileged'. Subordination here means treating people as if they are below you in position or status, while privilege here means having an advantage over another person. This means we can refer to oppression as where a group or a member of a group is treated in a way that denies them access to resources, rights or inclusion which directly results in another group benefitting. Oppression relies on there being some difference in power between the individuals, with the individual with the most power typically being the oppressor (Robbins, 2017). A key point about privilege is that it can often be unearned, meaning that a person has not had to do anything to earn the privilege, it occurs simply from how they are. This **unearned privilege** (Learning Box 15.1) is often unseen, but works to maintain the oppression of other groups (McIntosh, 1998).

Taylor (2016: 521) argues that a crucial difference between oppression and discrimination is that while discrimination is usually targeted at the individual, 'The target of oppression is a group, the entities privileged by oppression are also groups, and individuals are marked or picked out for the oppressive treatment in virtue of

Learning Box 15.1: Unearned privilege

The concept of unearned privilege refers to how the characteristics of certain groups are automatically accepted by others, automatically thought of as good, automatically respected by others and automatically treated with admiration by others (Nzira and Williams, 2008). As an example of this, consider the different ways in which a male single parent is viewed in comparison to a female single parent. Mcintosh (1998) provides a list of 46 unearned privileges that occur simply from being a white female, in comparison to her black female colleagues.

their group memberships' (Taylor, 2016: 521). This does not mean that oppression does not affect individuals, it simply means that the oppression is not specifically targeted at the individual, it is targeted at the group to which the individual belongs, in order to oppress the group as a whole. As an example of this, consider working in a place where the workforce is mainly female, but the managers of the workforce are mainly male. One reason for this could be a deliberate policy not to employ women as managers. Here, the oppression occurs not because there is a dislike of any single particular women, but because the target of the oppression is women in general, in order to maintain the privilege that the men as managers have. Oppressive practice also occurs where the conduct of an individual can negatively influence the treatments of others. An example of this is the Employment Tribunal case of *Rimmer v The Secretary of State for Work and Pensions* (2024), which is where the individual treatment of an hearing impaired individual was deemed to be oppressive from the fact that the actions of the Disability Employment Advisor were able to influence other employees to treat other hearing impaired service users in a similarly negative way. Ultimately, the outcome of oppression is inequality between groups, leading to similar outcomes as for discrimination.

We can now define AOP as a practice which works to understand, reduce and eliminate the status and privileges that groups have and use over another. The first key part of AOP is understanding what the status and privileges are, and that these occur from the power relations that can occur in practice. This may not be readily apparent, because often we carry these power relations without realising. For example, consider the power relations that can occur between you as an able-bodied practitioner and a non-able-bodied service user. The most obvious power relations that exist between you are in providing care, in terms of what is provided and how it is provided. This care can be provided in a way that maintains the status and privilege that you have over the non-able-bodied service user, so that they remain dependent on care and their position as a service user is maintained. This is an oppressive practice as it works to maintain the dominant position of one group over another. On the other hand, you can provide care in a way that seeks to limit the dependence on care and increase the independence of the service user to the extent that their status within society is improved. This is AOP, as it works to limit the effect that the disadvantages status the individual has.

Anti-discrimination and anti-oppressive practice legislation

Due to the negative effects that discrimination and oppression can have, there is specific legislation in place against them. These legislation seek to limit these negative effects. They mean that as a health and social care practitioner, you are required to be aware of these and follow them, as not doing so can lead to legal sanctions. However, a serious limitation of these ADP and AOP legislation is that they are **civil legislation not criminal legislation** (Learning Box 6.1). This means that the police are not responsible for investigating them when they occur, and it is the responsibility of the individual or group to pursue a case where they feel that discrimination and oppression occur. This limits the deterrence effect of the legislation.

Anti-discrimination practice legislation

The main legislation that concerns ADP is the *Equality Act 2010*, which legally protects certain individuals and groups with protected characteristics from discrimination in the workplace and wider society. It does this by banning **direct discrimination and indirect discrimination** (Learning Box 6.3) in most circumstances, although they are allowed in some circumstances. Individuals and groups can also use the *Human Rights Act 1998*, specifically *Article 14* which provides protection from discrimination for protected groups.

Anti-oppressive practice legislation

There is no specific legislation concerned with AOP. In some circumstances, the *Equality Act 2010* can be used where the rights of a protected group have been breached. Individuals and groups can use specific articles of the *Human Rights Act 1998*, such as *Article 3* to protect from bullying, harassment, abuse, discrimination, and *Article 5* to promote the independence, rights, choice and control over their own care, treatment and well-being.

The benefits of anti-discriminatory and anti-oppressive practice to health and social care

Having determined what ADP and AOP are, the chapter now focuses on explaining how these can benefit health and social care. There are three key ways in which ADP AOP are important to health and social care practice. These are improving the quality of care, improving the outcomes of care and enabling individuals and groups to positively contribute to wider society. It is important to make this link to practice as it makes ideas that are difficult to understand relevant to practice.

Improving the quality of care

When talking about improving quality of care, the focus is on how care positively improves the outcomes for individuals and groups. Care can have both a positive and a negative effect on individuals, an example of the former being the promotion of safeguarding, while an example of the latter is the unjustified deprivation of liberty. Discrimination and oppression limit the quality of care by treating people differently in a way that negatively affects their health and well-being.

Both ADP and AOP focus on how discrimination and oppression are interwoven into the daily lives of individuals with little awareness of how or why this is happening. To improve the quality of care requires an understanding of the needs that an individual or group has and then providing care that is equal to that provided to other service users. Where practitioners actively seek to understand the needs to service user, this can provide a more honest account of the issues that are affecting an individual or group, and therefore improve diagnosis and treatment (Aggarwal and Lewis-Fernández, 2020). For example, consider the circumstance of a working-class young person living with a clinically diagnosed mental health condition. From speaking to them and understanding their circumstances, it becomes possible to realise that at the core of their condition is loneliness, which is not a clinical mental condition but is actually a social issue. You realise further that this loneliness is made worse by the stigma that occurs from it, in terms of the expectation that someone of their age and in their social class should not be suffering from loneliness but should have lots of friends. This expectation means that there are very few services provided to overcome the loneliness, which makes the situation worse. Here we can see how discrimination based on age and oppression based on circumstances works to the limit the quality of care provided. It is only by understanding the circumstances that the quality of care can be improved, and this is possible through the focus of ADP and AOP through firstly understanding the needs of that a service user has, and then providing care that is equal to that provided to other groups or individuals.

Improving the outcomes of care

When discrimination occurs, it has significant negative mental health outcomes for the group that is being discriminated against, such as anxiety, depression, stress, anger, psychosis, low self-esteem, general anxiety disorder and post-traumatic stress disorder (PTSD) (Williams *et al.*, 2019). Oppression limits the quality of care by maintaining the privilege that one group has over another, leading to inequality between groups.

A key aspect of oppression and discrimination is the creation and maintenance of prejudicial beliefs between individuals and groups, which can lead to biases. For example, a person can have a prejudicial belief that people with mental health are dangerous, without having actually met a dangerous person with mental health, and this belief can bias the way that they act towards people with mental health in general. These biases have been shown to lead to some groups treated better than others, resulting in large health differences between groups. For example, Zestcott *et al.* (2016) have detailed how bias can negatively affects both the interactions that practitioners have with service users, and the judgements they make about service users, both of which can lead to negative care outcomes. In particular, practitioners have been observed to offer different treatments to individual based on their group identity and not on their need, which is a specific example of oppression in action. A particular observation is the assumption that particular treatments or care are more relevant to certain individuals or groups, and thereby providing this as the only option to them (Mateo and Williams, 2020). As an example of this, consider the historic focus on the treatment of mental health conditions primarily through medication or medical interventions, rather than with care with the family or in the community. We know that this medicalised approach has not only led to the stigmatisation of mental health, but also to treatment that is ineffective and unnecessary for many people (Lovell, 2015). Additionally, such treatments contribute to and sustain the discrimination and oppression of individuals and groups. Both ADP and AOP provide the possibility for alternative ways of treatments and care that may be more effective than the dominant model, thereby improving the outcomes for individuals and groups (Baines and Edwards, 2015). For instance, the move towards the social model of care (Chapter 9) occurred specifically from the desire by disabled people to move away from the oppression and discrimination that they were facing from care provided within the medical model of care (Beresford, 2007).

Enabling individuals and groups to positively contribute to wider society

In seeking to improve both the quality of care and the outcomes of care, ADP and AOP can be said to enable a wider positive change within society that benefits wider society in general. This is from the change that occurs not just within the group and individuals but also within society. Consider where a group or individual has been oppressed or discriminated against. This limits what they can do and how they can do it. Ultimately, it limits the potential that they have to benefit wider society. However, where discrimination and oppression are eliminated or limited, this enables individuals and groups to make a positive contribution to society. A good example of this is in relation to Professor Stephen Hawkin, who lived with a degenerative motor neurone disease which initially paralysed him and ultimately led to his death. Hawkin became the world's most famous physicist and his works are celebrated academically and socially. Hawkin was clear that the care that he received was significant in enabling him to contribute to society in the way that he did, stating 'I have had a lot of experience of the NHS and the care I received has enabled me to live my life as I want and to contribute to major advances in our understanding of the universe' (Triggle, 2017). This shows providing ADP and AOP care that enables people to overcome discrimination and oppression can benefit wider society.

The reason for this is the emphasis within ADP and AOP on equality (Thompson, 2020), in contrast to the emphasis within discrimination and oppression on inequality. Inequality prioritises the uneven distribution of resources and goods, which in turn leads to ill health, limited well-being and unhappiness (Hood, 2023). Moreover, these effects become multiplied over time, meaning that they worsen the circumstances and life chances of individuals and groups. This makes it hard for them to contribute positively to society.

In contrast, Wilkinson and Pickett (2010) outline several clear positive links occurring from equality, such as increased life expectancy, lower infant mortality, higher educational outcomes, higher social mobility, less poverty and lower rates of mental illness. Here, Maslow's (1943) 'Hierarchy of needs' becomes relevant, as it argues that it is only possible for individuals and groups to achieve their highest possible potential when such specific needs as those detailed above are met. To refer back to the example of Stephen Hawkin above, it is likely to be the case that without the NHS meeting his needs, he would have been able to achieve his potential. The focus within ADP and AOP on meeting the specific needs of all equally, as opposed to meeting the needs of some unequally, enables these foundational needs to be met and therefore for individuals and groups to positively contribute to society in general, regardless of their circumstances. This emphasises what Heffernan (2015:3) terms a 'just culture', which 'tap[s] the ingenuity, initiative, and sheer cleverness of every single individual' meaning that 'every single person counts', and every small change contributes to society.

Strategies to provide and promote anti-discriminatory and anti-oppressive practice: ACT

Having outlined the benefits of ADP and AOP, this section suggests a model to enable ADP and AOP in your practice. The best-known model to promote ADP and AOP is Thompson's (2020) Personal, Cultural, Social (PCS) model. In this model, Thompson argues that discrimination and oppression work at through the personal beliefs, cultural norms and structural institutions that exist in specific contexts. Thompson's model has been very influential, however, there have been criticisms of it such as its focus on the knowledge of the experts to work and how this may itself contribute to oppression (Wilson and Beresford, 2000). I propose an alternative model below to build on the strengths of the PCS model but also to overcome some of these criticisms.

The model I outline uses the mnemonic of ACTion, which refers to:

- Awareness of discriminatory and oppressive practices
- Challenging discriminatory and oppressive practices
- Transforming discriminatory and oppressive practices

Awareness of discriminatory and oppressive practices

Awareness refers to the process of firstly reflecting on our position within society to consider how this contrasts with the position in society of the groups and individuals we work with. This allows us to identify and confront the privileges that we have based from the perspective of our own position in society. As a practitioner, it is very likely that the position you hold is privileged in terms of status and power, and this may lead us to hold beliefs, attitudes and values about the groups and individuals that you work with which reinforces this status and power. The important point is that these privileges can and do affect the way that we interact with groups and individuals, and hence the outcomes for them from our practice.

Typically, we are so unaware of our privileges that we do not even notice they are there or question the effect that they have. A good example of this is the privileges that can occur from our gendered roles, and how these affect our interactions with service users in different ways. For instance, a male practitioner has the privilege of being seen as having more authority than women which can limit the inclination for service users to challenge what they say, while a female practitioner has the privilege of being seen as more caring than men which can limit the inclination to challenge the care being provided. These privileges inevitably have an impact even when we are not aware of it. This is important as it enables us to consider whether the focus of our practice is either on how the outcomes for individuals and groups are dependent on whether they do what we tell them to do, or on how our privileges affect what we tell them to do.

An important aspect of awareness of how discrimination and oppression are affecting groups and individuals is understanding the context within which they are operating. Discrimination and oppression do not operate in a vacuum, they are socially constructed concepts that require specific circumstances and contexts to operate. If this was not the case, then instances of discrimination and oppression would be the same wherever we were. However, we know that this is not the case. In some countries, discrimination and oppression occur to lesser or greater extents, anti-Semitism being a good example of this, and in some cultures, discrimination and oppression occur to greater or lesser extents,

Learning Box: 15.2: 'Being woke'

The term being woke is typically used negatively to refer to attempts to tackle discrimination and/or oppression. Being woke is considered an insult by a significant proportion of the population (Duffy *et al.*, 2021). However, its original and literal meaning is to be awake and aware to, as opposed to being asleep and unaware of, social problems and issues that negatively affect individual groups. It originated in America as a way to signify being well-informed or and sensitive to issues of social justice, such as discrimination and oppression. The more recent use of the term as an insult to signify weakness is the complete opposite of its original meaning as being aware of and working to tackle discrimination and oppression.

violence against women and girls being a good example of this. While discriminated and oppressed individuals and groups may understand this context and how it operates, as this is a necessity for it to operate, it is unlikely that you as a practitioner will also do so, and this can limit the effectiveness of your practice. Indeed, this lack of understanding of the context may actively contribute to the continued discrimination and oppression of the individual or group, if it ignores it or acts in ways that seeks to undermine it (Karim, 2023). As an example of this, consider where an individual is experiencing domestic abuse in the form of coercive control as opposed to physical abuse. A factor that would compound this is the stigma that exists in relation to such abuse, especially if the abuse occurs in an atypical context, such as between middle- or upper-class individuals. Without an understanding of this context, it would be possible for the practitioner to ignore or actively dismiss the signs and symptoms, as has occurred (Gowar and Unwin, 2021). Where this happens, it limits the beneficial outcomes for individual and groups in significant ways. To enable the possibility of ADP and AOP to be beneficial, an understanding of the context is very necessary.

Becoming aware of discrimination and oppression reflects the true meaning of the term **being woke** (Key Learning Box 15.2), not the negative way it is often used when talking about those seeking to tackle or angered by discrimination and oppression, as this denies the reality of how widespread they are, and the harmful effect that they can have.

Challenging discriminatory and oppressive practices

To progress our practice from awareness requires being prepared to challenge both the basis of the privileges that we have identified as owning, and the notion that they are neutral and/or harmless.

As identified above, health and social care practice can be limiting in terms of the type of care provided. For example, we identified that care for mental health is often medicalised, meaning that it is focused on providing care that aims to treat the condition that the person has through the use of medicine and medical treatments, such as antipsychotic medication. It assumes that the cause of mental ill health lies solely within the person and ignores the effect that social issues such as discrimination and oppression can have on mental health. For example, Harvey Head and Fillingham (2021) outline how having undiagnosed dyslexia during school years contributed to the discrimination that

Harvey Head faced at school, which ultimately led to the intensification of her mental health and medicalised treatment following this intensification. It was only after the use of non-medicalised, social treatment in the form of psychology and art therapy that Harvey Head's condition improved.

This suggests that challenging established and taken for granted approaches to mental health specifically and health and social care in general is relevant to tackling discrimination and oppression. This means recognising that care can be considered to be as wide as is appropriate, and that alternative approaches may be more fitting, such as **social prescribing** (Learning Box 8.1). Indeed, providing limited care can obscure and exacerbate the discrimination and oppression that may be contributing to individuals and groups circumstances. Doing this invites individuals and groups to challenge what we say and do in practice, which as we identified above has the potential to deliver beneficial outcomes. This is because when decisions are challenged with openness and honesty, there is less potential for misunderstandings and mistakes (Quick, 2022). Furthermore, as Baines and Edwards (2015: 28) argue, remaining neutral in discriminatory and oppressive situations means enforcing establishment values and laws that can work to reinforce such discrimination and oppression. For instance, Smith *et al.* (2023) identified how the unthinking use of special schools contributed to the low expectation of pupils who attended them, which in the long term made worse the disadvantages and inequalities that they experienced in trying to contribute meaningfully to society in later life. This is an example of how a narrow and limited application of care can lead to further and wider discrimination and oppression, which ultimately limits the recovery and participation of groups and individuals. This supports ADP and AOP practice that considers the possibilities for care in a comprehensive way that increases the possibility of reducing discrimination and oppression.

Transforming discriminatory and oppressive practices

Very often, what is key to discrimination and oppression happening is the difference in status between practitioners and service users, in terms of who they are and what they are allowed to do. This can result in an implicit or explicit divide between practitioner and service user, and this divide often expresses itself in the establishment of the traditional 'doctor knows best' situation (Dempster, 2023), which results in care 'on' service users. This can and does lead to unfriendly and/or authoritarian relationships between practitioner and service user, which then increases the possibility of discrimination and oppression either directly or indirectly (Sealey *et al.*, 2021). Such care 'on' service users reduces the possibility of full and meaningful engagement between practitioners and service users, which as we discussed above limits the outcomes of care.

The opposite of care 'on' service users is care 'with' service users. This is where care occurs as a consequence of practitioners working 'with' service users, which is often called co-production (Learning Box 15.3). Co-production is a practice that prioritises an equal relationship between practitioners and service users (Sealey *et al.*, 2021a). This transformative approach involves working together to design and deliver care, sharing strategic decision-making about care, as well as planning the best way to deliver care. This is an approach that actively draws on both expertise of the practitioner *and* the lived experiences and knowledge of service users as individuals who are able to make a meaningful contribution to their own care and needs. This limits the possibility of care that simply reinforces the expertise of the practitioner, thereby limiting the possibility of explicit or implicit discrimination or oppression.

Learning Box 15.3: Co-production

Co-production is defined as 'when an individual influences the support and services received, or when groups of people get together to influence the way that services are designed, commissioned and delivered' (Department of Health and Social Care, 2025: 2.20). From this definition, we can see that the focus of co-production is the design, choice and delivery of services with the specific engagement and involvement of these that it affects, such as service users, carers and the community that they live in. This means that co-production is about services with relevant groups, rather than on relevant groups, and treating all relevant parties as equal partners and co-creators (Sealey, 2021a).

As a simple example of this, consider where an individual goes to the doctor with high blood pressure. The doctor as an expert may think that prescribing blood pressure medication at a high dosage 'on' the individual is the logical way to treat this condition. However, the individual knows that there are specific circumstances that have occurred that have led to the high blood pressure, and explains this to the doctor. Having discussed this, the doctor and patient work 'with' each other to create a plan that includes a willingness to prescribe a lower dosage of medication on the part of the doctor, but also a willingness to make changes to their lifestyle on the part of the individual. This transformative approach actively embraces both the professional experience of the doctor *and* the lived experiences of the individual as a way towards more meaningful diagnosis and treatment, as it 'explicitly recognises that the lived experiences of service users and carers complements and enhances professional expertise and vice versa' (Sealey *et al.*, 2021: 3). This transforms practice away from discrimination and oppression to practice that enables individuals and groups to positively contribute to society, which reflects the specific benefits of ADP and AOP as identified above.

Summary

The focus of this chapter has been on discrimination and oppression, and specifically on encouraging practice that is not discriminatory and not oppressive. The chapter began by arguing that discriminatory and oppressive practices are bad for health and social care because they can have negative outcomes individuals and groups. The legislation that is in place seeks to limit these negative effects. The definitions of both discrimination and oppression reinforce their negative outcomes, as well as their exclusionary and unequal outcomes. In contrast, both ADP and AOP can have positive outcomes for health and social care in specific ways. For instance, ADP and AOP can improve the quality of care, improve the outcomes of care and enable individuals and groups to positively contribute to society. The chapter concluded by proposing ACTion as a strategy to provide and promote ADP and AOP. This involves Awareness of discriminatory and oppressive practices, Challenging discriminatory and oppressive practices, and Transforming discriminatory and oppressive practices. Both in isolation and together, this strategy seeks to limit the effects of discrimination and oppression and equalise the negative balance, or imbalance, of power that exists in society and is often reproduced in practice.

References

Aggarwal, N.K. and Lewis-Fernández, R. (2020) 'An introduction to the cultural formulation interview', *FOCUS*, 18(1), pp. 77–82. Available at https://doi.org/10.1176/appi.focus.18103

Bachman, C.L. and Gooch, B. (2018) *LGBT in Britain. Health Report*. London: Stnewall. Available at https://www.stonewall.org.uk/system/files/lgbt_in_britain_health.pdf (Accessed 14 May 2024).

Baines, S. and Edwards, J. (2015) 'Considering the ways in which anti-oppressive practice principles can inform health research', *The Arts in Psychotherapy*, 42, pp. 28–34. Available at https://doi.org/10.1016/j.aip.2015.01.001

Beresford, P. (2007) 'The role of service user research in generating knowledge-based health and social care: From conflict to contribution', *Evidence & Policy*, 3(3), pp. 329–341. Available at https://doi.org/10.1332/174426407781738074

Dempster, J. (2023) 'The "doctor knows best" model is no longer enough', *Nursing Times*. Available at: https://www.nursingtimes.net/cancer/the-doctor-knows-best-model-is-no-longer-enough-20-07-2023/

Department of Health and Social Care (2025) *Care and support statutory guidance, GOV.UK*. Available at https://www.gov.uk/government/publications/care-act-statutory-guidance/care-and-support-statutory-guidance (Accessed 16 April 2025).

Duffy, B. *et al.* (2021) *Culture Wars in the UK: How the Public Understand the Debate*. London: Ipsos/Kings College London. Available at https://www.kcl.ac.uk/policy-institute/assets/culture-wars-in-the-uk-how-the-public-understand-the-debate.pdf (Accessed 21 May 2024).

Fibbi, R., Midtbøen, A.H. and Simon, P. (2021) 'Concepts of discrimination', in R. Fibbi, A.H. Midtbøen, and P. Simon (eds.) *Migration and Discrimination: IMISCOE Short Reader*. Cham: Springer International Publishing, pp. 13–20. Available at https://doi.org/10.1007/978-3-030-67281-2_2

Gowar, D.J.S. and Unwin, P. (2021) 'Lived experiences of domestic abuse, domestic violence and intimate partner violence', in C. Sealey, J. Fillingham, and P. Unwin (eds.) *Social Policy, Service Users and Carers: Lived Experiences and Perspectives*. Cham: Springer International Publishing, pp. 177–192. Available at https://doi.org/10.1007/978-3-030-69876-8_11

Harvey Head, C. and Fillingham, J. (2021) 'Mental health: Services and struggles', in C. Sealey, J. Fillingham, and P. Unwin (eds.) *Social Policy, Service Users and Carers: Lived Experiences and Perspectives*. Cham: Springer International Publishing, pp. 163–175. Available at https://doi.org/10.1007/978-3-030-69876-8_10

Heffernan (2015) *Beyond Measure: The Big Impact of Small Changes*. First TED Books hardcover edition. New York; London: TED Books, Simon & Schuster.

Hood, R. (2023) *Inequality and Social Work*. 1st edn. Thousand Oaks: SAGE Publications Ltd.

Jackson, S.E., Hackett, R.A. and Steptoe, A. (2019) 'Associations between age discrimination and health and wellbeing: Cross-sectional and prospective analysis of the English longitudinal study of ageing', *The Lancet Public Health*, 4(4), pp. e200–e208. Available at https://doi.org/10.1016/S2468-2667(19)30035-0

Karim, S. (2023) 'Power-informed practice in social work', *Journal of Social Work*, 23(6), pp. 1062–1079. Available at https://doi.org/10.1177/14680173231180307

Lane, P. (2017) 'Conceptualising ageing and anti-discriminatory practice', in P. Lane and R. Tribe (eds.) *Anti-Discriminatory Practice in Mental Health Care for Older People*. London: Jessica Kingsley Publishers, pp. 19–47.

Lovell, B. (2015) 'Frontal lobotomy: A vanishing but important radiological finding', *Case Reports*, 2015, p. bcr2014208767. Available at https://doi.org/10.1136/bcr-2014-208767

Maslow, A.H. (1943) 'A theory of human motivation', *Psychological Review*, 50(4), pp. 370–396. Available at: https://doi.org/10.1037/h0054346

Mateo, C.M. and Williams, D.R. (2020) 'Addressing bias and reducing discrimination: The professional responsibility of health care providers', *Academic Medicine*, 95(12S), p. S5. Available at https://doi.org/10.1097/ACM.0000000000003683

McIntosh, P. (1998) *White Privilege: Unpacking the Invisible Knapsack*. New York, NY, US: The Guilford Press (Re-visioning family therapy: Race, culture, and gender in clinical practice), p. 152.

Nzira, V. and Williams, P. (2008) *Anti-Oppressive Practice in Health and Social Care*. London: SAGE.

Quick, O. (2022) 'Duties of candour in healthcare: The truth, the whole truth, and nothing but the truth?', *Medical Law Review*, 30(2), pp. 324–347. Available at https://doi.org/10.1093/medlaw/fwac004

Raineri, M.L. and Calcaterra, V. (2018) 'Social work strategies against crisis in everyday practice: An anti-oppressive case study', *International Social Work*, 61(1), pp. 130–142. Available at https://doi.org/10.1177/0020872815606793

Rimmer v Secretary of State for Work and Pensions (2024) 1802885/2022. Available at https://assets.ctfassets.net/y26owwfe9yxn/4zIaiDASoP9n1mbTz7dwtq/87e08d51a4cfda30d68ec2f6de9f889e/Judgement.pdf

Robbins, S. (2017) 'Oppression theory and social work treatment', in F.J. Turner (ed.) *Social Work Treatment: Interlocking Theoretical Approaches*. Oxford: Oxford University Press, pp. 377–387.

Sealey, C., Fillingham, J. and Unwin, P. (2021a) 'Co-production: Rationale, processes and application to this book', in C. Sealey, J. Fillingham, and P. Unwin (eds.) *Social Policy, Service Users and Carers*. Cham: Springer International Publishing, pp. 15–28. Available at https://doi.org/10.1007/978-3-030-69876-8_2

Sealey, C., Unwin, P. and Fillingham, J. (2021) 'Introduction', in C. Sealey, J. Fillingham, and P. Unwin (eds.) *Social Policy, Service Users and Carers*. Cham: Springer International Publishing, pp. 1–14. Available at https://doi.org/10.1007/978-3-030-69876-8_1

Silverio, S.A. *et al.* (2023) 'Inside the "imperfect mosaic": Minority ethnic women's qualitative experiences of race and ethnicity during pregnancy, childbirth, and maternity care in the United Kingdom', *BMC Public Health*, 23(1), p. 2555. https://doi.org/10.1186/s12889-023-17505-7

Smith, J. *et al.* (2023) 'Lived experiences of special schools in England: Key considerations for social work practice', *The British Journal of Social Work*, 53(3), pp. 1341–1351. Available at https://doi.org/10.1093/bjsw/bcac230

Taylor, E. (2016) 'Groups and oppression', *Hypatia*, 31(3), pp. 520–536. Available at https://doi.org/10.1111/hypa.12252

Thompson, N. (2020) *Anti-Discriminatory Practice*. 7th edn. London: Bloomsbury. Available at https://www.bloomsbury.com/uk/antidiscriminatory-practice-9781352010947/ (Accessed 14 May 2024).

Triggle, N. (2017) *Stephen Hawking: I'm worried about the future of the NHS - BBC News*. Available at https://www.bbc.com/news/health-40967309 (Accessed 22 July 2022).

Wilkinson, R.G. and Pickett, K. (2010) *The Spirit Level: Why Equality Is Better for Everyone* [with a new chapter responding to their critics]. Publ. with a new postscript. London: Penguin Books.

Williams, D.R. *et al.* (2019) 'Understanding how discrimination can affect health', *Health Services Research*, 54(Suppl 2), pp. 1374–1388. Available at https://doi.org/10.1111/1475-6773.13222

Wilson, A. and Beresford, P. (2000) '"Anti-oppressive practice": Emancipation or appropriation?', *The British Journal of Social Work*, 30(5), pp. 553–573.

Zestcott, C.A., Blair, I.V. and Stone, J. (2016) 'Examining the presence, consequences, and reduction of implicit bias in health care: A narrative review', *Group Processes & Intergroup Relations*, 19(4), pp. 528–542. Available at https://doi.org/10.1177/1368430216642029

16 'Healthy ageing'

The future of health and social care?

Clair Rees

The aims of this chapter are to:

- **Outline current and future projections of ageing, and its implication for health and social care**
- **Explore the impact that misconceptions of ageing and ageism have on older people.**
- **Outline the potential beneficial outcomes of polices and strategies that promote 'healthy ageing' for health and social care**

Introduction

This chapter considers how continued 'growth' throughout the life course, especially in older age, can have a beneficial impact on the future of health and social care. It challenges the traditional notion of inevitable decline into old age, and the increased demands this, in turn, places on the economy as our population ages. It outlines how a negative perception of ageing, and of an ageing population, often leads to stereotypical labels and ageist attitudes, which can impact the lived experience of the individual. It argues that embracing the concept of 'growing in age' as the norm, and recognising older adults as a diverse group with varying health and social care needs, are key elements to altering the perception of ageing. The chapter highlights the work of the Older Peoples Commissioners in Wales and Northern Ireland, along with the World Health Organization, to demonstrate how alternative approaches to ageing can foster inclusive, collaborative, and innovative benefits for health, social care, and broader society, promoting intergenerational support and social cohesion. As the ageing population grows, older adults are increasingly recognised for their potential contribution to societal development, ensuring their voice is incorporated into policies and programmes is essential for fostering inclusive growth.

Current and future projections of ageing in the population

Population ageing refers to the growing number and proportion of older individuals in the global population. Nearly every country is experiencing this shift, making it one of the most profound social changes of the 21st century. Data from the World Population Prospects (United Nations, 2022) highlights that the population aged 65 and older is expanding more quickly than younger age groups. By 2050, those aged 65+ are projected to make up 16% of the global population, up from 10% in 2022, highlighting the urgency to address the challenges and opportunities of an ageing society. All countries face major challenges to ensure that their health and social care systems are ready to make the most of this demographic shift.

DOI: 10.4324/9781032619309-18

In the UK, the situation is similar, as data from the Office for National Statistics (ONS, 2023) shows:

- In 2022, approximately 19% or 12.7 million people were aged 65 years or over in the UK. Projections estimate that this will increase to 22.1 million or 27% of the population by 2072.
- In 2021, approximately 1.2 million people aged 65 years and over in England and Wales were classed as unpaid carers. Almost half of these provided more than 50 hours of unpaid care per week.

These key data provide an insight into the changing population ratios worldwide and in the UK. The benefit of having rich demographic evidence offers us the opportunity to plan and prepare through targeted policy making for the potential health, social and care needs of distinct groups. Statistical data alone does not provide the whole picture though. Thinking about these changes more broadly, in different ways and from different perspectives can help policymakers prioritise key issues, such as identifying current health drivers, or highlighting growing inequalities.

This trend has widespread implications across various sectors, including labour markets, financial systems, and the demand for essential goods and services such as housing, healthcare, and accessible public spaces. It also affects family dynamics and relationships between generations. For example, with increased life expectancy, there is a growing 'sandwich generation' of middle-aged adults caring for both elderly parents and their own growing children. Universally adopted models, such as the Dahlgren and Whitehead's (2021) 'Rainbow model' of health determinants, and more recent adaptations of this, help identify the key factors that contribute to population health. This is shown in Figure 16.1.

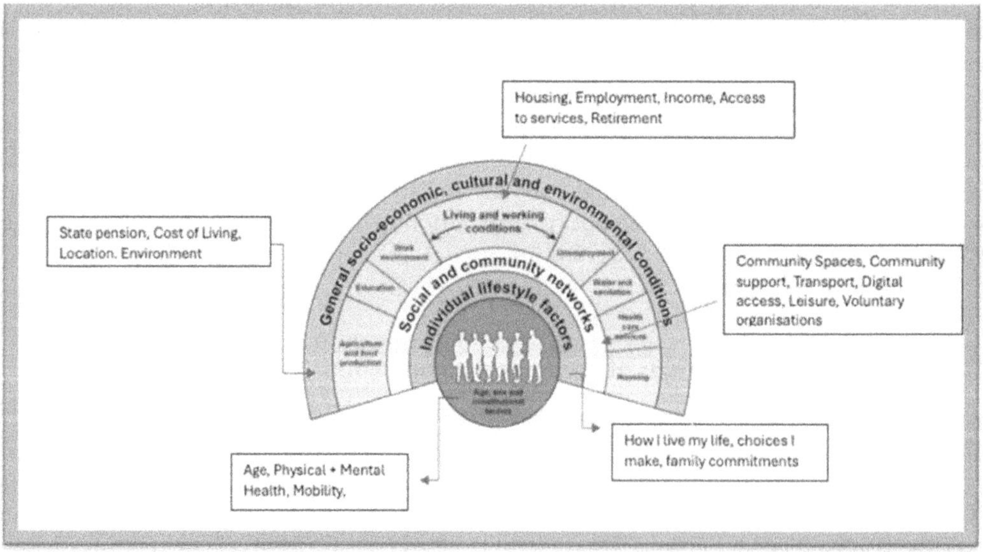

Figure 16.1 Key factors that contribute to older people's 'health'.

Source: Adapted from Dahlgren and Whitehead's (1991) Rainbow Model.

Figure 16.1 illustrates the relationship between the individual, their environment and their health, as applied to the older population. Models like these can significantly contribute to effective policy development when used to help define and identify the range of influences that contribute to the individual health and wellbeing of older persons (Jahnel *et al.*, 2022).

Understanding the misconceptions of ageing and ageism

Ageing is a universal process, i.e. it happens to everyone, regardless of structural and social differences (Finlay, 2021). This means that recognising and challenging some of the misconceptions of ageing and ageist perceptions held about 'old people' is necessary as society moves towards increasing population ageing (Johfre and Saperstein, 2023). This is especially relevant as life expectancy increases and people remain healthier and more active into their older years. As older adults remain active participants in their respective communities, and contributors to the economic and social fabric of society, they are, in turn, a 'visible' reminder of the presence of ageing individuals, and very much part of our shared life spaces. Social norms are changing as populations begin to age. For this reason, it may be more useful to think of ageing as a continuum as suggested throughout the Welsh Government literature whereby the 'older population' refers to those individuals that are 50 years and older.

Misconceptions of ageing

Many perceived negative issues are commonly associated with an ageing population. However, these concerns are often rooted in misconceptions rather than reality. Table 16.1 highlights some of the key negative issues attributed to an ageing population and demonstrates how these concerns are frequently based on misunderstandings or stereotypes.

Table 16.1 shows that when we begin to question some of the beliefs held about what it is to age, then our perception of older people begins to shift. Inaccurate and

Table 16.1 Key identified negative ageing issues from misconceptions of ageing

Identified negative issues from ageing	*Explanation of issue*	*Misconception of issue*
Care Dependent	The assumption that an ageing population is primarily dependent on care services fosters the misconception that older adults are a burden on families and healthcare systems.	While some older adults will require care as they age, most will continue to live independently and actively contribute to society. 97.3% of the older population reported living in private households with the remaining 2,7% living in communal residences, e.g. nursing homes (Office for National Statistics (ONS, 2023)
Increasing H/C costs	It is often argued that an ageing population leads to unsustainable healthcare costs due to higher medical needs.	Healthcare costs rise with age, but investment in long-term social care reform can mitigate these expenses. Better management of health issues and the ability to maintain independence can significantly impact the costs long term (Centre for Ageing Better, 2023)

(*Continued*)

Table 16.1 (Continued)

Identified negative issues from ageing	*Explanation of issue*	*Misconception of issue*
Absence of Disease	That being disease-free is the only measure of good health, ignoring the broader definition of wellbeing.	Good health in older adults does not necessarily mean the absence of disease. Many older individuals live with multiple health conditions, by focusing on improving their mental and physical capacities, better outcomes overall can be achieved (Welsh Government, 2021: 44–45)
Jobs for the younger generation	A common fear is that older adults remaining in or re-entering the workforce take jobs away from younger workers.	Mandatory retirement ages do not necessarily create opportunities for the youth, age should not determine an individuals' ability or eligibility to contribute to the workforce (Allen, 2023)
Economic Drain	The belief that older people are a financial burden on society ignores their economic contributions.	The spending power of older adults offers considerable contribution to the country's economy. Older consumers are often overlooked for both spending power and supporting the wider needs of community and society through time given freely for care duties and volunteering (Sealey, 2015)

misrepresented opinions relating to older persons as a homogeneous group limit our ability to capitalise upon the human resource that the older population contributes. Defining 'old age' or 'older persons' inevitably lead us to challenge our perception of what we define as 'old'. For example, the previous retirement age of 60 years for women and 65 years for men might have been a milestone age to determine the transition into older adulthood. However, retirement ages now vary from 55 years to over 75 years – a difference of 20 years, as there is no longer a default retirement age (*Equality Act, 2010*). Arguably, this traditional 'marker' for transitioning into 'old age' is no longer relevant.

The ability for individuals to remain in the workforce, stay active, have purpose, and maintain reasonable health all indicate that this is a varied and diverse generation. Using chronological age can be a limiting means of defining age groups. Attempting to categorise or define 'old age' can serve to promote generational divide, fostering misunderstandings, and ignoring the diverse experiences and contributions of older people. When considering how older people themselves define what it means to be 'old' it is important to recognise the determining factors that inform individual views, as these can vary. Examples of such differing concepts of ageing might include:

- An 80-year-old with unimpaired cognitive function who continues to live independently, engage socially, has some reduced mobility, and who does not label themselves as having reached 'old age' yet.
- A 65-year-old who has recently recovered from a heart attack and is now undergoing rehabilitation through a G.P. referral scheme, who deem themselves as 'over-the-hill' and old.

Additionally, the characteristics of older age are diverse and unique, likewise the needs of individuals in this age group. Table 16.2 shows the diversity of experiences in the older population.

Table 16.2 Diversity in the older population

Example	*Key statistic/Information (UK)*
Increase in Older People with diverse Ethnic Backgrounds	The number of people aged over 60 with ethnic backgrounds other than white has increased by 80% in ten years (ONS, 2023)
Bisexual and Gay men aged 65+ Living alone	More than half of bisexual and gay men aged 65+ live alone (ONS, 2023)
Total number of people aged 50+ living alone	Almost 5 million people aged 50 and over live alone (ONS, 2023)
Disability Rates among Older Adults (ages 70–74)	By the age of 70–74, one in three women and a quarter of men are classified disabled (ONS, 2023)
Sexual Orientation and Gender Identity among Older People	Over 4 x as many people aged 45–64 identify as LGB+ and over 2 x as many identify as Trans within the age group as for those aged 65+ (ONS, 2023)
Employment of Adults aged 65+	The number of people in employment aged 65 years and over rose to a record high 2022, working an average of 21.7 hours per week (ONS, 2022)
The number of people in England aged 50 and over.	An increase by almost 7 million in 40 years to 21.4 million –four in ten of us are now aged 50 and over (ONS, 2023)
Number of Female London Marathon runners 50 – 70 years	In 2022 a 65% increase in female runners aged 50 and older finished the race since 2018, plus a 91% increase in female runners registering to run aged 60–69 years (Hill, 2022)
Owner occupied homes in persons over 65 years	80% (5.5 million) of people aged 65 years and over live in their own homes, 75% of are owned outright with no mortgage (English Housing Survey: Older peoples housing, 2020–21)
Number of older adults living in care homes	The number of adults over 65 years living in care homes 2021 was 278,946 in England and Wales, 56.4% of residents were aged 85 years and over (ONS, 2023)

Table 16.2 shows that there is not one type of older person, but that older people live diverse lives. Older adults are not a single, undifferentiated group but encompass individuals with diverse backgrounds, identities, lifestyles, and health statuses. Actively seeking to understand this in relation to the ageing population drives change and challenges the often long held misconceptions that shape the societal narrative. Recognition of this fosters a more inclusive and person-centred approach to ageing, which considers the unique needs, preferences, and strengths of everyone.

Ageism

The negative perception of ageing and having an ageing population can lead to stereotypical labels and ageist attitudes. This can significantly impact the lived experience of the individual. Butler (2008) suggested that the social construction of ageing (thinking about what it is to age) is rooted in ageism – the systemic labelling and discrimination against older adults.

Ageism in the UK presents several societal and structural challenges, as older individuals report experiencing stereotyping, discrimination, and exclusion in various sectors such as employment, healthcare, and social engagement (Independent Age, 2023). Ageist attitudes or assumptions held about older individuals can have significant effect on the person experiencing such behaviour.

For example, older people may be subject to some of the following:

- *Direct Discrimination* – when an individual is treated differently or unfairly disadvantaged due to a particular characteristic, e.g. a travel insurance company has a policy that refuses to offer coverage to anyone over the age of 70, regardless of their health or medical history; an active and healthy 72-year-old applies for coverage but is automatically denied solely because of their age. These are clear cases of direct age discrimination, as the refusal is based purely on age rather than individual circumstances.
- *Indirect Discrimination* – when a policy or rule applies to everyone but can disadvantage a person with a protected characteristic, e.g. in 2009, the BBC decided to reposition its programme 'Countryfile' to a prime-time slot, resulting in the dismissal of four female presenters – all in their 40s and 50s. The BBC cited the need to appeal to a younger audience as the reason for this change. This case underscores how policies, even if not overtly discriminatory, can inadvertently marginalise older people, based purely on age.
- *Harassment* – behaviour that is deemed offensive by the recipient, e.g. humiliation and degradation. An older employee is regularly subjected to derogatory comments from colleagues, such as 'You're too old to keep up' or 'When are you going to retire?' This creates a hostile work environment.
- *Victimisation* – where one person treats another less favourably because they have asserted their legal rights or helped someone to do so, e.g. an older resident of a local community centre reports ageist behaviour after younger members repeatedly make dismissive remarks during group discussions, such as 'You're too old to understand social media trends'. After filing the complaint, the community centre staff respond by excluding the older resident from future workshops and social events, claiming they are 'not a good fit' for modern topics. This victimisation occurs because they were penalised for standing up against discrimination.

As highlighted above, ageism can have profound and multiple impacts on the lives of older individuals, undermining their rights, wellbeing, and sense of belonging in society. Addressing ageist attitudes and stereotypes is essential for fostering a culture of respect, inclusion, and equity across all ages. Challenging discrimination in any form through social consciousness is necessary to uphold societal values and foster community cohesion.

Challenging ageism and promoting opportunity

As the population ages and older people increasingly remain 'present', the marginalisation and often ingrained age bias linked to age is a destructive force and can have negative impacts upon health, (Levy *et al.*, 2018). Social consciousness is necessary to uphold societal values, foster community cohesion and commitment to the promotion of continued life course development and wellbeing.

Table 16.3 presents some key issues related to ageism, and potential actions to overcome ageism and promote opportunity.

Table 16.3 suggests that instead of rigidly defining 'old age', it might be necessary to challenge or question our personal beliefs or views of this age group. In doing so, we begin to gain the level of awareness and understanding required to truly promote diversity and inclusion of all. Welcoming diversity and respecting differences are an essential aspect

Table 16.3 Issues and actions related to ageism

Issue	*Action*
Limited Opportunities: Ageist attitudes may result in older individuals being overlooked for employment, promotion, or participation in certain activities based on stereotypes about their abilities, productivity, or relevance (Centre for Ageing Better, 2020). This can lead to feelings of exclusion, diminished self-worth, and financial insecurity.	***Education and Employment***: Offer choice and opportunity for older individuals to remain engaged in the workforce, contributing their experience, expertise and insight in a shared multi-generational environment. Enable continued learning, skill development, and employment opportunities for older adults that include access to training programmes, re-employment services, and flexible work arrangements.
Healthcare Disparities: Ageist assumptions about older adults' health and vitality can result in disparities in healthcare delivery and treatment options. Older patients may receive less aggressive or comprehensive care, be undertreated for certain conditions, or face age-based discrimination in accessing medical services, leading to poorer health outcomes and diminished quality of life.	***Education and Awareness***: National and community campaigns to raise awareness about ageism and its impact on individuals and society (Centre for Ageing Better, 2021, 31). Promoting and celebrating the diversity and value of older adults' contributions can challenge stereotypes and strengthen positive attitudes towards ageing.
Social Isolation: Ageist attitudes can contribute to social isolation and loneliness among older adults, as the need to facilitate social engagement and inclusion may not be prioritised. This can result in reduced social support networks, fewer opportunities for meaningful social engagement, and increased risk of mental health issues such as depression and anxiety.	***Age-Friendly Environments***: Creating age-friendly communities and public spaces that accommodate the needs and preferences of people of all ages. Designing accessible infrastructure, transportation systems, and recreational facilities promotes inclusivity and enhances quality of life for older adults (WHO, 2023)
Internalised Stereotypes: Older individuals may internalise ageist stereotypes and negative perceptions about ageing, leading to self-limiting beliefs, diminished self-confidence, and reluctance to seek out new opportunities or experiences (Centre for Ageing Better, 2021). This can have detrimental effects on mental and emotional wellbeing, as well as hinder personal growth and fulfilment in later life.	***Representation in Media and Advertising***: Promoting accurate and positive portrayals of older adults in media, advertising, and popular culture through representation of older individuals in diverse roles and contexts can combat internalised stereotypes and reinforce the richness of ageing experiences.
Erosion of Dignity and Autonomy: Ageist attitudes that portray older adults as dependent, frail, or burdensome can undermine their sense of dignity, autonomy, and agency. Older individuals may feel disempowered, patronised, or marginalised in their interactions with others, leading to feelings of frustration, resentment, or resignation.	***Advocacy and Empowerment***: Active empowerment of older adults to advocate for their rights and participate in decision-making processes that affect their lives. Supporting grassroots initiatives, advocacy groups, and community organisations amplifies older voices and promotes social change (Age NI, 2021)

(*Continued*)

Table 16.3 (Continued)

Issue	*Action*
Intergenerational Relationships: Ageist stereotypes can strain relationships between different age groups, fostering misunderstanding, resentment, and mistrust. Younger generations may perceive older adults through a lens of ageist assumptions, while older adults may feel undervalued or dismissed by younger counterparts, leading to intergenerational tensions and social fragmentation.	***Promoting Intergenerational Interaction & Reciprocity***: Facilitating opportunities for meaningful interaction and collaboration between different age groups has proven to be successful as a means of bridging the generational divides. Encouraging intergenerational activities, such as mentorship programmes, community projects, and cultural exchanges, promotes understanding, empathy, and mutual respect across generations (Webster *et al.*, 2023)
Policy outcomes: Ageist attitudes can influence public policies and resource allocation decisions, perpetuating systemic inequalities and barriers to social participation and inclusion for older adults. Lack of access to age-appropriate services, support programmes, and infrastructure can further exacerbate disparities and limit opportunities for older individuals to age with dignity and autonomy.	***Legislation and Policies***: Strengthening anti-discrimination laws and policies such as the *Equality Act (2010)* to explicitly prohibit age-based discrimination in employment, housing, healthcare and other areas.

of working within health and social care and relates to all groups within society – older adults are not an exception. Limiting our ability to 'see' individuals beyond stereotypical norms or labels minimises our capacity to consider the needs of all equally.

By challenging traditional norms or expectations of retirement years, older adults are empowered to explore opportunities in employment, entrepreneurship, creative pursuits, and civic engagement. This approach enables individuals to share their skills, wisdom, and talents, enhancing their sense of autonomy, self-worth, and identity. Embracing these themes fosters a supportive environment that values the contributions of older adults, enabling them to flourish as essential members of society and enjoy a fulfilling, high-quality life in their later years.

Towards 'healthy ageing'

The previous section outlined that adopting positive action in relation to life span development is pivotal in creating a shift to drive policy and behaviour change (Centre for Ageing Better, 2021). One way that this can be done is by embracing the concept of growing old as the norm, as this encourages a proactive approach to promoting 'healthy ageing' and preventing age-related decline. The WHO (2020) have used the idea of 'healthy ageing' to describe the functional ability to maintain wellbeing into older age. It recognises that ageing is a dynamic process influenced by lifestyle factors, social determinants, and environmental conditions.

What is 'healthy ageing'?

The aim of healthy ageing is to facilitate and support the continued good health of individuals as they progress throughout the older adulthood years, and recognising that older adults continue to grow and contribute meaningfully helps ensure they are valued and respected in society. It focuses on understanding and thinking of older adults as a diverse group with individual needs, as opposed to referring to 'old people' as a single sweeping statement that refers to all old people, leading to inclusion and recognition. By valuing older persons as participative members of society, this can help maintain and foster positive frameworks of ageing that may challenge age norms and stereotypes.

Within the UK, Wales and Northern Ireland have appointed a commissioner for older people who independently champion the rights of older people. The role is to ensure the needs of the older population are recognised and considered at both national and community levels, raising awareness, and creating an inclusive approach to targeted policy making and transformative change. The voice of older people is heard through participative engagement with community groups to protect and promote the views of older people themselves.

Healthy ageing can be supported through several key actions, including promoting wellbeing, a focus on life course development, encouraging intergenerational engagement, and implementing targeted policies. These are outlined in more detail below.

Promoting wellbeing

Viewing ageing as a natural and normal part of the life course encourages a more holistic or whole person perspective on health and wellbeing. Instead of focusing solely on medical needs or deficits associated with ageing, it acknowledges the importance of social, emotional, and environmental factors in shaping older adults' experiences and outcomes. This holistic approach recognises that successful ageing involves not only managing health conditions but also fostering social connections, maintaining independence, and pursuing meaningful activities. Age UK's *Index of Wellbeing* (2017) captured the concept of 'wholeness' when considering the experience of older persons as an expression of 'how well older people are doing', as shown in Figure 16.2.

As Figure 16.2 shows, living well into the older adulthood years is dependent upon multiple factors from environment, social inclusion and connectivity to housing and income, all of which may facilitate the opportunity to continue to thrive independently. However, physical health is the single common factor that influences the extent to which people age healthily.

The 'Men's Shed's' is an example of successful targeted intervention with an overarching aim of promoting older men's health and wellbeing. The UK Men's Sheds Association (2023) report suggests that there are over 1,130 projects within the UK equating to approximately 30,000 people attending each week. The Men's Sheds has taken the traditional idea of pursuing garden shed activities from a lone pastime to one that brings men together to reduce isolation and loneliness through social connection, friendship building and skills sharing. The Men's Shed movement actively engages in a diverse range of community projects, from restoring village landmarks to maintaining local parks and green spaces. Shed projects often collaborate with schools, libraries, and support individuals in need by building or repairing essential items. While activities vary widely, a typical Shed might feature woodworking, metalworking, electronics, and model building, and some even include car restoration projects, creating an inclusive space for skill-sharing, creativity, and community contribution. Mcgrath *et al.*'s (2022) study has cemented the reputation of Men's Sheds 'as settings that are inherently health promoting for men, with Sheds increasingly being seen by health and social policy makers as an exemplar for the promotion of men's health and well-being'.

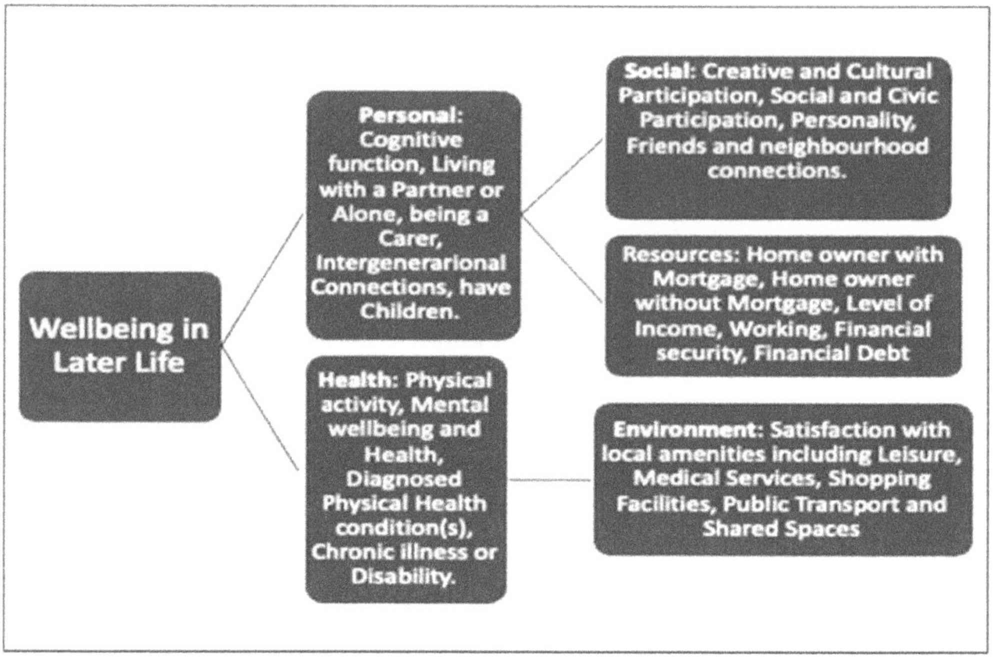

Figure 16.2 Issues affecting the wellness of older people.
Source: Adapted from Age UK's Index of Wellbeing in Later Life (Green *et al.*, 2017).

A focus on life course development

The relevance of considering life course development as a continuous and evolving developmental life journey is key to respecting individual growth across the life span – beginning to end, conception to death. Increasingly, western society has hailed youth and youthfulness as being the 'gold standard' point of the life course, linking youthfulness to societal worth, meaning individual value continues if one is deemed 'young or youthful' as opposed to old and redundant. The **life course approach contrasts with life span approach** (Learning Box 16.1) – through its focus upon growth as a lifelong process rather than one that is chronologically or age defined as promoted by Baltes' theory of development (1987). This outlines ageing as being a lifelong, multidirectional process that is dependent upon transitions and adaption, and later in Elder's (1994) work relating to life course theory.

Several main themes emerge when considering life course development into older adulthood:

1 **Healthy Ageing**: The focus is on prioritising key aspects of physical and mental wellbeing as individuals age to include promoting healthy lifestyles, regular exercise, nutritious diet, and access to healthcare services. It also includes encouraging preventive measures and early intervention can help individuals maintain independence and quality of life as they grow older.

Learning Box 16.1: Life course v lifespan approach

Life course and lifespan are often used to mean the same thing, but they have different meanings

Life course refers to the sequence of socially defined events and roles that individuals experience throughout their lives that shape personal growth and transitions. This concept highlights how life stages such as childhood and adulthood plus major life events such as marriage and career choices influence individual development over time.

Lifespan refers to years lived and the biological stages form birth to death. This typically focuses on biological ageing, longevity and the stages of physical growth and decline from birth to death.

2 **Active Engagement:** The development of opportunities for older adults to stay actively engaged in their communities through social, cultural, and recreational activities. This may include access to public transport, suitable communal spaces, volunteering, and participation in community events. It also includes encouraging social connections and meaningful relationships that can combat loneliness and isolation, enhancing overall wellbeing and continuing engagement, employment opportunities that offer similar engagement advantages.
3 **Lifelong Learning:** This is focused on recognising the value of continued learning and personal development throughout the lifespan. It also includes providing access to educational programmes, workshops, and skill-building initiatives enables older adults to pursue their interests, stay mentally stimulated, and adapt to changing circumstances as well as maintaining cognitive vitality.
4 **Financial Security:** Targeting and addressing concerns related to financial stability and retirement planning. It also includes promoting financial literacy and offering support services for managing finances empower older adults to maintain their independence and dignity.
5 **Intergenerational Exchange** (Learning Box 16.2): Being proactive in encouraging mutual support and interaction between different age groups. It also includes facilitating opportunities for intergenerational relationships, such as mentoring programmes or shared activities, promotes understanding, empathy, and a sense of community cohesion. Breaking down age-related stereotypes and fostering respect for diverse perspectives enriches societal bonds.
6 **Cultural Inclusivity:** Recognising and celebrating the diversity of experiences, backgrounds, and identities within the older population. It also includes promoting inclusivity and accessibility in services, policies, and public spaces ensures that all individuals can participate fully and enjoy a sense of belonging, regardless of age, ethnicity, gender, or other factors.
7 **Purpose and Fulfilment:** Focusing on supporting older adults in finding continued meaning, purpose, and fulfilment in their lives.

By challenging traditional norms or expectations of retirement years, older adults are empowered to explore opportunities in employment, entrepreneurship, creative pursuits,

Learning Box 16.2: Intergenerational terminology explained

Intergenerational: Relating to or involving people of different generations, typically focusing on connections, interactions, or influences between younger and older individuals.

Intergenerational Exchange: The sharing of knowledge, skills, or resources between different generations, often benefiting both parties (e.g. grandparents teaching traditional skills to grandchildren while learning about new technology in return).

Intergenerational Engagement: Any interaction between people of different generations that fosters connection, communication, and understanding, but without necessarily requiring a mutual exchange (e.g. young people volunteering in care homes to socialise with older adults).

Intergenerational Integration: The process of actively including and connecting different generations in shared spaces, communities, or activities to create a cohesive society (e.g. multi-generational housing projects or community centres designed for all age groups).

and civic engagement. This approach enables individuals to share their skills, wisdom, and talents, enhancing their sense of autonomy, self-worth, and identity. Embracing these themes fosters a supportive environment that values the contributions of older adults, with the opportunity to continue to flourish as essential members of society and enjoy a fulfilling, high-quality life in their later years.

Intergenerational engagement

Intergenerational engagement and continued connections between age groups within families, social settings, the workplace and through community spaces serves to facilitate respectful transition throughout the life course stages. The inter-connections created when barriers to intergenerational integration are removed help provide the space to nurture a culture and environment that enables dignity and respect to be reciprocated across the age boundaries and build bridges across divides that may exist.

The notion of a generational division between age groups has become significantly more acute (Carney and Nash, 2020: 97), due in part to social media and ageist attitudes, which can be used to reinforce negativity aimed at this age group. Together with more tangible examples being highlighted, as shown in Table 16.1 such as a lack of affordable housing for younger people or altered value systems, these can be presented as a negative result of having an ageing population. However, when considering how the social inclusion and mixing of age groups appears to be the accepted norm within some settings, such as greater integration of generational groups at mass gathering such as festivals, concerts or sporting events, this means that the reality might be that the divide is less embedded than we think or are led to believe.

Actively generating solidarity between generations can become a driving force for change when considering breaking down ageist stereotypes (of all ages). Harnessing the notion of shared values, and equal position within society whereby all can grow and develop is a concept that is captured through strategies such as 'Age Friendly Cities and Communities programmes' (AFCC), (World Health Organization, 2023) and the *Wellbeing of Future Generations Act (Wales) 2015*. Both seek to create environments that are age inclusive and facilitate positive life course development through the pursuit of establishing cities that are 'age-friendly'. Through considerate planning and focused attention on specific issues such as housing, health and social care, transport, and access to outdoor spaces as well as broader aspects of the wider community, innovative planning can drive generational connections.

Fostering healthy environments that are responsive to the needs of all age groups is in its nature inclusive, as all citizens benefit from such long-term sustainable planning for the future. Similarly reinforcing intergenerational shared experience, integrated spaces and tolerant communities undoubtedly offers richer lived experiences and wider wellbeing benefits for all. Below are examples of innovative intergenerational engagement, exchange, and integration schemes:

1. **Intergenerational Skill-Sharing schemes** – Retired professionals share expertise in areas, such as coding, business, and creative writing, mentoring students on school projects and future careers.
2. **Home Sharing Affordable Living** – pairing university students with seniors for affordable living and support for both the student and older person.
3. **Designing public libraries for use as community intergenerational hubs,** such as the HIVE library in Worcester.

Promoting intergenerational dialogue and inclusive policies can foster mutual respect, reduce stigma, and build a society that values individuals for their abilities, experiences, and contributions rather than their age.

Targeted policy making and support of the older population

In addressing the support needs of older persons, it is essential to create an integrated and adaptable approach that enables continued independence and community involvement. The goal of an integrated service approach is twofold: to support older adults in maintaining their health and independence for as long as possible, and to effectively manage the complexities of care as health declines. This requires a focus in policy making, where health and social care services are interconnected to respond to individual needs holistically. By aligning healthcare support with community resources and social services, we can create a responsive framework that enables timely interventions, promotes active lifestyles, and provides care continuity as older adults transition through varying levels of need.

Therefore, the focus of policy needs to be on:

a. Promoting good health and supporting independence.
b. Prioritising the wellbeing and sustainability of future generations
c. Establishing integrated services to offer sustainable person-centred health and social care provision.

Community level projects emerge through the implementation of national policies. These apply the overarching policy aim and objectives, to meet the specific needs of the community, often through targeted interventions and localised schemes.

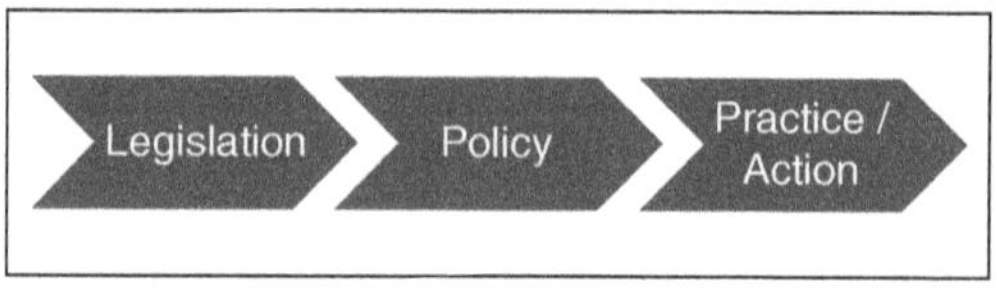

Figure 16.3 From legislation to policy to action.

It is important to remember that legislation set the rules and overall direction of policies (see Chapter 6). Policies are created based on these laws to guide decisions and actions as shown in Figure 16.3. These policies then shape what happens in real life, influencing how things are done in communities and organisations.

Implementation of strategies and policy that plan for future care needs of our older populations will aid the continuity of sector commitment and ongoing resource requirements. For instance, digital health solutions can be harnessed to monitor health remotely, thereby reducing the frequency of hospital visits and enabling proactive care. Community-based initiatives, such as social clubs and volunteer programmes, can help address social needs, reinforcing the sense of belonging and reducing isolation. Integrating these aspects within a robust service model can lead to healthier, more engaged ageing populations who can continue contributing to and participating in their communities. However, it will be reliant on continued investment into the life course approach to health and ageing.

Innovative projects such as the *Healthy ageing challenge* is funding research into diverse determinants, such as the need for creating healthy active spaces, supporting social connections, living well with cognitive impairment, and design for age-friendly homes is an example of such investment by the UK government. The aim is to enable people to remain active, productive, independent, and socially connected across generations for as long as possible.

Examples of key policies and strategic plans which are being used to enable such approaches:

- The UN Decade of Healthy Ageing (2021–2030)
- WHO Global Strategy and Action Plan (2016 – 2020)
- The Strategy for Older People in Wales (2013–2023)
- Age Friendly Wales: Our Strategy for an Ageing Society (2021)
- The NHS Long Term Plan (2019)
- *Care Act 2014*
- UK Digital Strategy (2022)
- The Healthy Ageing Challenge (2019)

Strategic goal setting on international, national and community levels is the result of the emerging awareness that the changing demographic profiles of populations requires sustainable provision and resources.

Summary

Ageing, specifically into the older adulthood phase, involves a level of physical decline – this is an inevitable result of 'years lived'. The human body is not a machine that will continue forever even if we are able to replace worn out parts. However, the uniqueness of individuals, shaped by factors such as health, lifestyle, and personal choices, underscores the diversity in ageing outcomes. Ensuring healthy ageing is not only essential for individuals and their families but also critical for community welfare and socio-economic stability. Supporting the journey of growing older, with a commitment to fostering independence and wellbeing, involves embracing the value of lifelong development. It calls for challenging views on ageing, understanding the factors that promote healthy ageing, and advocating for policies and strategies that ensure older adults can age sustainably and with robust support.

References

Age NI (2021) *The lived experience 2021: What matters to older people in Northern Ireland.* Available at https://www.ageni.org/the-lived-experience-2021 (Accessed 28 June 2024).

Allen, S.G. (2023) 'Demand for older workers: What do we know? What do we need to learn?', *The Journal of the Economics of Ageing*, 24, p. 100414. Available at https://doi.org/10.1016/j.jeoa.2022.100414 (Accessed 8 January 2025).

Butler, R.N. (2008) *The Longevity Revolution: The Benefits and Challenges of Living a Long Life.* New York: Perseus Publishing.

Carney, G.M. and Nash, P. (2020) 'Why do older people have it so good?: The myth of intergenerational conflict', in *Critical Questions for Ageing Societies.* Bristol: Bristol University Press. Available at https://doi.org/10.51952/9781447358312.ch007 (Accessed 29 April 2024).

Centre for Ageing Better (2020) *An old age problem? How society shapes and reinforces negative attitudes to ageing.* Available at: https://ageing-better.org.uk/publications/old-age-problem (Accessed: 28 October 2024).

Centre for Ageing Better (2021) *Reframing ageing: Public perceptions of ageing, older age and demographic change.* Available at https://ageing-better.org.uk/resources/reframing-ageing-public-perceptions-ageing-older-age and-demographic-change (Accessed 13 April 2024).

Centre for Ageing Better (2023) *Our ageing population*, in *State of Ageing 2023-24.* Available at https://ageing-better.org.uk/our-ageing-population-state-ageing-2023-4 (Accessed 17 December 2024).

Dahlgren, G. and Whitehead, M. (2021) 'The Dahlgren-Whitehead model of health determinants: 30 years on and still chasing rainbows', *Public Health*, 199, pp. 20–24.

Department for Digital, Culture, Media and Sport (2022) *UK digital strategy 2022.* Available at https://www.gov.uk/government/publications/uk-digital-strategy (Accessed 28 October 2024).

Department for Levelling Up, Housing and Communities (2021) *English Housing Survey: Older people's housing 2020 21*, p. 20. Available at https://assets.publishing.service.gov.uk

Elder, G.H. (1994) 'Time, human agency, and social change: Perspectives on the life course', *Social Psychology Quarterly*, 57(1), pp. 4–15. Available at https://doi.org/10.2307/2786971

Equality Act 2010, c5. Available at https://www.legislation.gov.uk/ukpga/2010/15/contents (Accessed 20 October 2024).

Finlay, J. (2021) 'Intimately old: From an embodied to emplaced feminist approach to aging', *Hypatia*, 36(1), pp. 80–100. https://doi.org/10.1017/hyp.2020.5

Green, M., Iparraguirre, J., Davidson, S., Rossall, P., and Zaidi, A. (2017) *A summary of Age UK's Index of Wellbeing in Later Life.* Available at https://www.ageuk.org.uk/siteassets/documents/reports-and-publications/reports-and-briefings/health--wellbeing/ageuk-wellbeing-index-summary-web.pdf (Accessed 20 March 2024).

Hill, A. (2022) 'A sea of positivity: older women boost London Marathon numbers', *The Guardian*, 30 September. Available at https://www.theguardian.com/sport/2022/sep/30/a-sea-of-positivity-older-women-boost-london-marathon-numbers

Independent Age (2023) *Who wants to listen to me? Why England needs a Commissioner for Older People and Ageing.* Available at https://www.independentage.org/commissioner-report (Accessed 15 July 2024).

Jahnel, T., Dassow, H.H., Gerhardus, A. and Schüz, B. (2022) 'The digital rainbow: Digital determinants of health inequities', *Digital Health*, 8, pp. 1–10. Available at https://doi.org/10.1177/20552076221129093

Johfre, S. and Saperstein, A. (2023) 'The social construction of age: Concepts and measurement', *Annual Review of Sociology*, 49, pp. 339–358. Available at https://doi.org/10.1146/annurev-soc-031021-121020 (Accessed 10 February 2024).

Levy, B.R., Slade, M.D., Pietrzak, R.H. and Ferrucci, L. (2018) 'Positive age beliefs protect against dementia even among elders with high-risk gene', *PLoS ONE*, 13(2), p. e0191004. Available at https://doi.org/10.1371/journal.pone.0191004

McGrath, A., Murphy, N., Egan, T., Ormond, G. and Richardson, N. (2022) 'An economic evaluation of "sheds for life": A community-based men's health initiative for men's sheds in Ireland', *International Journal of Environmental Research and Public Health*, 19(4), p. 2204. https://doi.org/10.3390/ijerph19042204

Michaelson, J. (2012) *Measuring Well-Being: A Guide for Practitioners*. London: New Economics Foundation.

Mortimer, J.T. and Moen, P. (2016) 'The changing social construction of age and the life course: Precarious identity and enactment of "Early" and "Encore" stages of adulthood', in Shanahan, M., Mortimer, J., and Kirkpatrick Johnson, M. (eds.) *Handbook of the Life Course*. Cham: Springer. Available at https://doi.org/10.1007/978-3-319-20880-0_5

National programmes for age-friendly cities and communities: A guide (2023) Geneva: World Health Organization.

NHS (2019) *The NHS Long Term Plan*. Available at https://www.longtermplan.nhs.uk/publication/nhs-long-term-plan/ (Accessed 29 April 2024).

Office for National Statistics (2022) *People aged 65 years and over in employment, UK: January to March 2022 to April to June 2022*. Available at https://www.ons.gov.uk/ (Accessed 1 May 2024).

Office for National Statistics (ONS) (2023) *Profile of the older population living in England and Wales in 2021 and changes since 2011* (Accessed 1 May 2024).

Sealey, C. (2015) *Social Policy Simplified: Connecting Theory with People's Lives*. London; New York, NY: Palgrave Macmillan. Available at http://find.shef.ac.uk/openurl/44SFD/44SFD_services_page?u.ignore_date_coverage=true&rft.mms_id=9983301999601441 (Accessed 19 July 2022).

UK Government (2014) *Care Act 2014*, c.23. Available at https://www.legislation.gov.uk/ukpga/2014/23/contents/enacted (Accessed 28 September 2023).

UK Men's Sheds Association (UKMSA). (2023) Report submitted to the Health and Social Care Committee. (online) Available at: (https://menssheds.org.uk/wp-content/uploads/Written-evidence-V8-04-Sep-2023-Video-supplement.pdf)

UK Research and Innovation (2019) *The healthy ageing challenge framework*. Available at https://www.ukri.org/what-we-do/browse-our-areas-of-investment-and-support/healthy-ageing/ (Accessed 10 August 2024).

United Nations Department of Economic and Social Affairs, Population Division. (2022) *World Population Prospects 2022*. Available at https://population.un.org/wpp/Graphs/ (Accessed 20 September 2024).

Webster, M., Norwood, K., Waterworth, J. and Leavey, G. (2023) 'Effectiveness of intergenerational exchange programs between adolescents and older adults: A systematic review', *Journal of Intergenerational Relationships*. Advance online publication. Available at: https://doi.org/10.1080/15350770.2023.2267532

Welsh Government (2013) *The Strategy for Older People in Wales 2013–2023*. Cardiff: Welsh Government. Available at https://www.cymru.gov.uk Accessed 5 May 2023).

Welsh Government (2014) *Ageing Well in Wales: A Framework for Action 2014–2019*. Cardiff: Welsh Government. Available at http://www.cpa.org.uk (Accessed 5 April 2023).

Welsh Government (2021) *Age friendly Wales: Our strategy for an ageing society*, p. 15. Available at https://www.gov.wales/age-friendly-wales-our-strategy-ageing-society-html (Accessed 15 March 2023).

Welsh Government (2021) *Age friendly Wales: Our strategy for an ageing society*, p. 44, 45. Available at https://www.gov.wales/age-friendly-wales-our-strategy-ageing-society-html (Accessed 15 March 2023).

World Health Organization (2017) *Global Strategy and Action Plan on Ageing and Health (2016–2020)*. Geneva: World Health Organization. Available at https://www.who.int/publications/i/item/9789241513500 (Accessed 5 May 2024).

World Health Organization (2020) *The UN Decade of Healthy Ageing (2021–2030)*. Available at https://www.who.int/initiatives/decade-of-healthy-ageing (Accessed 10 August 2023).

World Health Organization (2023) *National programmes for age-friendly cities and communities a guide*. Available at: https://www.who.int/publications/i/item/9789240068698 (Accessed 24 September 2025)

Part 3

Essential practice skills for health and social care

17 Being a reflective practitioner within health and social care settings

Naomi Blaikie

The aims of this chapter are to:

- Define reflective practice and discuss its importance to health and social care practice
- Examine the purpose and features of reflective writing and exemplify how to do this effectively
- Explore barriers to reflective practice and provide tips to start the process of reflective practice

Introduction

Reflection is a vital part of health and social care practice. From the very start of your student journey to the end of your professional career, the ability to reflect on your practice and on workplace situations allows you to evaluate and improve your decision-making (Guy *et al.*, 2020). It also develops empathy (Chen and Forbes, 2014) and increases your own resilience and emotional wellbeing (Koh *et al.*, 2022), ultimately leading to the ability to care for people as effectively as possible – 'striving for excellence' (Bassot, 2016: 3).

This chapter provides a broad overview of reflective practice for students starting on health and social care courses but is equally valid for professionals and other professions, in helping you to understand the basics of the reflective process and guiding you towards the skills and resources needed to reflect effectively. The chapter argues that reflection is a key component to professional practice, and that everyone can and should reflect as part of their development.

This chapter is divided into three main sections. The first section focuses on what reflective practice is, and how it will help you as a student. Here the concept and importance of reflective practice are introduced, and how this relates to your professional journey. In the second section, we look at reflective writing and how it can be done effectively, by examining features of reflective writing and the types of written reflections you might be expected to submit at university. It also discusses models of reflection and examples of reflective writing. Finally, the third section looks at what you can do to develop and improve your reflective practice.

This chapter helps you to understand the importance of reflection, be able to structure your reflective practice by using recognised models, understand how to write reflectively for university assignments, identify barriers to being able to reflect effectively, and engage in exercises to enable you to start reflecting.

DOI: 10.4324/9781032619309-20

What is reflective practice and what practical use is it to me?

You may already be familiar with reflective practice – perhaps you have had professional experience previously, or maybe you have a personality which is naturally reflective and analytic. For others, the idea of reflecting might feel unfamiliar, uncomfortable or even a bit scary. To provide reassurance about this process, Koshy *et al.* (2017: 1) point out that we have been used to reflecting for our entire lives in everyday situations and that it is just 'thinking about and learning from past experiences to avoid things that did not work and to repeat things that did'.

If we consider the concept of reflection in everyday life, this can take different forms and can help to explain how reflection on our practice might be beneficial. Below are four ways that reflection literally occurs in everyday life:

- A magnifying mirror can give you a clear and accurate reflection of the minute details of your face.
- A dentist might use an angled mirror in a patient's mouth to allow access to a view they cannot see ordinarily.
- A lake on a sunny day might reflect the sunlight hitting its surface illuminating the environment around it.
- A rear-view mirror in a car allows you to see where you have been, and the side mirrors help you to orientate yourself and assess where other people are in relation to your position.

We can use these examples to illustrate why reflecting on our practice is important. It might be that the reflection process helps us examine our thoughts, feelings and experiences in finer detail like a magnifying mirror, or it might be so that we can see a different angle in terms of our perspective. Alternatively, reflection can be illuminating in the sense that we can get clarity about a situation, or, as with a rear-view mirror, it helps us see where we have come from and where we are going as we develop personally and professionally. Returning to the specific idea of reflective practice in a health and social care context, this can therefore be described as '... [providing] an opportunity for health professionals and students to learn from their mistakes, successes, anxieties, and worries that otherwise would remain disjointed and worthless ...' (Artioli *et al.*, 2021: 1). Boud *et al.* (1985: 19) also describe reflection as 'those intellectual and affective activities in which individuals engage to explore their experiences in order to lead to new understandings and appreciations'.

In addition to the benefits of reflective thinking mentioned earlier, it also allows you to increase your confidence (Davies, 2012), evaluate and develop your practice and professional skills (Bassot, 2016), increase your self-awareness (Contreras *et al.*, 2020), and help you process difficult situations and events (Curry and Epley, 2022).

So what does reflection practically require you to do? Well, reflection involves taking time to think analytically about your practice (this is likely to be evaluating a particular event on placement) either on your own, with your mentor, or with another trusted person. It is about looking back at a situation and asking yourself questions about it to gain a full understanding of what was happening at the time, to evaluate what was successful and what needs to be improved next time. Reflection is continuous, so while you may focus on an incident in detail at any one time, the action of reflecting will occur again and again as you continue in your practice.

While the next section looks at reflective models and writing in more detail, Nicol and Dosser (2016: 39) suggest some initial prompt questions that can be used when thinking reflectively. These may provide a helpful starting point as you think back and analyse a situation in practice. The questions are:

1 What happened?
2 How did I feel?
3 What are the main points?
4 What do I need to explore further?
5 What are my initial thoughts were this to happen again?

You will notice that while the first question here seems to be asking you to recount the situation, the other questions encourage you to think in a deeper way about your experience. Reflection should be more than describing an event, it needs to include analysis, evaluation, and ultimately move you forward in your practice.

Becoming a reflective practitioner through reflective writing as a student

This section summarises the purposes and features of reflective writing, highlights the types of reflective writing you may be asked to put together for your assignments, and examines how reflection can be structured through a reflective model using fictionalised examples.

What are the purposes of reflective writing?

Reflection is noticeably different to other forms of academic writing as has been mentioned. As Bassot (2020: 18) highlights, it is **analytical rather than purely descriptive** (Learning Box 17.1), it allows a chance for you to unburden yourself as a type of

Learning Box 17.1: Reflective writing – analytical versus descriptive

If we revisit the idea of the reflective process as 'those intellectual and affective activities in which individuals engage to explore their experiences in order to lead to new understandings and appreciations' (Boud *et al.*, 1985: 19), then we can see that 'engaging' and 'exploring' require deeper thinking than just reporting back on something that happened.

Examples of analytical versus descriptive writing in reflection are excellently demonstrated in 'The Park' by Jenny Moon (2004), a writing exercise which is included in the third section of this chapter, showing differing levels of analysis from a single event.

According to Moon, a purely descriptive account is written from one perspective, tells the story but not much else, is sequential, contains no exploration of feelings or viewpoints, and no questioning of ideas or opinions (2004).

In contrast, a piece of analytical reflective writing is far more effective in helping you process your thoughts. Moon describes such an account as being purposeful, involves you standing back from the event, often includes the presence of your internal dialogue asking and answering questions of yourself, includes looking from other perspectives, and recognising the effect of your own emotions on your viewpoint (Moon, 2004).

'self-supervision', it can provide you with a written account of how you felt at various points and is an 'investment of your time in your own learning and development'. It could be argued that any form of academic work is a similar investment, but the nature of reflection means that it will be individualised and personal to you and will allow you to continue to learn from it in a functional and meaningful way.

Spencer and Healey (2022) emphasise the very practical fact that it is more effective to write our reflections down so that we do not forget them, and to help us focus and analyse the event. Whether you are keeping a more informal reflective diary over your placement that only you read, or whether you are submitting a reflective assignment, the act of writing down the thoughts and experiences you have had allows you to evidence your development as you go through the course.

What are the specific characteristics of reflective writing?

Reflective writing has a number of specific characteristics. Four key aspects have been highlighted below:

1 It is written in the first person, so use 'I', 'me', and 'my' statements in your reflective accounts, rather than the third person ('the author decided', etc.) as you might do for an academic assignment.
2 If you are fully reflecting, it is likely to include some aspect of your personal feelings. Depending on how expressive a personality you have, and which reflective model you are using (see later in the chapter), it might contain quite emotive language as you analyse your reactions and responses to a given situation.
3 Linked very closely to this, reflection needs to provide an opportunity where you can write in an honest and open way. Although your reflective account might include underpinning literature if it is an academic assignment, you should still be writing in an authentic manner. Hopefully, you will find it a dynamic and cathartic experience as you process your emotions and experiences, with some personal revelations as you write and reflect.
4 Effective reflection includes positives and negatives – rather than beating yourself up or denying that there are no improvements you can possibly make – and should avoid 'absolute judgements' (Williams *et al.*, 2020: 64).

When might I be asked to write reflectively on my course or at placement?

This will depend on the exact requirements of your course, but you are likely to be asked to write reflectively in a reflective journal and/or in reflective assignments. These are described below.

Reflective journal

You may be asked to keep a reflective journal throughout your placement. Some examples of this might be:

- writing notes at the end of the day in a book or on a device
- recording voice notes on your phone
- using one of the many different reflective journalling apps available
- writing quick reminder notes throughout the day to remind you of the experiences later
- drawing a mind map with prompt words and linked reflections.

It's possible you will be given a particular template or model to do this, but unless you need to submit anything to university, it makes sense to use the method you find most effective.

Reflective assignments

You may be asked to write a reflective account of an incident on placement. Again, you might be given a template or model to unpick a particular event or scenario. As these are university assignments, you will need to underpin your analysis with relevant academic literature, which will allow you to understand more about what was happening in the situation – for you, and others – and will inform your practice going forward.

It is vital that you follow your university or organisation's confidentiality policy when writing reflectively about your practice. Use initials, use anonymised names, but do not allow anything you write to be identifiable in terms of a client, relative, staff member or placement setting.

How do I structure a reflection?

One way of structuring your reflective writing is by using a model. There are a number of models that have been developed which provide prompts for you to reflect effectively on an event in practice. Usually, these models are structured as a cycle, with the idea that reflective practice is a continuing process. Many of these models form the same sort of arrangement – the first stage begins by prompting you to describe an event or situation, then encourages you to analyse and evaluate the various aspects of this, and then finally to consider what resolutions you might take forward for future practice. After this, the cyclical model feeds back into the first stage where you continue reflecting on your practice with this newly acquired learning.

For the purposes of this chapter, we are focusing on two widely used models:

- Driscoll's Model of Reflection (2007)
- Gibbs' Reflective Cycle (1998)

Driscoll's Model of Reflection (2007)

A simplified version of Driscoll's 'Model of Reflection' is shown in Figure 17.1.

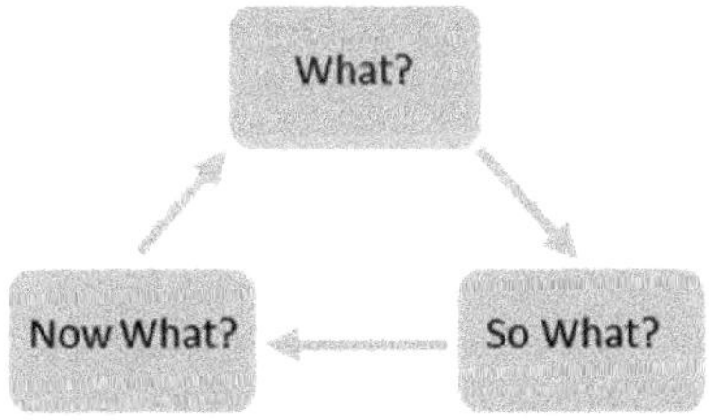

Figure 17.1 Driscoll's model of reflection.

Source: Adapted by author.

As shown in Figure 17.1, Driscoll's model is a three-stage process that uses three key questions to act as prompt questions to aid reflection:

- The 'What?' stage is a factual description of the event or situation.
- The 'So What?' stage is the part where the analysis takes place, and this where the person reflecting is prompted to think about the implications of what happened, and what the conclusions of this learning might be.
- The 'Now What' stage then examines what actions might be taken forward in practice with this new learning; and then the cycle continues from the 'What' stage as the learning is applied.

Below is an example of reflective writing using Driscoll's Model of Reflection (2007):

What?

Today I started my placement at the youth club. I felt nervous, and despite enjoying my local youth club when I was younger, I felt out of place and awkward as I realised I was no longer a young person attending, but one of the adults supporting them. I introduced myself to two of the young people who attend and tried to make a joke, and as I walked away, one of them said something to the other and they both laughed to themselves whilst looking in my direction. I've no idea if it was about me, or just coincidental, but it dented my confidence.

So what?

I questioned why it bothered me so much. It doesn't seem as though it was that long ago that I was attending a youth club myself, and while I know it's not my place to try and be a 'friend' to these young people, I don't yet feel mature or respected enough to feel like a leader. It has made me feel a bit flat and vulnerable and I'm already dreading next week. That said, from the perspective of the young people I talked to, perhaps I came over a bit over-friendly, or weird, even. I don't feel like I have found my feet yet with my identity and role in this setting. I know that in terms of ethical practice, I need to ensure that I understand and maintain appropriate boundaries with these young people. It would be unprofessional and potentially unsafe for both me and the young people to try and support them without knowing where the boundaries lie between being friendly and being in a leadership role. The National Youth Agency highlight the importance of age-appropriate and healthy boundaries in a youth setting, which, when maintained correctly, should build the confidence of all involved, including the workers (National Youth Agency, 2021). Hart (2016) asserts that young people are often very willing to work within these boundaries and respect them, which is reassuring to me. I think establishing and maintaining clear roles and boundaries will be important to everyone, especially the young people I will be working with, and this will help manage everyone's expectations. In terms of confidence, I am hoping that the more I work here, the more confident and 'at home' I will feel. One thing I identified with my personal tutor before I started placement was about increasing my resilience. Benaton et al. (2022: 49) describe emotional resilience as like wearing a 'multi-functioning coat' that can give some protection as you work in a challenging setting, and this is what I would like to begin to develop on placement. I am hoping that gaining a clear sense of professional boundaries in my behaviour (in terms of how to relate to the young people; knowing the limits of my role, etc.) will help with this sense of confidence and resilience.

Now what?

While I feel like I am just at the start of this journey, this initial reflection has led me to identify two big aspects that I would like to develop – an understanding of effective boundaries, and emotional resilience. I have arranged to speak to my mentor next week and get some advice about establishing clear boundaries (even while I don't feel like a leader) and will be looking into how to increase my emotional resilience. The youth club have also suggested some training which they offer to volunteers in terms of roles and responsibilities in the setting which will also help. I still feel nervous, but at least I can go back into the setting knowing what I can start focusing on, and to be aware of how I interact with the young people in an appropriate and effective way.

Using Driscoll's model as a continuous cycle means that the new knowledge that this student might gain about boundaries and how to increase resilience will feed back into the model as they move forward in practice. The next time they use the model, their 'What' section will be a situation which is informed by their new learning, their next 'So What' section will analyse and evaluate their knowledge and examine what else they might need to learn or develop, and their subsequent 'Now What' section will have a new set of actions to take forward. How does using this model add to our learning? Well, by using a template in this way, we have a systematic order of prompts to follow, allowing us to structure our thoughts and aid reflection in an effective way, always looking towards improving our future practice. To get even more from the reflective experience using this framework, consider looking at the specific cue questions that Rolfe added to their revised version of Driscoll's model (Rolfe *et al.*, 2011: 45).

Gibbs' Reflective Cycle (1998)

A simplified version of Gibbs' Reflective Cycle is shown in Figure 17.2.

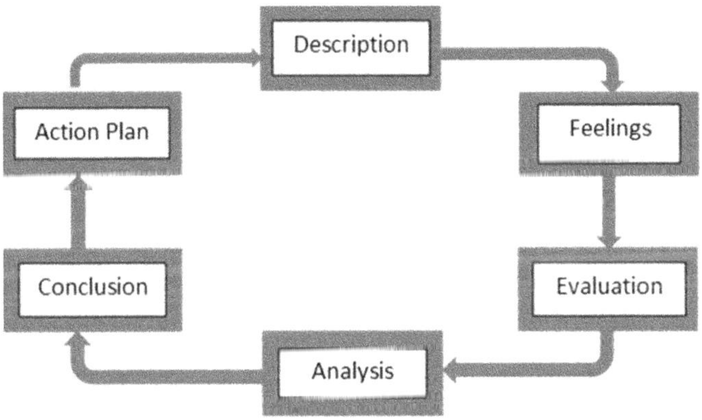

Figure 17.2 Gibbs' reflective cycle.

Source: Adapted by author.

Similarly to Driscoll's model above, Gibbs' reflective cycle encourages the same process in terms of describing an event, evaluating it, and having actions, or learning, to take forward. It is a more structured model with six steps rather than three and considers personal feelings as a distinct stage. As with every model, there are pros and cons of using it. These extra stages can be both beneficial to those wanting more structure, but potentially unhelpful to those who don't necessarily want to focus on all these aspects in a quick reflection. An example of the Gibbs' model in action is set out below.

Description

Today on placement, one of the residents at the care home, Joan, became very distressed and said she didn't like the dog barking in the lounge. There was nothing there that I could see, so I tried to comfort Joan by telling her she didn't need to worry, but she continued to cry, and the senior carer intervened.

Feelings

I felt upset that I couldn't comfort Joan, confused about what was going on, and frustrated that I couldn't help. I felt relief when the senior carer came over but pretty rubbish for not being able to make things better for Joan. I know this is my first placement and I don't know everything, but I wanted to be able to sort the situation out. I guess it made me feel like a failure, and I didn't understand what was happening.

Evaluation

My instinct to show empathy and concern was correct – Joan was clearly frightened, and I felt upset for her. My approach to this was not successful though. Ultimately though, Joan was comforted, which was the most important thing, even if I couldn't help her.

Analysis

I have spent some time talking to my mentor and placement tutor about this. I know that people living with dementia can experience auditory and visual hallucinations, and this has been particularly linked to certain types of dementia, such as Lewy body dementia (Eversfield and Orton, 2019; Mehraram et al., 2020) which might explain Joan's actions. In terms of reacting to this in a positive way, research has shown that validating the person's reality is an important step in supporting them if they are experiencing a distressing hallucination (Blackhall et al., 2011). I found it upsetting to see Joan so distressed, and I guess this is part of the job, and something I either need to talk through with my mentor, or something that will get easier with time and experience. I am hoping I can admit how uncomfortable this made me, and not feel guilty for it.

Conclusion

I now understand that the residents I work with, such as Joan, may experience hallucinations, and that if they are distressed, I need to ensure I validate their reality and emotions, rather than trying to tell them the situation is not real.

Action plan

In order to allow me to support residents more effectively if this situation arose again, I will spend time looking at the VERA framework (Blackhall et al., 2011) and Validation Therapy (Feil, 1992) to gain a further understanding of the suggested steps to take if I need to comfort someone experiencing a hallucination in the care home.

In terms of carrying this forward using Gibbs' cycle, the aim is to put your new-found knowledge and skills into practice. The next time that you work with Joan, you would then consider the **VERA framework** (Learning Box 17.2) in your communication with her, and the reflective cycle continues from the beginning again. How does using this model add to our learning? Well, similarly to Driscoll and other models, the framework allows you to reflect in a structured way, leading – hopefully – to more effective and thorough reflections than if you were just thinking about the situation. What I like about the Gibbs' model is that the stages take a specific focus each (for example, the emotional reactions you may have had to the situation, and the conclusions you have reached), helping you to process different aspects of the event. That said, some may disagree and argue that these specific headings may prove too prescriptive and limit the amount of freedom and flexibility that you need to reflect openly, but I find the framework helpful as a starting point to consider different angles.

It is worth saying that academic literature has been included in both reflective examples to provide the sort of evidence-based account you might need to submit for university. When you are writing reflections in a journal for yourself, you would not necessarily need to do this, although still consider where theory can be linked in.

Learning Box 17.2: VERA Framework

The VERA Framework (Blackhall *et al.*, 2011) is a person-centred communication strategy designed to support people living with dementia. Originally developed by Amanda Blackhall and colleagues in 2011 to assist student nurses, the framework is built around four key concepts: Validation, Emotion, Reassure, and Activity (VERA).

- *Validation* – involves acknowledging and accepting the feelings, experiences and reality of the person living with dementia, even if they seem irrational or incorrect.
- *Emotion* – focuses on recognising and responding to the emotional content of what the person is communicating. By addressing the emotions behind their words, caregivers can provide comfort and understanding.
- *Reassure* – involves offering comfort and security to the person living with dementia. Simple actions like holding their hand, smiling, or verbally assuring them that they are safe can significantly reduce anxiety and agitation.
- *Activity* – involves engaging the person in meaningful activities to help distract them from distressing thoughts and provide a sense of purpose.

Barriers to reflective practice and practical considerations

By now you should have an understanding of why reflection is so important in your practice and have an idea of some of the models you can use when writing reflectively. Is it a straightforward, seamless process though? Not always, particularly as you start the reflective process. In this section, possible barriers to reflection are identified, and suggestions given as to how to tackle these barriers. In addition, tips and exercises are also provided in this section to help you develop your reflective skills.

Barriers to developing reflective practice skills

There are several barriers that can affect your ability to reflect effectively. These can be very roughly grouped into external and internal boundaries.

External barriers to effective reflection

TIME

As you start placement for the first time with all the new experiences and logistics that this involves (or indeed, continue in your existing workplace while juggling studies, university life, and potentially caring responsibilities) time can feel in very short supply. Spending time on an exercise such as reflection, on top of other assignments and tasks might feel like a luxury you do not have, but if you can identify a regular short time slot as soon as possible once you have finished your placement or work day, this will help to set a routine where you give yourself time to review your experiences clearly. Bassot (2016) emphasises the positive results that can be achieved with even just 15 minutes reflecting.

SPACE

Another practical consideration that can act as a barrier is your physical environment. If you have managed to identify a suitable time to reflect but are attempting to think and write in a room at home full of other people, or at the staffroom at work when you are still being asked questions despite clocking off, this is unlikely to be helpful or conducive for effective reflection.

Internal barriers to effective reflection

MOTIVATION

This can be one of the biggest personal barriers to almost anything challenging in life! Similarly to the external aspects above, it can be difficult to discipline yourself when you are tired and busy, but needs to be prioritised as an important personal and professional development area.

FEAR

This might seem a strong word to describe the feelings of discomfort or unfamiliarity that may surround writing reflectively for the first time, but I am using it empathically.

Some of us are naturally reflective and emotionally aware, where others are more pragmatically or philosophically minded and find reflection very difficult. A colleague of mine who is a scientist by background described the 'weird' experience of writing a reflective assignment for the continuing professional development course she was doing, as it did not have the quantitative data that she was so used to recording and analysing in the lab. It can also feel very exposing and vulnerable to commit your feelings in writing, so it is important to work out the boundaries that you will maintain in your own personal journal, and those you will maintain for reflective assignments that a marker will read. You do not need to bare your soul!

MINDSET

There can also be an uncomfortable vulnerability with appraising your own abilities – be it not wanting to boast, or conversely to admit your weaknesses or limitations. The good news is that reflection does not need to be either of these polarised ideas but can be a gentle balance of good practice and areas of improvement. Having a mindset where you commit to looking for, and celebrating areas of good practice, while being aware of your areas for development is healthy.

Ideas and exercises to overcome barriers to reflective practice

Here are some ideas for some short exercises to start getting you reflecting on situations, and to develop your understanding of writing reflectively.

Hopes and fears

Think about the course you are about to start, or perhaps your first placement. If you have already started these, you can think about your future career plans, or another aspect of your professional experience. For this example, I am going to discuss anticipating a placement at a care farm working with adults with learning disabilities, as shown in Table 17.1.

Table 17.1 Example of hopes and fears exercise

Hopes and fears	*Example*
What are your hopes for this placement?	I hope that I will learn a lot, and I hope I get on with everyone I am working with. I hope it will increase my knowledge and skills of working with people who have learning disabilities.
What are your fears?	That it will feel uncomfortable or nerve-wracking as I have not worked in this area before, and I am worried I might say the wrong thing or feel unsure of myself.
What might you need to do to address those fears?	I think it would be helpful for me to do some research about the setting, and find out a bit more about learning disabilities, perhaps by looking at the Mencap website for example.
Who might be able to help?	I may not know specifically until I start working at the placement, but I am hoping my mentor will be supportive. I know I can also talk to placement staff and the teaching team at the university too.

Prompt questions about your day

Using Nicol and Dosser's prompt questions (2016: 39) in the first section of this chapter, look back to a recent notable scenario, and answer the questions using a sentence for each one. This exercise is about getting you to reflect generally, so it does not need to be related to your course, placement or health or social care at this point.

For example, although I am writing this at midday, I am still thinking about yet another stressful morning trying to get my daughter out of the house to school several hours ago. What can I learn from this situation to improve things for the future?

- *What happened*? The house was chaotic, we were already running late, my daughter was being uncooperative, and we had lost her school bag and drinks bottle.
- *How did I feel*? Frustrated with my daughter's unhelpful behaviour, anxious about time, and angry with myself for not being organised.
- *What are the main points*? Everything is rushed and in a mess. It puts me and my daughter in a bad mood before the day begins. We end up late for school and work and I feel guilty.
- *What do I need to explore further*? Why does this happen so regularly? What routines can I put in place to avoid it? How can I deal with this better emotionally? Are there deeper issues at play? What effect might this have on the two of us?
- *What are my initial thoughts were this to happen again*? I don't want it to, so I will spend time tonight preparing school items, and setting alarms 15 minutes earlier. I will also be aware of what I am feeling and take a deep breath before getting angry so that we both have a positive start to the day.

Keyword spider diagram

Using the headings from Gibbs' reflective cycle discussed earlier in the chapter, create a spider diagram with keywords and short sentences to help you reflect about a specific event. This could either act as an aide memoire for a longer written reflection later, or just an exercise in itself to allow you to start reflecting. In Figure 17.3, I have returned to my earlier reflection about Joan in the care home to complete a shortened version as an example.

'Letter to a friend'

Based on Sandra Waddock's (1999: 193) work with undergraduate business students in setting them a reflective task that helped them to 'find their own personal voice' in an assignment, this exercise takes some of the awkwardness away from reflecting on your own practice to yourself.

By imagining that you are writing to a close friend, you can bring an authentic, and perhaps less self-conscious tone, to your reflective writing. As Waddock says, this can provide 'an opportunity for an energetic, active, and coherent voice to emerge' (Waddock, 1999).

You could write an imaginary letter to your friend about any aspect of your life, but some reflective prompt questions might be:

- Think about your talents, skills and past experiences, and what these could bring to a health and social care course

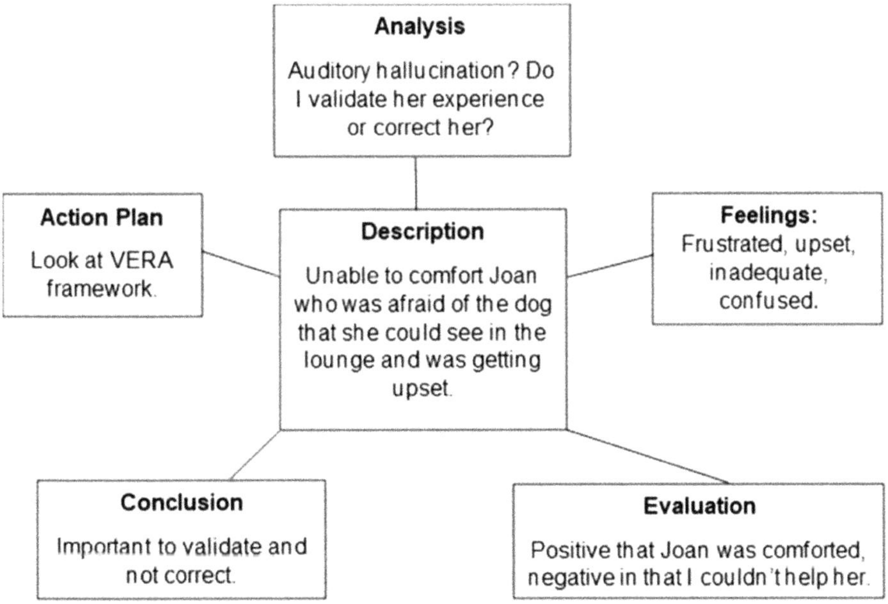

Figure 17.3 Example of reflective keyword spider diagram.

- What dreams do you have for your future career and how do you plan to achieve these?
- What difficulties do you anticipate completing the course?

The Park

This activity from Jenny Moon *(Moon, 2004: 172)* is particularly helpful to allow you to gauge different levels of reflective writing. Moon provides four accounts of a fictional scenario written by 'Annie' that range from purely descriptive to an account that is analytical and dynamic in terms of learning from a situation reflectively.

The resource can be used in different ways – you can read the examples and explanations in one go and reflect on your own level of writing. Or you could take one account at a time and critique each for their detail and reflection, adding your own notes about what else 'Annie' could have discussed. Alternatively, you could work with a friend and taking turns in pretending to be 'Annie', reading out the first account and using the other to identify questions that could be asked in the writing to deepen the level of reflection.

Summary

In this chapter, we have explored different aspects of reflective practice, and how this might be used in a number of different health and social care settings – initially as a student on placement but with the aim of developing reflective skills over your career as a professional.

The importance of reflection has been discussed in terms of improving practice, developing your skills, increasing your confidence, allowing you to see different perspectives and viewpoints, and to help process challenging situations. We have looked at reflective writing in more detail, examining different models and how these can be used to provide a clear structure for reflecting.

In addition, some of the challenges relating to reflective practice have been identified, from time constraints to barriers that we can put up internally due to fear. Helpful tips and hints have been provided as an aid to starting the reflective process.

Whether you are at the start of your career or developing your skills as a professional, reflection is vital at every stage in order to assess where you have been and to guide you to where you are going in your future practice.

References

Artioli, G., Deiana, L., De Vincenzo, F., Raucci, M., Amaducci., Bassi, M.C., Di Leo, S., Hayter, M. and Ghirotto, L. (2021) 'Health professionals and students' experiences of reflective writing in learning: A qualitative meta-synthesis', *BMC Med Education*, 21, p. 394. https://doi.org/10.1186/s12909-021-02831-4

Bassot, B. (2016) *The Reflective Practice Guide: An Interdisciplinary Approach to Critical Reflection*. London: Routledge.

Bassot, B., (2020). *The Reflective Journal*. 3rd edn. London: Red Globe Press.

Benaton, T.-M., Green, P. and Fuller, F. (2022) 'Emotional resilience' in Williams, S., and Conroy, D. (eds.) *A Student's Guide to Placements in Health and Social Care Settings: From Theory to Practice*. London: Critical Publishing.

Blackhall, A., Hawkes, D., Hingley, D. and Wood, S. (2011) 'VERA framework: Communicating with people who have dementia', *Nursing Standard*, 26(10), pp. 35–39. https://doi.org/10.7748/ns.26.10.35.s49

Boud, D., Keogh, R. and Walker, D. (1985) *Reflection: Turning Experience into Learning*. London: Kogan Page.

Chen, I. and Forbes, C. (2014) 'Reflective writing and its impact on empathy in medical education: Systematic review', *Journal of Educational Evaluation for Health Professions*, 2014(11), p. 20. https://doi.org/10.3352/jeehp.2014.11.20

Contreras, J.A., Edwards-Maddox, S., Hall, A. and Lee, M.A. (2020) 'Effects of reflective practice on baccalaureate nursing students' stress, anxiety and competency: An integrative Review', *Worldviews on Evidence-Based Nursing*, 17(3), pp. 239–245.

Curry, A. and Epley, P. (2022) '"It makes you a healthier professional": The impact of reflective practice on emerging clinicians' self-care', *Journal of Social Work Education*, 58(2), pp. 291–307.

Davies, S. (2012) 'Embracing reflective practice', *Education for Primary Care*, 23(1), pp. 9–12.

Driscoll, J. (ed.) (2007) *Practicing Clinical Supervision: A Reflective Approach for Healthcare Professionals*. Edinburgh: Elsevier.

Eversfield, C. and Orton, L. (2019) 'Auditory and visual hallucination prevalence in Parkinson's disease and dementia with Lewy bodies: A systematic review and meta-analysis', *Psychological Medicine*, 49(14), pp. 2342–2353. https://doi.org/10.1017/S0033291718003161

Feil, N. (1992) 'Validation therapy', *Geriatric Nursing*, 13(3), pp. 129–133. https://doi.org/10.1016/S0197-4572(07)81021-4

Gibbs, G. (1998) *Learning by Doing: A Guide to Teaching and Learning Methods*. Oxford: Oxford Brooks University.

Guy, L., Cranwell, C., Hitch, D. and McKinstry, C. (2020) 'Reflective practice facilitation within occupational therapy supervision processes: A mixed method study', *Australian Occupational Therapy Journal*, 67(4), pp. 320–329. https://doi.org/10.1111/1440-1630.12660

Hart, P. (2016) 'Young people negotiating and maintaining boundaries in youth work relationships: Findings from an ethnographic study of youth clubs', *Journal of Youth Studies*, 19(7), pp. 869–884. https://doi.org/10.1080/13676261.2015.1112881

Koh, D., McNulty, G. and Toh-Heng, H.L. (2022) 'Reflective practice through clinical supervision: Implications for professional and organisational sustainability', *British Journal of Guidance & Counselling*, 50(6), pp. 879–896. https://doi.org/10.1080/03069885.2021.1978056

Koshy, K., Limb, C., Gundogan, B., Whitehurst, K. and Jafree, D.J. (2017) 'Reflective practice in health care and how to reflect effectively', *International Journal of Surgery Oncology*, 2(6), p. e20. https://doi.org/10.1097/IJ9.0000000000000020

Mehraram, R., Taylor, J.P., Murphy, N., Peraza Rodriguez, L., Cromarty, R., Graziadio, S., O'Brien, J., Killen, A., Colloby, S. and Kaiser, J. (2020) 'The visual ventral network is disconnected in Lewy body dementia with visual hallucinations', *Alzheimer's & Dementia*, 16(S5). https://doi.org/10.1002/alz.040350

Moon, J.A. (2004) *A Handbook of Reflective and Experiential Learning: Theory and Practice*. London: Routledge Falmer.

National Youth Agency (2021) *Guidance on personal professional and environmental boundaries*. Available at https://www.nya.org.uk/wp-content/uploads/guidance-on-personal-professional-and-environmental-boudnaries.pdf

Nicol, J.S. and Dosser, I. (2016) 'Understanding reflective practice', *Nursing Standard*, 30(36), pp. 34–42.

Rolfe, G., Jasper, M. and Freshwater, D. (2011) *Critical Reflection in Practice: Generating Knowledge for Care*. 2nd edn. London: Red Globe Press.

Spencer, M. and Healey, J. (2022) *Surviving Your Placement in Health and Social Care: A Student Handbook*. 2nd edn. London, England: Open University Press.

Waddock, S.A. (1999) 'Letter to a friend: a personal reflection exercise', *Journal of Management Education*, 23(2), pp. 190–200.

Williams, K., Woolliams, M. and Spiro, J. (2020) *Reflective Writing*. 2nd edn. London: Red Globe Press.

18 Communication skills for practice

Rebecca Weston

The key aims of this chapter are to:

- **Outline important theories of communication relevant to health and social care practice**
- **Identify key verbal skills, non-verbal skills and active listening skills for effective communicators**
- **Identify potential barriers to communication in practice**

Introduction

Communication is something that we take for granted. Until we are faced with a situation where we have left an exchange thinking, 'I don't know what just happened there', or 'I didn't understand a word of that', we do not tend to think about how we communicate or how we like to be communicated with. In health and social care practice, developing effective communication skills is key to ensure that we speak, write and behave with clarity, unambiguity, respect and empathy in our interactions with service users, patients, clients, children and young people, family members, care givers, colleagues and other professionals.

One of the most significant reasons for this is that it helps to improve the quality of care (Pentland *et al.*, 2021). This significance is echoed in professional regulatory bodies' statements or ethical principles concerning effective communication for social work, nursing and midwifery and health and care professions, as shown in Table 18.1.

Table 18.1 Professional regulatory bodies' statements on communication

Professional regulatory body	*Statement on communication*
British Association of Social Workers (BASW)	Social Workers should communicate effectively and work in partnership with individuals, families, groups, communities and with public bodies and other agencies' (BASW, 2021: 10)
Nursing and Midwifery Council (NMC)	'(7.3) Use a range of verbal and non-verbal communication methods and consider cultural sensitivities to better understand and respond to people's personal and health needs' (NMC, 2018: 10)
Health and Care Professions Council (HCPC)	'(2.5) You must use all forms of communication responsibly when communicating with service users and carers' (HCPC, 2024: 11)

DOI: 10.4324/9781032619309-21

Another reason to have a better awareness of our communication skills in practice is that recognising that the 'skill' of effective communication is something to be learned, and that there are differences between how we communicate on an interpersonal level with our friends and family and how we communicate professionally within a workplace setting, which is what this chapter focuses upon.

This chapter explores a range of communication skills that are used in health and/or social care. This chapter introduces some of the underpinning theories of and about communication. This is designed to help both emerging and experienced practitioners develop their communication skills for use in their practice, as well as develop their own understanding of what makes good communication.

By the end of this chapter, you will have an understanding of key communication theories that inform practice within health and social care settings. You will be able to identify important and evidence-based communication skills that you can use in your own practice as well as identifying aspects of both good and poor communication.

What is communication?

Communication tends to mean different things to different people within different settings and contexts. It is, therefore, a very broad term that can cover a very wide range of behaviours, means of communication and definitions. At its core, it can simply mean the 'transmission of information from one source to another' (Thompson, 2018: 12) and one of the models of communication we look at in this chapter is as straightforward as that. However, communication in any context is more complexed and nuanced than that simplistic definition, which ignores questions such as 'was the transmission intentional?'; 'was the transmission accurately sent?'; 'was the transmission accurately received?' and many more. This complexity is reflected by Pavord and Donnelly (2015: 13) in their exploration of Wood's definition of communication that considers the importance and use of symbols in how understanding can be formed and processed in a multi-layered way. This complexity is discussed within the second model of communication later in this chapter.

Theories of communication

To help us better understand how communication works, and therefore help us define it more clearly, this part of the chapter focuses on two models of communication. The first model is the *Transmission Model of Communication* (Shannon and Weaver, 1949). This model outlines basic transmission or interaction between two people, and supports Thompson's core meaning of communication (2018: 12). It is considered 'linear', meaning that it moves from one stage to another in that order. The linear nature of the model implies that it only moves in one direction, highlighting the core nature of communication.

The second model that the chapter explores is the *Transactional Model of Communication* (Wood, 2004), which examines how communication is multi-faceted and can operate on different, multiple levels simultaneously. This helps us to explore the more nuanced complexity of our communications and interactions.

Transmission model of communication

The *Transmission Model of Communication* (Shannon and Weaver, 1949) indicates that communication occurs as a simple, straight line (linear) process, starting with a person

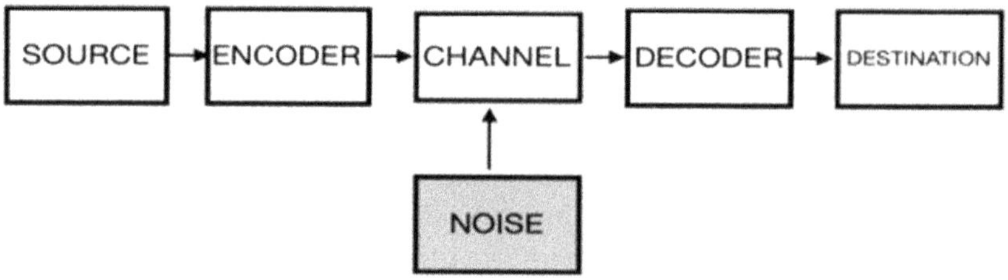

Figure 18.1 Shannon and Weaver's Transmission Model of Communication.

sending a message and ending with another person successfully receiving the message. This is shown in Figure 18.1, which starts when someone creates a message (Source), such as when someone speaks. This message is sent through the air by sound waves (Encoder), and is received by the ear (Channel). The message is sent from the air to the brain to be understood (Decoder), and once understood, is then sent to the correct part of the body for action (Destination). For example, a request to 'Pass the Ketchup' would be made by one person to another through speech, this is transmitted through the air, received by person audibly, processed by the brain and a signal is sent to the arm to action.

The model also depicts 'noise' as a force that disrupts or breaks the line of communication, most obviously occurring at the midpoint of the transmission. Noise is explored more fully later on, and there is a reflective activity at the end of the chapter to encourage you to think about the role of 'noise' in communication transactions.

Whilst this model does not really capture how we might think of communication in any setting, it is quite effective in illustrating the process of communication, which is useful for helping practitioners to reflect when communication is not successful or there are breakdowns in communication. For example, if the information needed to be conveyed is overly technical or complicated (the first point on the model), then the person communicating it (the encoder) may have to adapt it to ensure the successful receipt and decoding (understanding) of it.

However, because of the linear nature of the model, it risks oversimplifying communication and can feel mechanistic as it does not consider any internal experiences, values, attitudes and beliefs, cultural experiences or context to the communication in question. It implies, therefore, that whilst a person is talking, the recipient is very passive, merely waiting to receive the information before beginning to process (decode) it. This is where a transactional model offers a different perspective.

Transactional Model of Communication

Wood's *Transactional Model of Communication* (2004) captures the more complex and multi-faceted nature of human communication, as well as what Barnlund terms the dynamic and continuous nature of communication (1970). This is shown in Figure 18.2.

In contrast to Shannon and Weaver's model above, this model outlines communication as a dynamic rather than static process, with messages, interpretations and understandings being sent and received and created simultaneously and adapted as needed. In this model, both parties are labelled as 'communicators', recognising the role of listening as communication, and how the constant exchange of spoken words and listened-to responses contribute to a shared understanding and interpretation of what is being

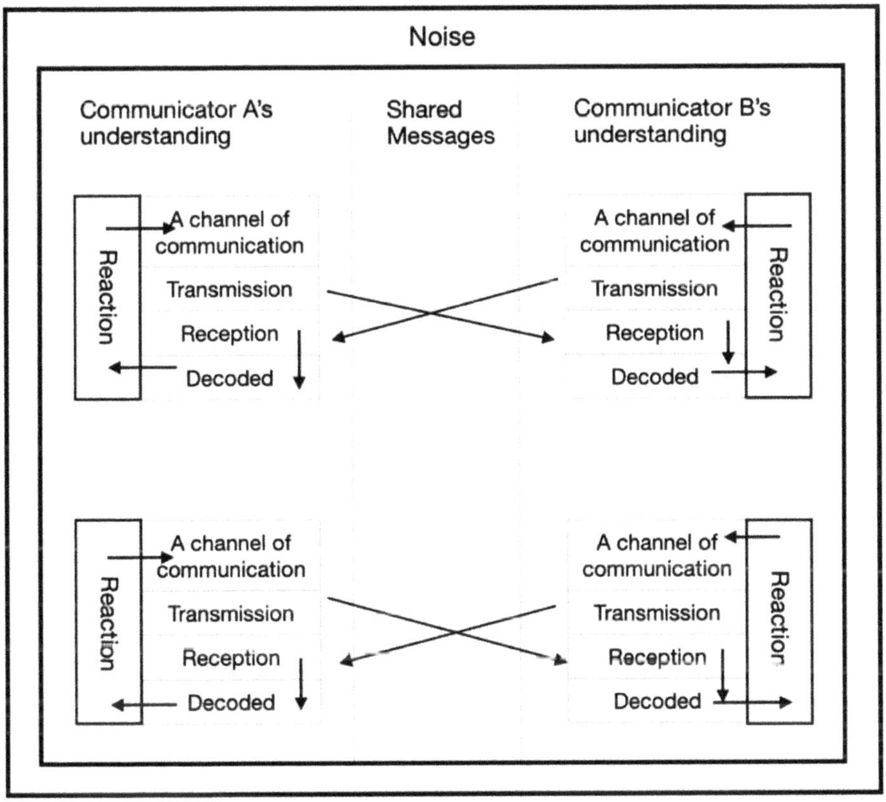

Figure 18.2 Wood's Transactional Model of Communication.

communicated. It also highlights that there are many different events occurring simultaneously within one transaction or 'unit' of communication and that both communicators are involved in these events before, during and after the communication. Wood's model also acknowledges 'noise' as an ever-present source, not necessarily merely as a disruption, but as something that human beings can co-exist with whilst communicating.

However, a criticism of Wood's model is that it can look overly complicated as it does not acknowledge that some transactions rely upon both verbal and non-verbal methods of communication. This is partially addressed by the 'reaction' section of the model, which indicates an acknowledgement, or response from one communicator as the message is received and decoded, however it is not made clear that the 'reaction' may be verbal or non-verbal. Furthermore, there is no explicit consideration that 'reactions' can be cultural, psychological, environmental and/or unintentional.

The differences between the models are that Shannon and Weaver provide a clear and linear model of transmission, where communication is viewed as a one way process, with 'noise' featuring as a purely disruptive force. Conversely, Wood's transactional model captures the complex and simultaneous nature of communication between people, where 'noise' is ever-present but not necessarily only disruptive. When trying to understand how effective our communication skills are, Shannon and Weaver's model is excellent at giving a clear, non-ambiguous overview, but it is Wood's transactional model that allows us to better understand why, when and how communication has been, or not been, effective.

Communication skills for practice

This section identifies important communication skills for practice. It discusses verbal and non-verbal communication skills, as well as active listening skills, which are often referred to as 'soft skills' and are skills that you may either already use in your practice or be thinking about as you start practice.

Verbal communication skills

When we talk about verbal communication skills, we are talking about spoken communication and any form of communication involving words at its core. There are therefore different types of verbal communication styles to consider, such as written, spoken, formal, informal, 'slang' or colloquial. The intended audience or recipients of the verbal communication style often dictates the style of communication required.

Thompson (2021: 100) outlines that verbal communication falls into two distinct parts: what is said (output) and what is heard (input). This section focuses on the first part of that, the 'output' or what is being said.

Spoken communication skills

In our everyday personal lives, our speech carries its own pattern and qualities of tone, based upon some of the paralinguistic features discussed below. Our spoken voice carries a natural speed, falls into a particular pitch, and has a natural volume, and all of these factors are enhanced by our language, education and geography (such as accent).

In our practice settings, Thompson (2021) suggests that having an awareness of these qualities of our spoken language can improve our clarity of communication and of our listening skills. For example, if we take the pitch our voice naturally holds, and then consider how we vary it to communicate differences and emphases in our words and exchanges, it can be noticed that this can affect how people understand us. One use of pitch or intonation is to discern between making a statement and asking a question. This can be indicated by a rise in intonation at the end of a statement, making it more like a question. For example, consider the difference in meaning between 'You are going out' said with a flat voice throughout, and 'You are going *out*' with a rising intonation on the word out. Likewise, little variation in intonation over a sentence or more, can feel quite monotone and often difficult to listen to. Overuse of the constant rise in intonation, or indeed, the lack of variation in intonation can become a barrier to effective communication.

Written communication skills

Words that are written down carry their own style or 'etiquette' of meaning and interpretation. Some written communications need to be accurate, factually based and devoid of any personal comment. This is because, under *the Data Protection Act 2018*, for 'professional' emails sent between colleagues that relate to third parties, there exists the right to see any/all communication within a professional setting, or where email content may be used in court or legal proceedings (Jenkins, 2017).

Other written communications can still be quite formal but more open to opinion and acknowledge familiarity between people. Work emails between colleagues may fall into this category, their formality may be unconscious, for example if we have a 'work signature' that is automatically generated, or the communication may start off in a formal manner but develops into a more fluid email 'conversation'.

The increase in various technology platforms to improve communication in work settings can further blur the line between formal and informal, professional and personal. For example, using a group chat function for work might mix rules of communicating with work colleagues (it is a work group chat) with rules of communicating with friends or family (it is on a social media platform and often accessed via a personal smart phone).

Non-verbal communication skills

Non-verbal communication refers to how we present information about ourselves, often before we have had the chance to speak. According to Mehrabian (1972), the words we use to communicate are less prominent than other factors such as body language, or paralanguage. These two factors often acting as signals or indicators of what kind of communication may be received can prepare an individual for an appropriate response. For example, if a kindly colleague approaches you at work, but they are striding across the room to you, swinging their arms slightly and holding your eye contact as they do so, this body language may feel out of kilter with their usually friendly disposition. Figure 18.3 shows that according to Mehrabian's Model of Communication (Mehrabian, 1972), a mere 7% of what we communicate is through the words we speak, whilst 55% of is through body language alone, and the remaining 38% is through how we say those words, or *paralanguage* (Figure 18.3).

It is important, therefore, that as practitioners, we are aware of our non-verbal communication styles and the potential implications of what they may communicate to service users, patients and others, who may already be feeling vulnerable or apprehensive about their interaction with us. Through awareness of our styles, we can develop the skills to present in a way that promotes empathy, patience, care and calmness, rather than say, authority, power, abruptness or irritability.

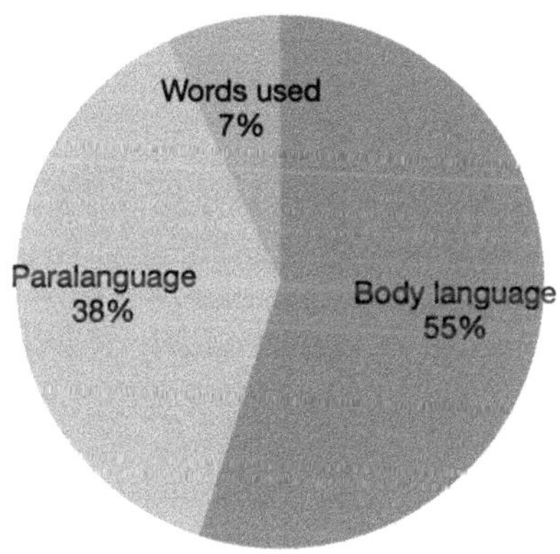

Figure 18.3 Mehrabian's Model of Communication.

Source: Mehrabian (1972).

We use paralinguistic skills all the time, without even realising it. To exemplify this, invite a friend, colleague or family member to help you with this activity. For 90 seconds, talk to your 'listener' about a neutral topic that you are comfortable with. Throughout that time, whilst you can both make eye contact with each other, avoid using any other paralinguistic skills. This means, adopting a neutral facial expression and body language, no gesturing or touch during the conversation. Afterwards, reflect on how it felt to not utilise any of those skills but also how it felt to not receive any paralinguistic cues from your listener.

Below are various non-verbal communication skills or paralanguage that we use.

Body language

How we stand or sit, distribute the weight throughout our bodies, or where our arms and hands are can all communicate different messages. Ideally, a welcoming 'neutral' body language can convey the desired skills, so sitting without crossing legs or slouching. If standing, ensure that the weight is distributed equally, so you are not giving the sense of standing with a hand on your hip (this can communicate impatience or insolence).

Eye contact

Where possible, maintaining regular but quite short intervals of eye contact is considered beneficial, and communicates that the speaker is being listened to and 'held'. Pavord and Donnelly (2015) acknowledge that levels of eye contact may vary depending upon situation, but more eye contact does demonstrate that the practitioner is present and listening than avoiding it.

Facial expression

We use our faces to communicate emotion. Initially, there were six expressions of human emotion identified (happy, sad, disgust, fear, surprise, anger); however, research conducted by Du *et al.* (2014) includes combinations of these leading to more nuanced facial expressions. As practitioners, we are probably likely to witness these facial expressions, rather than display them, so our facial expressions should be open, relaxed and aim to communicate calm and empathy.

Haptics (touch)

This refers to the concept and appropriateness of touch – when/if we should and if so, how? Think of the way in which smart watches and smart phones can give a small pulse or vibration to indicate a notification to you. Similarly, sometimes a gentle hand on the shoulder or upper arm can communicate far more than any empathic response, but we must be aware of the reception of this, particularly if working in a trauma-informed way, with people with different cultural experiences and expectations and of course, in children and young people settings.

Kinesics

This refers to our gesturing and movement in our communication style. Whilst standing or sitting rigidly still would not convey effective or positive communication, consider how much you use your arms and hands in communication – as this can sometimes give the sense of 'driving a point home'.

Some skills related to kinesics can be used to validate experiences or de-escalate situations. In the first instance, Nelson-Jones (2013) recommends that mirroring an individual's body language can be seen as affirmative, if done with sensitivity and can convey empathy. An example of this may be mirroring (copying) a gesture made when an individual is communicating emotively, such as tucking their hair behind their ear. Psychologically, this can convey a shared experience or empathic understanding of what is being communicated (Nelson-Jones, 2013). Conversely, if an individual is angry, Moss (2017) suggests that using posture to model desired communication may ameliorate a potentially aggressive interaction. For example, repositioning oneself by adopting a more open body language and facial expression can model this. It is important to ensure that safety is maintained at all times in these situations.

Proxemics (closeness)

This relates to the distance between two people and how close we get to them. You may be aware of aware of the concept of 'social distancing', which was initially developed by a mathematician, who looked at ideal zones for different types of communication. Hall (1968) felt that there were broadly three different zones of communication as shown in Table 18.2.

This can be used in conjunction with both kinesics and touch, often to achieve similar outcomes. For example, in the communication to de-escalate, stepping out of a very close proximity to one where there is more distance can reinforce feelings of safety and reduce vulnerability. Likewise, if using touch, one would need to be reasonably close to the individual for it to not look forced, but not so close that it can feel threatening.

Active listening skills

Active listening skills are a range of communication skills designed to demonstrate that the person talking is being truly heard, understood, and valued. They draw from both verbal and non-verbal forms of communication discussed above and were developed from Carl Rogers' (1957) core conditions of counselling which are often used as the foundations of building effective therapeutic relationships in counselling and psychotherapy. When we listen in our everyday personal life, to our children, partners, friends and others and to an extent, personal relationships in a workplace setting, we are listening whilst our minds are semi-occupied with multiple other thoughts, tasks, memories and distractions. For example, we can show that we are listening to a friend talk about work by making

Table 18.2 Hall's zones for effective communication (1968)

Zone	*Distance*	*Type of communication*
Social	1.7m–2.1m	Interactions where more than two people need to be included, or there are no confidentiality concerns within the content.
Personal	0.45m–1.5m	Conversations between two people, not designed to be overheard
Intimate	0–0.45m	In healthcare settings may be whispered, but this also may not be appropriate!

non-verbal encouragers ('hmms', 'awws', etc.) and body language cues. However, our minds are also occupied with unrelated mental reminders and thoughts, or formulating an appropriate response to what our friend is saying. So although we 'hear' what is being said, it is fair to say, that our friend does not have our entire attention.

Active listening is a set of skills that helps us to train our minds to give that complete focus and attention, but more importantly to effectively communicate to that person that they have our focus and attention (Egan, 2010). Active listening skills can feel quite awkward when they are first practised, but once developed, do help us listen much more effectively and by reflecting some of that listening back to the individual, they are empowered to make the choices or decisions based upon their own understanding of their experience. According to Egan (2010), these are important skills to build positive relationships within a helping focus. Some important active listening skills are outlined below.

Reflecting

This is exactly as it sounds. When someone says something to you, an active listening response is to reflect it back word for word. This does feel very unnatural, as, like with many active listening skills, it is not part of our normal way of communicating with people. The aim of this skill, is that by reflecting back exactly what is said, you are firstly showing that you have heard what has been said and that secondly, by using their choice of words, you are giving the individual the chance to hear their own words, which can then allow affirmation or refute. On its own, it is quite limited, but used in conjunction with the other skills can be very powerful. An important feature of reflection is what Nelson-Jones (2013) describes as 'you feel ... because ...' which not only demonstrates your ability to actively listen but also to offer a reason why that feeling is important (validation).

Paraphrasing

The next active listening skill is 'paraphrasing' what has been said to you. When we paraphrase sections of communication, we do so by substituting their chosen words with some of our words. In doing this, we demonstrate that we have both internalised their words or comment and processed it by using our own choice of words which then can convey understanding and perception. As with reflecting, offering the speaker the chance to hear how their own words have been internalised and perceived by a listener can either validate their own experience or offer the opportunity to refute.

An example of both reflecting and paraphrasing what has been communicated to you could look like this:

- **Communication:** 'I have no time at all to complete these assignments and work full time, it's all too much and I'm completely stressed out'
- **Reflecting:** 'You have no time at all to complete your assignments and work full time. It's all too much and you are completely stressed out'
- **Paraphrasing:** 'I'm hearing that you are struggling with your assignment deadlines whilst working full time. The stress of it all is overwhelming'

Clarifying and open questions

Clarifying can be an active skill either on its own or one which develops through effective use of either other active listening skills, or as illustrated here, with open-ended questions.

Table 18.3 Examples of closed and open questions

Closed question	*Open question*
Did you have a nice day?	What was your day like?
Are you okay?	How are you feeling?
Was Katie involved?	Who was involved in that?

Essentially, this skill enables you to fact-check what is said and through this, develop both your own understanding of the important points for the person talking and allowing the person talking to provide you with additional information. In this application of the skill, it may be that you include open-ended questions to help further your understanding.

Open-ended, or open questions are questions that require an answer other than 'yes', 'no' or 'I don't know'. They can often be posed as statements. Table 18.3 shows examples of both closed and open questions.

Often, open questions are most effective when they start with words such as 'what?', 'where?', 'who?' because they require either more information than a 'yes' or 'no', or more specific information is needed.

Summarising

The skill of summarising is helpful at the end of conversations or where you, as the listener, feel there needs to be a point where you can help the person talking consider some of the key points they are making. Often, summarising may be required when the person talking is giving a lot of information in a condensed or rushed way, or they are in an emotive state and are struggling to convey things in a way that is easy to understand.

Summarising follows nicely from clarifying, as you may find yourself switching from one skill to another to help remind the person talking that you have heard them, you are aware of what you feel is important to them. However, in summarising, you would not usually include open questions, as this could start to elicit more or new information.

When using either clarifying or summarising skills, some of the words you use may help give the person talking cues as to the type of responses: 'So, just to check here ...' (clarifying); 'To summarise what I think are the key points ...' (summarising).

Giving and receiving feedback

This is a challenging skill in any situation or setting. Both can sometimes be perceived as criticism or judgement. In any healthcare setting whether communicating with colleagues, service users or families and carers, there is a fine art to giving feedback in a neutral, supportive and non-judgemental way. The following suggestions can also apply to how we receive feedback, when given, or offered in this way.

Firstly, when giving or offering feedback, practitioners should use words that indicate that it is their opinion and something to be offered rather than imposed. The easiest way to do this is to frame your feedback by using 'I language': 'I wonder if ...'; 'I felt that ...'. In this way, your feedback is coming entirely from the giver's perspective, rather than an indictment on the behaviour, action or choices of the receiver. Table 18.4 further illustrates these differences.

Table 18.4 Feedback: 'I' language versus judgemental comments

'I' language	*Judgemental comments*
I felt that the chair might be more accessible by the window	You shouldn't have placed that chair so close to the bed
I wonder if there had been the opportunity to ask about the dog, what the response would have been.	You should have checked about their dog – you knew it was unwell.

Barriers to communication

Moss describes a barrier to communication as 'any action, behaviour, attitude, world view or physical arrangement (such as room layout) that discourages the other person from feeling comfortable, accepted and valued, thereby reducing your and their ability to communicate positively and effectively' (Moss, 2017:39).

Returning to Shannon and Weaver's and Wood's theories of communication above, another way of thinking about barriers to communication is to consider them as 'noise', or something that impacts upon how effectively the communication is received and/or understood. Shannon and Weaver (1949) outline 'noise' purely as a disruption in the passing of and receiving of information through a chosen channel of communication. Whilst this is helpful to visualise the effect it has, it does oversimplify both the purpose of noise and the human capacity to tolerate a degree of 'noise' whilst communicating successfully. This nuance is captured more accurately in transactional models of communication, such as that of Wood (2004) and Barnlund (1970).

Table 18.5 gives some examples of types of 'noise' and how they can affect communication. The list is not a complete list, and there are very likely other types of 'noise' you find disrupting and which can impact your part in communication.

Table 18.5 Types of noise in communication

Type of noise	*Explanation*
Physical, literal noise	Being in a noisy environment, e.g. being talked over, or other secondary sounds interrupting the flow of communication
Psychological noise (our internal dialogue)	Intra-personal communication often runs parallel to our daily activities and does not disrupt; however, there are occasions where it can break our concentration or competes with the interpersonal communication to an extent that this becomes secondary, e.g. thinking about what we are going to make for dinner when we should be paying attention in a meeting.
Semantics	This is a broad type of noise, it can include vocabulary (jargon, technical language, age appropriate language), differences in language or accent, or the use of a common word that has more than one meaning which is not clear. For example, 'So, your husband's current observations are showing abnormal BP which will be discussed at his MDT meeting later'.
Physiological / somatic noise	This barrier refers to sensations experienced in our body, e.g. body temperature, presence of pain, a disability or an impairment that potentially impacts the processing of information.

(*Continued*)

Table 18.5 (Continued)

Type of noise	*Explanation*
Visual noise	Being distracted by seeing something, often unexpected can disrupt the flow of conversation, e.g. seeing another person appear unexpectedly in an online meeting.
Mismatch of what we hear and what we see	The example of asking someone how they are, and they respond 'fine', whilst looking down at the floor and avoiding eye contact. Further examples of this would be adopting an overly formal tone of voice when socialising with friends or being too informal or casual in a workplace setting may undermine our professional role (Thompson, 2021).

Summary on different types of noise

Different 'noise' can impact our ability to communicate differently. Some people will find certain types of noise explained in the table above more distracting than others. For example, trying to listen whilst in proximity to a contrasting secondary noise source such as running water can be challenging, whereas talking on the telephone in a busy office environment where the secondary 'noise' is similar may not cause problems. Sometimes 'noise' can aid communication, for example, under 'psychological noise' we can be receiving internal cues informing us that our communication is not as clear as it could be.

Summary

This chapter has outlined two key theories of communication and identified a range of communication skills that are of relevance to health and/or social care practice. These include paralinguistic communication skills which sit across both verbal and non-verbal communication styles, and active listening skills which can be used to great effect in verbal communication. Some specific barriers to effective communication have also been discussed, including the impact different types of 'noise' can have on how we process, understand and communicate effectively in the workplace. The chapter has also outlined how communication can limit effective communication. These communication skills are important for both the emerging and experienced practitioners. This is designed to help the development of your communication skills for use in practice, as well as develop your understanding of what makes both good and poor communication in practice.

References

Barnlund, D.C. (1970) 'A transactional model of communication' in J. Akin, A. Goldberg, G. Myers and J. Stewart (eds.) *Language Behaviour: A Book of Readings in Communication*. Boston: De Gruyter, Inc, pp. 43–61.

BASW (2021) *The BASW Code of Ethics for Social Work*. Birmingham: BASW.

Du, S., Tao, Y. and Martinez, A.M. (2014) 'Compound facial expressions of emotion', *Proceedings of the National Academy of Sciences of the United States of America*, 111(15), pp. 1454–1462. https://doi.org/10.1073/pnas.1322355111

Egan, G. (2010) *The Skilled Helper: A Problem Management and Opportunity-Development Approach to Helping*. 9th edn. California: Brooks.

Hall, E.T. (1968) 'Proxemics', *The University of Chicago Press Journals*, 9(2), pp. 83–109. Available at https://www.jstor.org/stable/2740724?seq=1#metadata_info_tab_contents

HCPC (2024) Standards of conduct, performance and ethics. Available at https://www.hcpc-uk.org/globalassets/resources/standards/standards-of-conduct-performance-and-ethics-2024.pdf

Jenkins, P. (2017) *Professional Practice in Counselling and Psychotherapy*. London: SAGE Publications Ltd.

Mehrabian, A. (1972) *Silent Messages: Implicit Communication of Emotions and Attitudes*. Belmont: Wadsworth Publishing.

Moss, B. (2017) *Communication Skills in Health and Social Care*. 4th edn. London: SAGE Publications Ltd.

Nelson-Jones, R. (2013) *Introduction to Counselling Skills: Text and Activities*. 4th edn. London: SAGE Publications Ltd.

NMC (2018) *Professional standards for practice and behaviour for nurses, midwives and nursing associates*. Available at https://www.nmc.org.uk/globalassets/sitedocuments/nmc-publications/nmc-code.pdf

Pavord, E. and Donnelly, E. (2015) *Communication and Interpersonal Skills*. 2nd edn. Banbury: Lantern Publications.

Pentland, D., Riddell, H. and Regan, L. (2021) 'Communicating and relating effectively', in B. McCormack, T. McCance, C. Bulley, D. Brown, A. McMillan and S. Martin (eds.) *Fundamentals of Person-Centred Healthcare Practice*. Oxford: Wiley Blackwell, pp. 80–91.

Rogers, C.R. (1957) 'The necessary and sufficient conditions of therapeutic personality change', *Journal of Consulting Psychology*, 21(2), pp. 95–103. https://doi.org/10.1037/h0045357

Shannon, C. and Weaver, W. (1949) *The Mathematical Theory of Communication*. Illinois: University of Illinois Press.

Thompson, N. (2018) *Effective Communication*. 3rd edn. London: Bloomsbury.

Thompson, N. (2021) *People Skills*. 5th edn. London: SAGE.

Wood, J.T. (2004) *Communication Theories in Action: An Introduction*. California: Wadsworth/Thomson Learning.

19 Placement skills for health and social care students

Daniel Howarth and Naomi Blaikie

The aims of this chapter are:

- To offer support and guidance for your placement journey, including before, during and after placement
- To introduce, explain and apply the five stages of the 'Benner Continuum' to your placement experiences
- To explore how to get the best quality learning from your placement experiences

Introduction

As a student studying health and social care at university, it is almost certain that your course has some form of work based learning (WBL) or placement experience. This is where instead of being in a classroom or lecture, you are out in some kind of work setting working with real service users or clients. There are different forms of placements, including online placements or simulations but the most common form, and the main focus for this chapter, are practical placements within a health or social care setting. This chapter takes you through the three main steps of the placement experience, which are:

- **Pre-Placement:** Some points for you to consider before you begin your placement
- **During Placement:** Some guidance and supportive suggestions to help you get the most learning from your placement experience
- **Post-Placement:** Some points to remember and carry forward once your placement has completed

The chapter uses Patricia Benner's (1984) five-stage 'novice to expert' theory as a way to explain the learning process of placements. This provides a good understanding of what is likely to be your experience while on placement. The chapter offers suggestions and guidance for you regardless of what stage of learning you are at, with the aim of helping you progress through the stages as your placement progresses and your knowledge and skills increase.

Overall, this chapter aims to encourage you to genuinely make the most of your placement experience and offers suggestions on how to get the most valuable learning from your placements as possible. This looks at how to approach placement, how to achieve in placement and how to carry your learning forward while trying to make the most of your opportunities as a student regardless of your level of prior experience.

DOI: 10.4324/9781032619309-22

The relevance of placements to your course

It is worth stating here that different specific settings and courses all tend to use slightly different terminology to mean essentially the same thing. When talking about placements, some use WBL, and when talking about those who you provide care for, some courses use either patient, service user or client. Mostly, these are all interchangeable and essentially mean the same thing, and so in this chapter, we use a variety of terms.

Before we start to look at the different aspects of completing a placement, it is helpful to consider why placements are an important component to a health and social care course. Placements can be beneficial to both students and placement providers.

Benefits of placements to students

From a university point of view, one of the most valuable reasons for students to have a placement experience is to allow you to link the theory you learn in your lectures to your practice. It is important to be able to see the connection between the theory learned in the classroom and the real human experiences of clients out in practice (Williams and Conroy, 2022). It is a key method for students to be able to develop professional skills, knowledge and understanding of working as a health and social care practitioner. In the words of Naish and Minton (2015: 142), you may even find yourself acting as an 'agent for change' in your workplace which might be truly transformative for you and the setting.

For a number of years, we have asked the students we work with for feedback on their placement experiences, and it has been helpful to gather their responses as to what they have gained during practice. They can be broadly categorised as follows:

- Skill development (communication skills, listening and empathising, quick thinking, problem solving, time management, creativity)
- Confidence building, self-belief and sense of pride ('I can see my potential')
- Developing resilience and overcoming challenges
- Specific professional knowledge about clients and settings, gaining a real insight
- Work with experienced practitioners – increase teamworking and 'people' skills/experience
- Interesting/rewarding/enjoyable experiences that have confirmed their choice of career

Benefits of placements to placement providers

There are also numerous advantages for the placement providers who offer placement opportunities for students. Some of the most obvious might be the economic benefit of having students work with them, and the potential of new and innovative ideas coming into the workplace (Ferrandez-Berrueco and Sanchez-Tarazaga, 2021). Speaking to the employers and placement mentors that we have worked with over the years, we would also add that many find teaching and guiding a new generation of students rewarding which allows them to develop their own skills in mentoring and sharing best practice. Other benefits mentioned are the support given to clients by students on placement, the different experiences and ways of working that students can bring to a setting, and the dedication they show to the team they are working with.

As you can see, placement experiences benefit both students and providers.

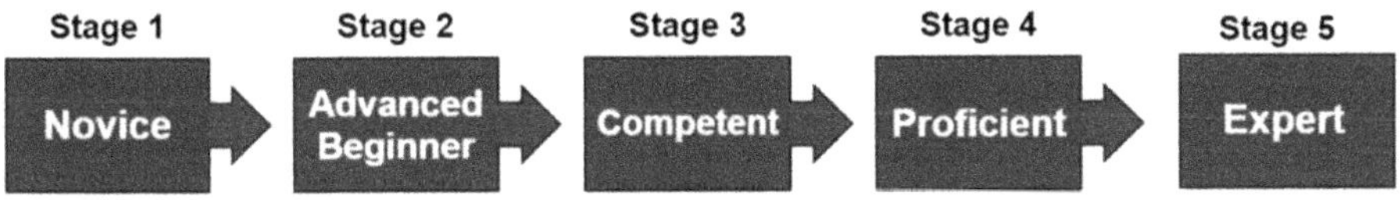

Figure 19.1 The five stages of the Benner Continuum.

Source: Created by authors based on Benner (1984).

The Benner Continuum

At this stage, it is relevant to introduce Patricia Benner's (1984) five-stage 'novice to expert' theory, which is often referred to as the *Benner Continuum*. The Benner Continuum is an explanation of the different stages that an individual goes through when they are learning a new role. The five stages of the Benner Continuum are shown in Figure 19.1. The stages are described below.

Stage 1: Novice – where everything is completely new and unfamiliar

Stage 1 of the Benner Continuum is *Novice*. Novice is defined by Benner as having 'no experience of the situations in which they are expected to perform' (1984: 20). Some of you may recognise this in yourselves as a student about to start placement for the first time ever. Benner describes this very early stage as there having been no practical or real-world situations encountered which means that the student has to essentially follow simple overarching rules until they have more experiences in the specific setting (Benner, 1984). In some ways as a student, everyone will be starting, or have elements of their placement experience, in this first Novice section. Even if you are using a setting you have worked in currently or previously, just being there now as a student is new.

Benner's suggestion that, at this Novice stage, people need to follow set and objective rules begins to illustrate the key rationale and importance for practical work-based learning. In terms of being a student this is where you will perhaps begin to see that some things taught to you in the relative safety and theoretical world of your lectures and classes do not match or work as smoothly out in your actual placement setting with real service users and clients. Benner states that this is because 'clinical practice is always more complex and presents many more realities than can be captured by theory alone' (Benner, 1984: 36). An example of this as a case study is that a student learnt about Makaton in class and was excited to use it with a service user who the student knew was non-verbal. The student tried to use Makaton with the service user who responded, but not with gestures the student knew from class. The student did not understand, and this seemed to upset the service user. The student spoke with their mentor who explained the service user did use gestures to communicate but had their own gestures as they did not have the fine motor control for BSL or Makaton. The student then learnt the specific gestures for the specific service user.

Stage 2: Advanced beginner – becoming more used to how things work

Stage two is the *Advanced* Beginner. This is where you have seen enough real-world situations to begin to notice, or have pointed out to you, the more context specific aspects of a situation. You begin to move on from context-free rules or lists and can begin to assess and understand contextual aspects specific to the individual situation (Benner, 1984). Benner discusses how these two earliest stages in particular can be somewhat overwhelming, and you may struggle to take in all of the new information and experiences while also having to remember the 'rules' of this new setting. This overwhelming feeling is the same for everyone. This is not because your previous experience disappears or becomes irrelevant, but because there are now new rules to learn and new experiences to encounter that need new context placed on them.

Stage 3: Competent – being able to work on your own

Benner's assertion is that someone who is a *Competent* practitioner might have been in the same job role, or same setting for a couple of years. In terms of being a student starting the course as a Competent practitioner, we would make the assumption that you are used to a health or social care environment, and are likely to be using your workplace for your placement experience (or if not, you are able to assimilate easily into a similar role in a similar setting). It is likely that you will be familiar with the professional language used in practice and have a clear sense of the roles of other colleagues and professionals. It is also likely that you will have a good understanding of the day-to-day duties and responsibilities of the role, as well as a good level of experience of client needs, and the situations that may arise in the setting. Benner details in nursing that 'the competent nurse lacks the speed and flexibility of the proficient nurse but does have a feeling of mastery... [and that] ...the conscious, deliberate planning that is characteristic of this skill level helps achieve efficiency and organisation...' (Benner, 1984: 27).

Stage 4: Proficient – becoming skilled in your role

A *Proficient* practitioner is an applicable description for those of you who are not just Competent in practice, but capable enough to be able to clearly evaluate your knowledge, skills and experience. This allows you to assess what it is you would like to develop in these areas, while (arguably) not having the challenges of those who are Novice going into a workplace for the first time. You are able to take your professional communication and understanding of your setting as a given, and perhaps not have to deal with some of the more uncomfortable feelings of starting completely afresh.

As a Proficient practitioner, you are in a comfortable, yet exciting, position point to be able to consolidate what you have already learned in your career so far as a strong foundation towards gaining those additional experiences and *Expert* skills.

At the same time, you are clearly hopeful to develop your knowledge, skills and experience, so as a student on placement (even as an employee in your own workplace), having a more experienced, senior mentor will be a really important component of your placement. We would advise you to 'put your student hat on' during your placement hours at work, and ask questions of yourself, your colleagues, your mentor and your manager. Examine why certain practices are done, and what is effective – or ineffective – about them. Start to link the theory that you are gaining at university to your practice, to further your understanding. Relish new experiences that are offered, and work with your mentor/manager to identify new learning opportunities for yourself – whether that is further training in a particular area, or a chance to shadow a different colleague, for example. Hone your skills of reflective practice (see Chapter 17) during placement, so that you can effectively evaluate your experiences in practice and develop your skills. As

Thompson and Thompson (2023: 10) explain, 'Learning will not take place and practice will not develop if no connections are made between the thinking and the doing – that is, if we are not able to understand what we are doing and why we are doing it as part of a broader, more holistic picture of our work'.

Stage 5: Expert – mastering a skill

As the final stage of the Continuum, Benner describes the *Expert* as having enormous background experience, an intuitive grasp of each situation and performing from a deep understanding (Benner, 1984). The question at this point in your journey is to consider how this Expert label fits your current situation, and whether you are an Expert yourself in any way. It is probable that as you are still a student, you are not yet an Expert in this kind of work overall, but there may be specific aspects where you might be. You may also be working alongside people who are Experts in the field, either in placement or in university.

We think you should be aiming to become an Expert but consider how you will manage to get there. You may not accomplish this by the end of this placement or even the end of this course. Benner does explore the idea that the experience you need to move through the stages is not about the amount of time you have spent, but rather the refinement of ideas based on the number of practical situations you have encountered (Benner, 1984). And that is an attitude you should take into whatever placements you do. You will likely have little control over its duration, but you can likely influence the number of practical experiences you encounter. Even if your placement is for a short time, you should still try to make it more valuable for yourself by trying to get as actively involved as possible.

If you recognise yourself in these stages, and we imagine that most if not all of you do at least to some extent, there are some things you can do to keep ahead of yourself. Firstly, hopefully there is some reassurance just in reading this section and recognising that anything you are feeling in yourself around being nervous, overwhelmed or drained by placement is absolutely normal. What we perhaps need to help you with at this point is to offer suggestions on how to cope with these feelings. Some general tips and advice we can offer are speaking to your mentor/placement supervisor, booking a tutorial with a tutor/lecturer, reaching out to friends or peers who are going through similar placement experiences or doing some wider reading around what you are seeing and dealing with in placement. These are all by necessity fairly broad as we do not know you as a specific student, so do try things out and see what is beneficial for you.

A key thing to appreciate with our use of the Benner Continuum, if considered genuinely and honestly, is that there will be movement back and forth through the different stages when things change. For example, even an experienced and Proficient staff member may suddenly shift to being an Advanced Beginner if moving jobs to a different organisation or new service users arrive with a diagnosis they haven't worked with previously.

Throughout this chapter, we have taken the base framework and stages from the Benner Continuum and slightly re-purposed it for a more general and varied use than the original intention. We are essentially suggesting its use as a framework, so how you use it is up to you. However, we would say it is best used with real consideration and honesty, requiring you to be clear and genuine about where you are on the continuum.

We provide more detail on the stages in the main sections below, moving from pre-placement through to post-placement. The next section of this chapter outlines important factors to complete and be aware of before your placement starts.

Pre-Placement

As a new student, you firstly need to find out how you get a placement arranged. Many courses send their students out on a specific set of placements that the university has pre-arranged. Other courses work completely differently, for example, by supporting their students to find their own placement, and some courses may use online or peer learning placements.

Finding a placement

If you are on a course that needs you to find your own placement, you should check if there is anyone from the university to support this. Also, check if they already know any potential placement providers. Some of the starter questions you can consider to help this process are:

- Could you use a current relevant job or volunteer work?
- Who are you interested in working with?
- Where geographically does your placement need to be?
- What work do you want to move into?
- What experience do you already have?

If you need to contact a potential placement yourself, the first step is to send a polite email outlining who you are, what your course is and why you want this placement setting specifically.

You may not get an immediate response back, and you may have to follow up on your initial email. Our suggestion is to try and be patient, as most settings are usually very busy, but if after a week you have had no reply, it might be best to make a phone call.

Administrative and practical aspects of placement

Whether you need to find your own placement or you get sent to pre-arranged settings, there is a broad list of administrative and personal considerations that you should try to get familiar with before starting your placement, or even the course itself. Some of these are likely to be a simple rule or policy that covers the course or all placements, and some need more specific input or discussion for you as an individual.

The administrative aspects to check likely include things like:

- **Paperwork** – Most courses with a placement need to get students cleared or approved with a **Disclosure and Barring Service (DBS) check** and an **Occupational Health check (OH)** (Learning Box 19.1) and possibly more. Check how these get sent to you, and what the timeframe is for you to complete them.
- **Uniform/Training** – check if you need to wear a uniform, and/or complete any mandatory pre-placement training. If so, check how this is provided and whether you need to pay for it yourself.
- **Assessments** – check what you will actually do on your placement. This is often about completing a set of competencies and then completing a portfolio or essay-based assessment. You should also check if you will need some kind of mentor or supervisor in placement.

Learning Box 19.1: DBS and OH checks

A Disclosure and Barring Service (DBS) check refers to a criminal records check, to establish if you have any criminal convictions that bar you from working with certain groups of people. It is mandatory for people working in health and social care settings to have a DBS check. There are different levels of DBS check, for example, basic or enhanced, and your placement or university should provide guidance on this. Once a check is undertaken, you should receive a certificate detailing the results of the check.

An Occupational Health (OH) check evaluates the health and fitness of students undertaking a placement. It usually includes an initial questionnaire completed by the student, but in some cases, may include medical assessments, screening, or further discussions about the student's physical and mental wellbeing to ensure they can safely undertake the placement. It is always focused on supporting the student, and its goal is to safeguard wellbeing, prevent workplace injuries or illnesses, and ensure students have a successful work-based learning experience.

- **Placement Policies** – check the policies that are in place for your placement. Most organisations have policies in place for **whistleblowing and safeguarding** (Learning Box 19.2) health and safety, disciplinary and equal opportunity. These policies detail what your responsibilities are while on placement and what to do when you are not sure in certain circumstances.

  The personal aspects to check likely include things like:
- **Reasonable Adjustments** – consider if you have any learning differences or physical conditions that might need to be taken into consideration or require some reasonable adjustments. If so, consider how you get this arranged – it usually connects in some way to any needs assessments or adjustments made for the lecture/academic side of your course but do not forget about your placement when completing this.

Learning Box 19.2: Whistleblowing/safeguarding

Whistleblowing is the term used when someone reports a concern about poor practice or risk, usually about their workplace (Rahman and Myers, 2019), so this may be a concern about poor care provided by a carer or the organisation.

Safeguarding is the general process of keeping anybody safe. You can get more information on safeguarding in Chapter 11.

As a student, there is a legal and moral requirement to whistleblow and declare or follow up any safeguarding concern. Placement settings and universities should have clear published guidelines and procedures to support you on placement. These should include how to report concerns.

Before starting your placement, you should make yourself aware of your university's and placement's policies and procedures and key contacts for whistleblowing and safeguarding.

- **Time Management** – consider factors such as travel time, caring responsibilities and any other work. Remember to also factor in and prioritise the more easily forgotten but important elements like self-care or time for socialising.

During placement

In this section, we focus on aspects of work-based learning that you might want to consider during your placement. We appreciate that as health and social care students you are going to be:

a based in a wide variety of care settings and working with different client groups;
b fulfilling a range of assessment briefs depending on your specific course requirements;
c arriving at university with a wealth of different experiences, backgrounds and skills.

For this reason, it is difficult for us to provide you with detailed, specific information about exactly how your placement might develop or the tasks you will be undertaking, but we have anticipated some general practical considerations – particularly around professionalism, communicating expectations, and maintaining boundaries. We focus specifically on the workplace related considerations in this chapter, but you will find much more information around theory and classroom-based aspects of work-based learning throughout this book.

Placement mindset

This section signposts you to three concepts to help you develop over your time on placement – professional attitude, reflection and person-centred care. As well as the important practical elements needed in terms of finding and starting a placement, it is also vital to think about the more theoretical aspects to preparing for practice, which form part of what Williams and Conroy (2022) refer to as a 'placement mindset'.

Professional attitude

Some of what is considered 'professional' is thought of in terms of behaviour (such as good time management and appropriate dress mentioned previously), but we have also identified three key themes in terms of what an effective professional attitude involves:

- ***Curiosity*** – Do not be afraid of asking questions in placement. This shows that you are keen to learn but also helps you to settle into the placement quickly, understand why certain tasks are done the way they are, and ultimately be able to link theory and improve your own practice. For example, a Novice might want to know how a hoist works in helping a resident in a care home. For a more Expert practitioner, the question asked might be a philosophical reflective question examining their values. *This professional curiosity and desire to continually learn and develop is integral to being an effective student on placement.*
- ***Capacity*** – Knowing your role and capabilities is another important aspect of being a professional. As before, wherever you see yourself on the Benner Continuum, an understanding of the responsibilities and boundaries of your role will allow you to work safely and effectively – this might be as a Novice, ensuring that you do not take on more

than you are equipped to deal with, or as an Competent practitioner, having additional learning development opportunities identified that are extra to your existing role.

- ***Collaboration*** – It should probably go without saying, but you will need to work effectively with other people on placement, whether they are fellow colleagues, other professionals, mentors, clients, families, university staff or peers. A willingness to work with – and learn from – other people, whatever their background, story or experience is key in practice. Not only will this help you to get to know people that you are working with and caring for, but will allow you to maintain effective professional communication, develop an understanding of person-centred care, and work well as part of a team.

Reflection

Reflective practice is covered in its own chapter in this book in Chapter 17, and it is an integral part of your placement and your assignments. Some of you who identify yourselves as Competent (or higher) on the Benner Continuum in terms of your professional skills and experience will likely be familiar with the idea of reflecting on your practice, while others may not have heard of this before. Either way, in terms of this area of preparation, you need to be willing to take time to look back at a situation in practice, analyse it, evaluate the positive and negative aspects of what happened, examine the situation through a theoretical lens, and be prepared to implement changes based on what you have learned.

Person-centred care

The notion of being person-centred can be attributed to the work of Carl Rogers (1957). Rogers proposed that in order to have a successful and effective counselling relationship with a client (and for the patient to thereby affect positive change in their situation), the counsellor needed to be congruent, empathic, and hold unconditional positive regard for their client.

Whether you are working with babies and young children, older people living with dementia, or any client group in between, the concept of person-centred care means 'ensuring that people's preferences, needs and values guide clinical decisions and providing care that is respectful of and responsive to them' (Health Education England, 2023). How person-centred care looks for your clients will depend on the setting you are in, and the wants and needs of the people you are caring for. You may experience barriers to being able to always provide full person-centred care – such as staffing and time constraints – that you are not able to control (Mackreth and Walker, 2021) but it is a vital component of caring effectively in practice.

Issues on placement

While it is exciting to consider all the learning opportunities that are due to come your way whatever your level of experience, from Novice through to Expert, we would be doing something of a disservice if we did not highlight that sometimes things do go wrong on placement. Issues often arise at the start of placements, and we often see issues around mismanaged expectations, communication between students and mentors and personality clashes. Difficulties on placements can be due to all sorts of factors, but the most important piece of advice we have is to talk to someone. If you cannot talk to your mentor at placement, you should talk to a member of staff at the university as soon as any issues arise. The worst thing is just to withdraw and isolate yourself and not seek support or practice self-care. University study and placement learning are likely to be, and perhaps indeed should be, challenging but they should never be crushing, so do be honest and pro-active with getting yourself supported through these new and potentially overwhelming experiences. You should make yourself aware of what policies and procedures your course and/or placement setting have to support you.

Post-placement

Once you complete your first placement, you may be concentrating on placement-related assignments or practice-based portfolios for university, reflecting on your placement experience and planning action steps for the next time. There are specific skills and services that you can use to help you with this, as detailed below.

Self-reflection

We hope by now you understand what reflection means and how you might process this using Benner Continuum – or that you can at least see the importance of thinking back over an experience. However you reflect, it is important to look back and see how far you have come during this placement. This is a time to give yourself a pat on the back, record all the successful or rewarding situations you experienced, and consider the skills you have developed during this time. This is important to give you confidence for your practice going forward, and to recognise your strengths both personally and professionally. As Ghaye and Lillyman (2014) assert, it is the positive interactions and successful experiences that need to be repeated, not the failures.

It goes without saying that you also need to think about the areas that you found challenging – perhaps these were interactions with staff or clients that did not go well, or maybe there was an obvious gap in your theoretical knowledge when you needed it on the spot. Whatever the areas for improvement, make a note of these, and think about how you might deal with them on your next placement.

Mentor feedback

Your reflections on the most recent experience you had need to go hand-in-hand with the feedback you received from your mentor. This may have been formal feedback you received at the end, or it may have been done throughout your placement. You may find there are areas you agree with in terms of the feedback, or you may find that there are aspects highlighted to you that you had not been aware of. If you can ask for further clarification from your mentor, this can be helpful. If not, these are areas that can be considered for development next time. This links to a theory known as Johari's Window that you may find useful to look up as a tool for understanding your self-awareness (Luft and Ingham, 1955). You can read more about this in Mackreth and Walker (2021), chapter 2.

Next placement?

If your course has multiple placements, it is worth considering how you get ready to move into a second or third placement, carrying forward what you learnt from your first placement considering the steps and guidance above. Some courses only have one placement, so this may not be relevant to everyone.

Longer term considerations

In some ways, the long-term considerations post-placement are the same as the short-term considerations. Importantly, you should reflect just how far you have progressed and grown and feel proud of what you have accomplished. In the longer term, once you have finished your course and all the immediate placement requirements, be aware of any new practical considerations or rules that may apply. Things to consider might include:

- If you need a reference, consider whether one of your placement tutors or mentors might be a good person to write it for you.
- If you are exploring new employment options, or even further post-graduate study, consider not just what you learnt from your placements but also any contacts you may have made. This kind of professional and inter-professional networking can be beneficial in helping you make career decisions and advance in employment. It can happen that placements take a student as a volunteer and be so impressed they encourage them to apply for a paid role within the organisation. When it comes to applying for jobs or further academic study there can be a tendency to focus on classroom learning and forget the richness of your placement-based learning. Do not discount those placement experiences just because you had them 'just on placement' or 'only as a student'. Your placement experiences and learning can be really rich and can form the basis for successful personal statements or interviews for a long time afterwards.
- If you would like to specialise in a specific area or kind of health and social care work, consider if there may have been a specific kind of work or patient or job role that really engaged and motivated you, that perhaps you were unaware of before starting placement.

As a final note, as you continue in this kind of work, it is likely that at some point you may end up supporting students as a mentor yourself. In some roles this is almost guaranteed and may happen very swiftly, so try your best to remember your own placement experiences. Consider how it felt on that first day, what your supervisors did that really helped you or that perhaps really did not help you. If, and when, you become a mentor yourself, remember that as every service user is different, so is every student, and remember the Benner Continuum. This new mentoring role may send you towards the Novice stage again where you rely just on your own rules and experiences. You may well make missteps learning this, but we still offer the same advice, keep a note on what you've done, reflect and learn, and keep moving towards becoming a fully rounded Expert.

Summary

In this chapter, we have examined the placement-based learning journey from the start of your course to the completion of your first placement, using the Benner Continuum.

We have used Benner Continuum to highlight the way that your placement experience may differ depending on whether you view yourself as a Novice, Advanced Beginner, Competent, Proficient or Expert, and have attempted to reassure you that there is no right or wrong stage to be at in your professional experience.

We have highlighted that there are practical arrangements that you may need to make before a placement starts, such as where to look for an opportunity, and what sort of paperwork you might need to complete. We have also outlined the importance of having a theoretical mindset before going out on practice that focuses on professional curiosity and a willingness to learn.

Finally, we have discussed the potential post-placement actions you could take. This can be in the short term, such as reflecting back on your experiences, and preparing for your next placement, or whether in the longer term, such as thinking about your career and how you might mentor less experienced colleagues.

Whatever your starting position as you read this book – whether you would deem yourself to be a Novice, Competent or Expert – remember that you always have something to offer, as well as something to learn. We hope this chapter has helped you to prepare well for your placements, and we wish you all the best with your work-based learning experiences.

References

Benner, P. (1984) *From Novice to Expert: Excellence and Power in Clinical Nursing Practice.* California: Addison-Wesley.

Ferrandez-Berrueco, R. and Sanchez-Tarazaga, L. (2021) 'Student work-placements from the company perspective: A case study', *Higher Education, Skills and Work-Based Learning*, 11(4), pp. 888–907.

Ghaye, T. and Lillyman, S. (2014) *Reflection: Principles and Practices for Healthcare Professionals.* 2nd edn. London: Quay Books, A Division of MA Healthcare Ltd.

Health Education England (2023) *Person-centred care.* Available at https://www.hee.nhs.uk/our-work/person-centred-care (Accessed 12 August 2024).

Luft, J. and Ingham, H. (1955) *The Johari Window, a Graphic Model of Interpersonal Awareness.* Proceedings of the western training laboratory in group development. Los Angeles: UCLA.

Mackreth, P. and Walker, B. (2021) *A Handbook for Support Workers in Health and Social Care: A Person-Centred Approach.* Milton: Taylor & Francis Group. Available from ProQuest Ebook Central (Accessed 18 December 2023).

Naish, J. and Minton, A. (2015) 'Support and guidance for work-based learning students' in Helyer, R (ed.) *The Work-Based Learning Student Handbook.* 2nd edn. London: Palgrave.

Rahman, S. and Myers, R. (2019) *Courage in Healthcare: A Necessary Virtue or Warning Sign?* London: SAGE Publications Ltd.

Rogers, C.R. (1957) 'The necessary and sufficient conditions of therapeutic personality change', *Journal of Consulting Psychology*, 21(2), pp. 95–103.

Thompson, S. and Thompson, N. (2023) *The Critically Reflective Practitioner.* Bloomsbury Publishing Plc. London ProQuest Ebook Central (Accessed 15 January 2024).

Williams, S. and Conroy, D. (eds.) (2022) *A Student's Guide to Placements in Health and Social Care Settings: From Theory to Practice.* St Albans: Critical Publishing. Available from ProQuest Ebook Central (Accessed 18 December 2023).

20 Leadership and teamworking – the foundations of organisational culture in health and social care practice

Lisa Porter and Clair Rees

The aims of this chapter are to:

- **Define leadership and identify leadership approaches for contemporary health and social care practice**
- **Define teamworking and identify types of teamworking for current health and social care practice**
- **Explain the importance of both leadership and teamworking to positive organisational culture in health and social care**

Introduction

Research shows that effective leadership and teamwork are vital for delivering high-quality health and social care services, directly influencing organisational culture which improves care (Ystaas *et al.*, 2023). Leaders who promote inclusivity help create robust and resilient teams who are equipped to learn from mistakes and adapt to challenges (Nembhard and Edmondson, 2006). Leadership in health and social care significantly influences patient outcomes, staff morale, and service quality. Successful leaders therefore understand the different approaches to leadership and management and recognise the need to adapt their approach based on team needs and organisational context (Yukl, 2013). Applying the skills and knowledge of effective leadership creates a more cohesive and adaptable staff team who are more resilient to the dynamic pressures within health and social care. Teamworking is equally crucial, contributing to better decision-making, efficiency, and quality of care. Effective teams improve health outcomes, reduce staff turnover, and enhance service user satisfaction (West *et al.*, 2014). This chapter explores leadership styles and teamworking. It examines their practical application in health and social care settings and highlights their role in enabling a positive organisational culture that supports enhanced patient and service user outcomes.

What is leadership?

Leadership in health and social care can be defined as the ability to inspire, influence, and guide individuals and teams towards delivering high-quality, person-centred care. It involves cultivating a culture of collaboration, ethical decision-making, and continuous improvement to enhance patient outcomes, staff well-being, and service delivery. Effective leaders in these sectors must possess adaptability, emotional intelligence, and a commitment to advocating for both service users and the workforce, ensuring care that

DOI: 10.4324/9781032619309-23

Table 20.1 The differences between leaders and managers

Leaders	*Managers*
Focus on **vision and change** – they inspire and motivate staff to improve services.	**Focus** on **organisation and efficiency** – they ensure day-to-day operations run smoothly.
Encourage innovation and adapt to new policies, technologies, and patient needs.	**Implement** policies, procedures, and regulations to maintain quality care.
Informal authority, influencing teams through personal qualities, respect, and expertise.	**Formal authority**, responsible for budgets, staffing, and compliance.
Prioritise long-term goals and service improvements for better patient outcomes.	**Prioritise short-term goals**, ensuring services meet standards and performance targets.

is safe, equitable, and sustainable (Birken *et al.*, 2018). The leadership approaches used in practice often align with a specific leadership style (for example, autocratic and democratic) or underpinning theory (for example, emotional intelligence, servant, or transformational leadership), as discussed below.

The leadership approach taken by an individual influences the team dynamics, staff morale, service efficiency, and ultimately, patient outcomes – demonstrating how important it is to get right. For healthcare students, understanding various leadership approaches and their influence on team cohesion and organisational culture is essential. This knowledge forms the foundation for recognising the diversity and relevance of leadership approaches, depending on the context, workforce, and organisational goals.

Leader vs manager

The terms 'leader' and 'manager' are sometimes used interchangeably to mean the same thing. However, they refer to different, focused roles and have distinct meanings. Recognising these differences is important for understanding the benefits and limitations of both roles and how they can be utilised effectively in health and social care. Table 20.1 summarises the key distinctions between leadership and management based on widely recognised principles.

As shown in Table 20.1, managers focus on processes, structure, and efficiency, using planning and organisation skills to help ensure order and maintain consistency. Leaders inspire, motivate, and drive change towards a shared vision (Swanwick, 2019). In recognition of the need for innovation and adaptability, the National Health Service (NHS) has invested in leadership development through initiatives like the NHS Leadership Academy (2025) while maintaining managerial roles to uphold policies, procedures, and operational efficiency. In some cases, the person responsible for a service may need to fulfil both leadership and management functions. This overlap explains why the terms are often used interchangeably and highlights the importance of understanding their distinctions. Leadership theories and styles are not exclusive in their uses, and they can be utilised by both managers and leaders.

Leadership approaches

Understanding leadership styles and theories provides the foundation for adopting specific approaches within the workplace. The leadership approach adopted directly shapes how staff are supported and how effectively services are delivered. For example, theories such as transformational leadership influence how a leader motivates staff and drives change. Increased knowledge of the diversity and adaptability of leadership models means individuals can increase self-awareness of their own skills, and practice different approaches that align with organisational goals and team needs.

Leadership styles

Kurt Lewin's work on leadership (1939) provided a foundational framework for understanding various leadership styles and their associated behaviours. Lewin identified three primary leadership styles: autocratic, democratic, and laissez-faire, extended later by others to include bureaucratic leadership. Table 20.2 summarises these core leadership styles, highlighting their differences and outlining the potential benefits and limitations of each approach in the workplace.

Current and emerging leadership theories

Lewin's leadership styles in Table 20.2 have been highly influential over the last 50 years. However, current and emerging leadership theories focus more on collaboration and

Table 20.2 Lewin's leadership styles

Leadership style	*Description*	*Potential impact on a team*
Autocratic e.g. Hierarchical/ Top-Down/ Authoritarian	*Tells*. One way communication is used. Lack of consultation with colleagues. Desire for control in decision-making. Limited delegation.	*Benefits*: Useful in the right type of setting or circumstance where tight control, clear direction and rapid decisions are needed, such as miliary/command and control situations or circumstances such as the COVID-19 pandemic. *Limitations*: Long-term use is likely to lead to lack of motivation, reduced job satisfaction and low morale. Potential for disconnection from the leader.
Democratic e.g. Transformational/ Compassionate/ Servant	*Asks*. Two-way communication is used. Promotes sharing of responsibility, consultation, delegation, and feedback. Creates, a culture of leadership development.	*Benefits*: Enhances involvement and shared decision-making. Open communication creates a motivated workforce that feels valued and committed. *Limitations*: Lengthy decision-making processes can be slow, causing frustration and increasing costs. May not be suitable in rapid change or high-pressure situations where there is insufficient time to involve and consult.
Laissez-faire e.g. Delegative	*Avoids*: Little or no direction. Employees have ultimate freedom because authority is given to staff who must establish goals, make decisions and resolve problems. Meaning the leader is in name only, providing little actual leadership.	*Benefits*: Effective when staff are highly experienced, competent and motivated. Staff can feel trusted and committed by the leader delegating power to them. *Limitations*: Can be overwhelming and potentially unsafe if staff feel insecure and need leadership. Oversight and involvement are still needed for staff to feel connected to leader.

(*Continued*)

Table 20.2 (Continued)

Leadership style	*Description*	*Potential impact on a team*
Bureaucratic e.g. Rigid Leadership/ Transactional	*Organises*: Ensures policies and procedures are in place, job roles are clear, and that staff follow the rules creating a sense of order and stability.	*Benefits:* Clear structures for service operation are in place, enabling safe practice and the maintenance of high standards. Useful to bring order to chaotic situations. A useful approach to maintaining safe standards within health and social care settings. *Limitations:* Can stifle creativity and autonomy, resulting in demotivated staff, and organisation which does not progress or adapt well to change. Can be limiting in an era of rapid change.

inclusivity. These modern approaches create an environment in which all individuals are valued and diverse perspectives contribute to decision-making and innovation (Department of Health and Social Care, 2022).

Consequently, contemporary leadership approaches that emphasise empathy, ethical decision-making, and the empowerment of others are being adopted. These qualities align with the core values of health and social care, enabling growth, innovation, adaptability, and resilience, which are important for the sector's future. This section outlines key features of current and emerging leadership approaches, including transformational, emotionally intelligent, servant, and sustainable ethical leadership, which are aligned with the future direction of health and social care.

Transformational leadership

The theory of transformational leadership, first proposed by Burns (1978) and later expanded by Bass (1985, 1990), focuses on inspiring and empowering followers to exceed expectations. Bass and Bass (2008) further refined this theory by emphasising the need for leaders to foster creativity, motivate and engage individuals through a shared vision, and support personal development. This leadership style promotes intellectual stimulation, encouraging innovation and enabling team members to reach their full potential.

Ultimately, transformational leadership drives change by shaping attitudes, values, and behaviours, creating an environment where individuals can grow and contribute to organisational success. Within healthcare, this approach is particularly relevant, as the sector relies on innovation, motivation, and continuous improvement to overcome the many challenges it faces. Transformational leaders lead by example, creating a culture where learning and evidence-based practice are central to service improvement and change.

Emotional intelligent leadership

Emotional intelligence is the ability to recognise, manage, and regulate emotions in ourselves and others (Goleman, 1995). It helps us stay in control of our feelings, respond calmly to challenges, and understand how others feel. Key skills include self-awareness (knowing our emotions), self-regulation (controlling our reactions), and empathy (understanding others). Goleman (1995) suggests that these skills are necessary to lead effectively inorder to aid adaptation in dynamic high-pressure demanding and changeable situations within healthcare. These leaders build trust, compassion and collaboration within the team, reducing conflict and building resilience to protect against challenges such as staff burnout.

Servant leadership

Through serving others as a priority, leaders act as a catalyst for the growth, well-being, and professional development of their teams (Blanchard and Broadwell, 2018). In healthcare settings, a servant leadership approach is increasingly valued as it prioritises team well-being, personal growth, and compassionate service delivery. This can improve staff morale, employee retention, and maintain good service quality. Emotionally intelligent and servant leadership approaches involve qualities that support improved patient satisfaction and enhanced care quality.

Sustainable ethical leadership

This leadership approach in healthcare integrates long-term ethical and environmentally responsible strategies into service delivery, considering both immediate patient needs and future societal and environmental impacts (McKimm and McLean, 2020). Sustainability in this context includes both environmental sustainability, such as reducing waste and lowering carbon emissions, and operational sustainability, ensuring that resources, staffing, and funding are managed effectively to maintain long-term service quality. It involves guiding teams with principles of integrity, fairness, and transparency, ensuring equitable access to care, fair resource distribution, and culturally competent care practices. Ethical leaders empower others, promote ethical decision-making, and embed sustainable practices to enhance resilience in a dynamic healthcare environment.

Sustainable leaders integrate both ethical and long-term environmental considerations into their decision-making (Wu and Zhu, 2022). The combination of sustainable and ethical leadership is an emerging focus – named 'eco-ethical leadership' by McKimm and McLean (2020). With this approach leaders balance individual needs and long-term societal responsibilities, promoting values that support sustainability in healthcare settings. This combined approach enables healthcare leaders to address economic, social, and environmental challenges effectively, while meeting both immediate and long-term responsibilities, including providing ethical care for patients and service users.

A summary of the key features of these current and emerging leadership approaches is provided in Table 20.3, along with examples of what this might look like in health and social care practice.

The summary of foundational leadership styles in Table 20.2 and current and emerging leadership theories in Table 20.3 demonstrates a wide range of approaches to leadership. While individuals may have the skills, experience and values aligned to a particular leadership style, Hersey and Blanchard (1969) argue that there is no single 'best' leadership style. Rather, leaders must adjust their approach based on the contextual situation, adapting to the needs and competency of the team or individual. This might mean, for example, adopting a bureaucratic leadership style to bring order to chaotic situations or transformational leadership during periods of significant change. Effective leaders often

Table 20.3 Current and emerging leadership theories

Leadership theory	*Key features*	*Example in practice*
Transformational Leadership	Creates vision. Leading by example, inspires and motivates promoting creativity and innovation, developing staff members skills	A senior doctor leads a project to improve patient safety in A&E. They inspire the team with a vision for better care, encourage innovative ideas, and implement new protocols that reduce waiting times and medical errors
Emotional Intelligent Leadership	Self-awareness, self-regulation, and empathy in self, and fostering these skills in others. Adaptability and resilience to withstand sector pressures.	A ward manager notices a nurse is overwhelmed after a difficult shift. They check in with the nurse, offer support, and adjust their workload to prevent burnout, ensuring staff well-being and patient care are prioritised.
Servant Leadership	Focuses on team wellbeing, team members' professional development, and personal growth. Compassionate service delivery enhances care for patients.	A social care team leader actively supports frontline staff by stepping in to help with complex cases, ensuring they have the right skills and resources, organising staff training to support this and prioritising staff well-being, demonstrating that their leadership role is to serve and empower the team.
Sustainable Ethical Leadership	Balancing patient needs with future societal and environmental responsibilities and promoting values that support sustainability in healthcare.	A care home manager implements a new policy, reducing waste by switching to reusable medical supplies. They also invest in staff development to ensure long-term workforce sustainability, benefiting both the environment and the quality of care.

combine multiple styles to enable efficient teamwork, ethical standards, and responsive decision-making. Whatever leadership approach is adopted, ensuring it is appropriate to the context is essential because effective leadership enhances team performance, supports ethical decision-making and improves patient care (Dye, 2023). Effective leadership is therefore not defined by a specific style or type, but by aligning the leadership approach with the needs of the team and the context of the setting.

What is teamworking?

West (2012) defines teamworking as working together collaboratively with others to achieve common goals. This is achieved through effective communication, coordinated activities, relying on each other's skills, and being mutual accountable for your part in the team. Successful teams rely on each member contributing skills and expertise, engaging in problem-solving, and adapting to challenges to achieve their objectives. The core purpose of teamworking is to deliver safe, high-quality, and person-centred care for the benefit of patients and service users. Teamworking must be effective in order to achieve this. However, effective teamwork in health and social care is not just about best practice – it is also a legal requirement, mandated by legislation, supported by policy and reinforced by regulation. When the Care Quality Commission (see Chapter 7) inspect services against the *Health and Social Care Act 2008 (Regulated Activities) Regulations 2014*, they are looking for effective teamworking within and across organisations, ensuring collaboration prevents duplication, enhances care coordination, and improves continuity for individuals (Care Quality Commission, 2022).

The NHS Constitution emphasises the importance of teamwork in delivering high-quality care, particularly through Principle 5, which states that '*The NHS works across organisational boundaries and in partnership with other organisations*' (Gov.uk, 2025). This principle highlights the need for collaboration not just internally, but also between NHS services, local authorities, public sector organisations, private and voluntary providers to improve patient outcomes and community health. Similarly, the core NHS value of working together for patients (Gov.uk, 2023) reinforces that effective teamwork ensures coordinated, patient-centred care, where professionals across different sectors share knowledge and resources. Strong effective teamworking is therefore essential for providing high-quality care within a setting, and for working in partnership with other professionals and organisations, enhancing communication, and delivering seamless, integrated care for the benefit of patients.

Types of teams in health and social care

All healthcare workers regularly work in teams within their practice settings. Since the core purpose of teamworking is to provide safe, effective, person-centred care for individuals who often have complex care needs, collaborating with other professionals across different organisations is essential. Various types of teams exist, distinguished by membership and function within the health and social care system. These teams vary based on professional background, purpose, and structure, but all maintain a focus on sharing specialist knowledge.

The benefits of working collaboratively across organisations and professions include resource sharing, improved communication, continuity of care, and the breakdown of silos to support integrated working. These factors contribute towards enhanced service delivery and service user satisfaction. Understanding different types of teams is therefore important, as it helps healthcare students recognise the roles, dynamics, and collaboration methods within each team, enabling them to communicate effectively and contribute meaningfully when working in practice. The types of teams you will most likely connect with across the health and social care sector are explained below.

Multi-Disciplinary teams (MDTs)

MDTs are also referred to as interdisciplinary or multi-professional teams. They bring together professionals from various disciplines to collaborate towards a shared objective (Dodkin, 2021). Each team member contributes their specific expertise to meet the varied needs of patients or service users. There is no single prescribed structure for MDTs, allowing them to adapt flexibly to different contexts and requirements. The composition of an MDT is often shaped by the specific goal it aims to achieve and may extend beyond the boundaries of a single service, setting, or professional role. For example, an MDT involved in hospital discharge planning for an individual patient may include a private speech and language therapist, a local authority social worker, a care home manager, a discharge coordinator, and an NHS hospital doctor, working collaboratively to ensure a safe and effective transition of care.

Integrated care teams (ICT)

This type of teamworking involves collaboration across different providers (such as healthcare, social care, voluntary organisations, and community services) to provide seamless, integrated care for patients and service users. The *Health and Care Act 2022* formalised integrated care systems in England, aiming to improve collaboration for joined-up care. By reducing bureaucracy, encouraging partnership working, and prioritising local decision-making, the Act aimed to make services more responsive and sustainable. Establishing shared objectives, effective communication methods are important for successful teamworking.

Networked teams

Networked teams are a collaboration of professionals that extend across more than one department or organisation, working together to share knowledge, resources, and expertise for a specific purpose such as a project, service, or policy. While some networked teams operate within a defined timeframe, others may evolve continuously depending on their function and setting. These teams play a crucial role in facilitating care coordination, improving patient outcomes, and supporting the adoption of innovations. By creating professional connections and bridging gaps between disciplines, networked teams contribute to more efficient, person-centred care (Rajamani and Iyer, 2023). For example, a networked team might be established to develop an integrated mental health outreach programme. This team, comprising representatives from a local hospital, community mental health services, the local authority commissioning team, and a mental health charity, collaborates under a formal agreement until completion. By sharing knowledge and resources, each member contributes their expertise to design and implement the community mental health outreach service successfully.

Communities of practice (CoPs)

Unlike networked teams, which are often outcome-focused, CoPs develop organically and persist beyond a specific remit. The CoP's scope is informal with a focus on knowledge exchange, professional growth and collaborative learning across boundaries. CoPs have no fixed timeframe and are sustained through shared interest and engagement. Wenger *et al.* (2002) describe CoPs as groups of professionals (the community) who share a common domain of interest (the practice) and engage in joint learning or develop a shared body of knowledge by exchanging ideas and best practices. This enables innovation and supports continuous professional growth. For example, a CoP in mental health might consist of clinicians, social workers, and researchers (which together make up 'the community') who regularly meet informally to share best practices, discuss innovative treatments or explore challenges in patient care (which makes up 'the practice'). Such communities are self-sustaining, continuously advancing their shared expertise, ideas and knowledge (Wenger *et al.*, 2002).

Establishing and sustaining cross-organisational collaboration can be challenging due to differing priorities, professional cultures, governance structures, and legal and policy frameworks. Misaligned IT systems and data-sharing protocols can further hinder teamworking. Overcoming these barriers requires strong, effective leadership and supportive organisational structures (Best and Holmes, 2010). Practical steps, such as establishing common goals, data-sharing agreements, and aligning policies, can help facilitate cross-organisational collaboration.

Models of teamworking in health and social care

Models of teamworking describe the ways teams collaborate by focusing on their structure, organisation, and methods of interaction. The various types of teams discussed in this chapter may operate according to any of the models outlined below. Over the past decade virtual and hybrid models have emerged in response to technological advancements, policy changes, and sector demands, with the COVID-19 pandemic acting as a major catalyst. During this period, teams rapidly adapted to new ways of working and service delivery, accelerating the adoption of virtual collaboration. These practices have since become embedded in the post-pandemic workplace and three primary models of teamworking are discussed below:

Co-located teamworking

This is a team of people who work in the same physical space, for example, a care home, hospital, GP practice, or any other type of shared workspace (Jelphs *et al.*, 2016). This type of setup allows team members to collaborate, interacting to share ideas, skills and support each other, while accessing the equipment and facilities they need to provide person-centred care. Co-located teams are particularly beneficial in care settings, where direct interaction with patients or service users in one physical setting is crucial. However, this approach also presents challenges such as power dynamics forming bringing conflict, or the eroding of role boundaries as staff support each other. There may also be logistical constraints such as different staff needing to use the same space at the same time. Successful co-location needs clear role definitions, respect for professional boundaries, and proactive conflict management to maximise effectiveness.

Virtual teamworking

Individuals who are geographically dispersed, yet collaborate across boundaries, which may include locations, time zones, or organisations. These teams usually rely on information technology to maintain connections and collaborate effectively (for example, online video meetings, virtual groups, and shared document access) to facilitate their work (Jelphs *et al.*, 2016). In practice, for example, virtual MDTs allow various healthcare professionals to coordinate care efficiently, while reducing travel time and improving accessibility. Telehealth enables remote patient assessments, increasing access to care, particularly for those in rural areas or with travel limitations.

Hybrid teamworking

This flexible approach blends in-person and virtual collaboration using technology, allowing professionals to adapt based on specific tasks, goals, and service needs. This approach helps overcome geographical barriers and enhance flexibility. For instance, social workers can attend important in-person visits while using virtual platforms for case reviews or attending training. The hybrid approach balances the benefits of co-location and virtual working. Face-to-face interactions help build trust, rapport, and enhance communication. Meanwhile, virtual collaboration reduces travel time, increases efficiency, and allows for more inclusive participation which is especially important for dispersed teams.

Virtual and hybrid teamworking models do however create challenges that must be addressed for effective collaboration to be established and maintained. Communication barriers such as technical issues and digital inequality (including disparities in technology access, internet speed, and digital skills) can hinder participation. Additionally, blurred work-life boundaries may impact staff well-being and productivity. There are strategies which can be used to overcome these challenges, including coordinated planning, staff training, clear communication, and shared digital resources (Myszkowska and Łużniak-Piecha, 2022). By working towards digital equity, organisations can promote inclusive, accessible, and diverse teams while maximising the benefits of hybrid and virtual working models.

Features of effective teamworking

Buljac-Samardzic *et al.* (2020) highlight that high-functioning healthcare teams are defined by clear objectives, ensuring a shared understanding of purpose, along with well-defined roles and responsibilities so that each member understands their contribution. Strong leadership is also fundamental, as it provides direction and support, needed for team cohesion. Table 20.4 sets out some of the most important elements of effective

Table 20.4 Effective teamworking factors

Teamworking factor	*Description*
Communication and Information Sharing	Clear and open communication ensures all team members understand patient needs and contribute effectively towards effective teamworking, for example during staff handovers. This includes verbal and written communication in all formats, including digital and electronic (for example, digital care plans and emails).
Collaboration and Interprofessional Working (internally or externally)	Through collaboration team members share expertise, learn from one another, and develop a shared understanding of patient needs. This enhances efficiency and ensures continuity of care, particularly in complex cases requiring multidisciplinary input from a range of professionals, for example, within MDT meetings.
Mutual Accountability and Trust	Effective teams distribute responsibility fairly, ensuring all members roles are clear and that they are accountable for their contributions and actions, for example ensuring understanding of roles is often part of induction for new staff. Building psychological safety and trust among team members creates a supportive working environment, reducing workplace stress and enhancing patient safety, creativity and innovativeness.
Adaptability and Problem-Solving	Health and social care settings are dynamic, requiring teams to respond to emergencies, policy changes, resource changes and individual patient needs with flexibility. Teams that engage in reflective practice and learning can continuously improve their effectiveness, and problem solve to overcome challenges. Having regular and timely team meetings, for example, is one approach which can support this.
Strong Leadership and Decision-Making	Strong leadership is not simply referring to authority but to empowering teams and team members, guiding effective decision-making, and creating a positive team culture which can promote collaboration and innovation. Using transformational leadership to overcome low staff morale, high sickness and regular patient safety issues in a hospital setting is one such example.

teamworking, based upon common themes within effective teamworking literature (Edmondson, 1999; Goleman, 2017; O'Daniel and Rosenstein, 2008; Reeves *et al.*, 2017; West *et al.*, 2014). It also describes what these might look like in practice.

Table 20.4 enables you to understand the factors involved in achieving effective teamwork in practice, highlighting the core skills and principles needed to work collaboratively. By developing strong communication, personal accountability, adaptability, and building leadership skills, you will be better prepared to navigate complex healthcare environments and contribute to high-functioning teams.

West and Lyubovnikova (2012) researched UK healthcare teams and identified three key features of 'real' teams, which are necessary for delivering high-quality care and creating positive work environments. These are:

1 **Clear shared objectives:** the team must understand the goals to be achieved, so they can work towards these
2 **Working closely:** communicating and coordinating to deliver effective, efficient and continually improving compassionate care
3 **Meeting regularly:** to review and reflect on their performance and consider any areas of improvement needed

While regular meetings may seem unrealistic in a high-pressure sector, even brief check-ins (such as huddles or time-outs), or virtual meetings help teams stay connected and adaptable. When these key features are met, teams become more effective, reflective and innovative, enabling them to adapt to challenges, improve practices and become more resilient. For staff, 'real' teams create a sense of purpose and support, reducing stress and enhancing employee wellbeing and job satisfaction. Organisationally, 'real' teams, reduce staff sickness and turnover, improve efficiency, facilitate collaboration and accountability, ensuring care services are adaptable and effective. For patients' 'real' teams can deliver timely, person-centred care that improves their outcomes.

The success of a team in health and social care therefore depends on its ability to coordinate, integrate, and collaborate effectively due to clear objectives, defined roles, enhanced trust, personal accountability and good communication (Baird *et al.*, 2020; Care Quality Commission, 2024). These factors not only enhance patient outcomes but also align with regulatory standards, ensuring high-quality, person-centred care.

Ineffective teamworking

Just because a healthcare team is named as such, it does not automatically mean that it will be able to perform as a team. Ineffective teamworking in health and social care refers to poor collaboration among staff, teams, and services. West and Lyubovnikova (2013) describe ineffective teams as those lacking clear shared objectives, role clarity, and mutual accountability. There are two main types of ineffective teams: 'pseudo' teams (West and Lyubovnikova, 2012) and dysfunctional teams (West, 2012). The definitions below help demonstrate their differences:

- **A pseudo team** appears to be a team but lacks genuine collaboration and coordination. Team members may work in the same setting, but operate in parallel, independently rather than collectively, leading to inefficiency, poor communication, duplication or neglect of tasks, and a failure to innovate or adapt (West and Lyubovnikova, 2012).

These teams may still complete work, but without efficiency, shared purpose, or a positive impact on patients or service users.

- **A dysfunctional team** is actively hampered by internal conflict, lack of trust, poor leadership and ineffective communication (Stoller, 2021). A dysfunctional team fails because of division, with tensions between members preventing progress and leading to disorganisation, stress, and poor patient outcomes.

While both pseudo and dysfunctional teams hinder effective teamwork, they fail in different ways, as pseudo teams suffer from lack of collaboration and poor coordination, whereas dysfunctional teams break down due to conflict and poor leadership. Ultimately, both contribute to a poor organisational culture, creating disengagement, mistrust, and compromising the standards of service provided.

Developing teamworking

Tuckman's (1965) model of team development is particularly relevant when considering the challenges teams face and how it can affect teamworking and patient outcomes. Tuckman suggests that teams progress through four distinct stages of team development in succession, starting at 'forming' and progressing through the stages to 'performing'. Figure 20.1 describes each stage and shows the progression through the stages.

The team development stages in Figure 20.1 can be identified in teamworking across health and social care practice. One such example is an MDT which is formed to plan the hospital discharge of a patient with complex needs. The team includes a doctor, nurse, social worker, physiotherapist, care home representative, and discharge coordinator. Figure 20.2 shows how this team may progresses through the stages of Tuckman's model.

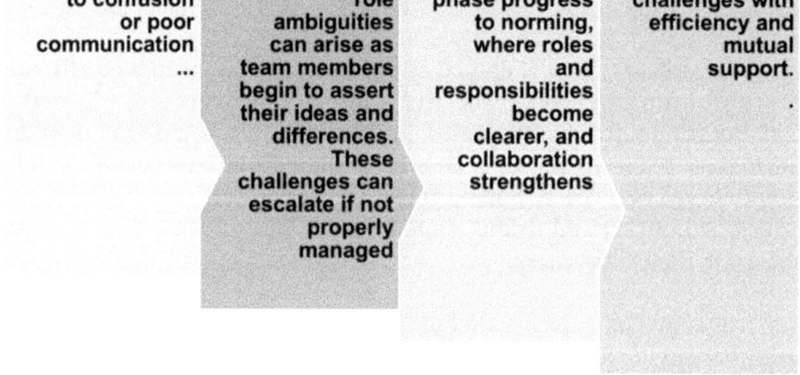

Figure 20.1 Tuckman's developmental stages.

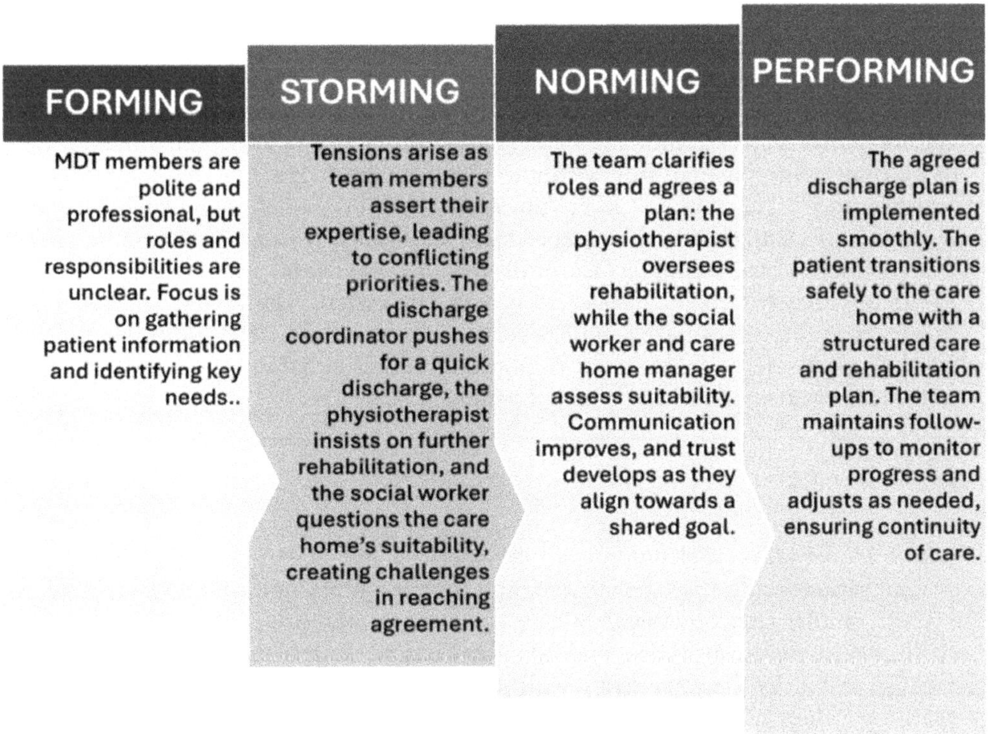

Figure 20.2 Tuckman's developmental stages applied to an MDT.

While the MDT team in the example above progress easily through each stage of team development, this is not always the case. Teams may become stuck in a particular stage and require support to progress. They can also revert to earlier stages due to factors such as the introduction of new team members, which may return the team to the 'forming' stage. Tuckman (1965) later added an 'adjourning' stage to the model which is relevant for teams working on specific tasks that come to an end, such as project teams. In the 'adjourning' stage teams reflect on achievements, celebrate contributions, and experience emotions such as sadness.

Recognising Tuckman's (1965) development stages enables teams to assess their current phase, identify obstacles, and take proactive steps towards more effective collaboration. Its enduring relevance attests to the model's robustness, helping leaders and teams to progress and achieve their full potential.

Leadership, teamworking, and organisational culture

Mannion and Davies (2018: 1) define organisational culture as 'the shared ways of thinking, feeling, and behaving in healthcare organisations'. This modern interpretation builds on traditional definitions that emphasise shared values and beliefs shaping working practices (Mannion and Davies, 2018; Schein, 2010). Organisational culture can be considered the 'personality' of a practice setting, shaped by the effectiveness of leadership and team collaboration. It determines how staff interact and ultimately influences how care is

Learning Box 20.1: The Winterbourne View scandal

The Winterbourne View scandal exposed the dangers of an abusive organisational culture, where poor recruitment, inadequate training, weak leadership, and a lack of accountability created an environment of fear and silence. A BBC Panorama investigation (2011) revealed severe physical and emotional abuse inflicted by staff on vulnerable individuals. The Department of Health review (2012) found that dysfunctional teamworking, a lack of professional oversight, and repeated failures to act on concerns enabled abuse to persist unchecked. The review stressed the urgent need for values-based, transparent, and accountable leadership, alongside psychological safety, professional responsibility, and collaborative teamworking, to prevent organisational cultures that enable abuse.

delivered. However, these definitions do not specify what constitutes a positive or negative organisational culture. A positive organisational culture in health and social care is one where mutual respect, ethical values, and best practice are consistently reflected in the collective mindset, attitudes, and behaviours that shape daily practices. A healthy culture is created by characteristics such as an inspiring leadership vision, shared organisational values, clear goals, and performance feedback, all of which support effective teamwork (King's Fund, 2025).

However, as past healthcare scandals have shown, ineffective teamwork can lead to errors and fragmented care for patients, while unclear roles create conflict, hierarchies, and exclusion which undermine the effectiveness of a team. This can be a recipe for a toxic team culture. If left unchecked, these issues can escalate into a 'culture of harm' where systemic failures and weak leadership normalise abusive practices (Borsay and Dale, 2018). An abusive culture in health and social care is a systemic pattern that normalises harmful behaviours such as discrimination, bullying, and blame, compromising both staff well-being and patient safety, as in the case of the **Winterbourne View scandal** (Learning Box 20.1), which highlighted what an abusive organisational culture looks like in practice.

Leadership and teamworking are interconnected, each shaping the other and both influencing the organisational culture of a healthcare setting as depicted in Figure 20.3. Leaders shape culture through their vision, decision-making, and interactions, which, in turn, influence team dynamics. West *et al.* (2014: 240) defines organisational culture in healthcare as 'the shared values, beliefs, and practices that shape how staff work together to provide patient-centred care, with a focus on collaboration, communication, and continuous improvement'. This definition demonstrates how effective healthcare teams engage well with one another and adapt to ever-changing challenges in providing care within a positive organisational culture.

Figure 20.3 illustrates that effective leadership is foundational for positive organisational culture and is essential for developing effective teamwork. Leaders set the tone within the organisation through their vision, decisions, and interactions, reinforcing the core values that shape the culture (Schein, 2010). Conversely, ineffective leadership can erode team collaboration, leading to a negative and toxic work environment. The key

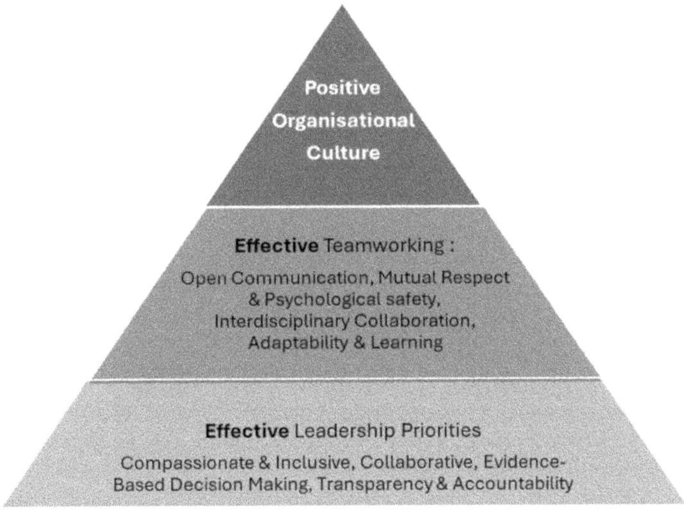
Positive
Organisational
Culture
Effective Teamworking :
Open Communication, Mutual Respect
& Psychological safety,
Interdisciplinary Collaboration,
Adaptability & Learning
Effective Leadership Priorities
Compassionate & Inclusive, Collaborative, Evidence-
Based Decision Making, Transparency & Accountability

Figure 20.3 The importance of leadership and teamworking to organisational culture.

takeaway from Figure 20.3 is that both leadership and teamwork are critical determinants of whether an organisational culture is positive or detrimental. A robust organisational culture, in turn, underpins sustained teamwork, which is vital for delivering high-quality, person-centred care. Consequently, fostering a strong organisational culture is instrumental in promoting the sustainability and resilience of health and social care services.

Summary

This chapter has demonstrated that effective leadership and teamwork are fundamental to shaping positive organisational culture and delivering high-quality, person-centred care in health and social care settings. Leadership drives vision and collaboration, while teamwork enhances service delivery and patient outcomes. A key distinction explored was between leaders who drive innovation and change, and managers who ensure stability and efficiency. An individual's leadership approach may be a distinct style, a modern leadership theory, or a blend of multiple styles and theories. Effective teamworking is equally vital, with 'real' teams having clear objectives, close collaboration, and regular reflection, leading to better adaptability, efficiency, and staff well-being. In contrast, 'pseudo' teams lack genuine teamwork, while dysfunctional teams suffer from conflict, poor leadership, and disorganisation). Both leadership and teamworking directly influence organisational culture, shaping whether a setting enables accountability and best practice or develops a toxic culture, highlighting the importance of understanding and practising effective leadership and teamworking.

References

Baird, B., Chauhan, K., Boyle, T., Heller, A. and Price, C. (2020) *How to build effective teams in general practice*. Available at https://www.kingsfund.org.uk/insight-and-analysis/long-reads/effective-teams-general-practice (Accessed 12 February 2025).

Bass, B.M. (1985) *Leadership and Performance beyond Expectations*. New York: Free Press.

Bass, B.M. (1990) 'From transactional to transformational leadership: Learning to share the vision', *Organizational Dynamics*, 18(3), pp. 19–31.
Bass, B.M. and Bass, R. (2008) *The Bass Handbook of Leadership: Theory, Research, and Managerial Applications*. New York: Free Press.
Best, A. and Holmes, B.J. (2010) 'Systems thinking, knowledge and action: Towards better models and methods', *Evidence & Policy: A Journal of Research, Debate and Practice*, 6(2), pp. 145–159. https://doi.org/10.1332/174426410X502284
Birken, S., Clary, A. and Tabriz, A.A. (2018) 'Middle managers' role in implementing evidence-based practices in healthcare: A systematic review', *Implementation Science*, 13, p. 149. https://doi.org/10.1186/s13012-018-0843-5
Blanchard, K. and Broadwell, R. (eds.) (2018) *Servant Leadership in Action: How You Can Achieve Great Relationships and Results*. Oakland, CA: Berrett-Koehler Publishers.
Borsay, A. and Dale, P. (2018) 'Cultures of harm in institutions of care: Introduction', *Social History of Medicine*, 31(4), pp. 679–687.
British Broadcasting Corporation (2011) *Undercover Care: The Abuse Exposed*. BBC One. 31 May. Available at https://www.bbc.co.uk/programmes/b011pwt6 (Accessed 31 March 2025).
Buljac-Samardzic, M., Doekhie, K.D., van Wijngaarden, J.D.H. (2020) 'Interventions to improve team effectiveness within health care: A systematic review of the past decade', *Human Resources for Health*, 18(1), p. 2. https://doi.org/10.1186/s12960-019-0411-3
Burns, J.M. (1978) *Leadership*. New York: Harper and Row.
Care Quality Commission (2022) *How staff, teams and services work together: good*. Available at https://www.cqc.org.uk/guidance-providers/adult-social-care/how-staff-teams-services-work-together-good (Accessed 28 February 2025).
Care Quality Commission (2024) *How staff, teams and services work together*. Available at https://www.cqc.org.uk/guidance-regulation/providers/assessment/single-assessment-framework/effective/staff-teams-work-together? (Accessed 15 February 2025).
Department of Health and Social Care (2012). *Transforming care: A national response to Winterbourne View Hospital*. Available at https://www.gov.uk/government/publications/winterbourne-view-hospital-department-of-health-review-and-response (Accessed 26 March 2025).
Department of Health and Social Care (2022) *Leadership for a collaborative and inclusive future*. Available at https://www.gov.uk/government/publications/health-and-social-care-review-leadership-for-a-collaborative-and-inclusive-future/leadership-for-a-collaborative-and-inclusive-future (Accessed 10 March 2025).
Dodkin (2021) *Working differently together: Progressing a one workforce approach Multidisciplinary Team Toolkit*. Available at https://www.hee.nhs.uk/sites/default/files/documents/HEE_MDT_Toolkit_V1.1.pdf? (Accessed 19 February 2025).
Dye, C.F. (2023) *Leadership in Healthcare: Essential Values and Skills*. 4th edn. Chicago, IL: Health Administration Press.
Edmondson, A.C. (1999) 'Psychological safety and learning behavior in work teams', *Administrative Science Quarterly*, 44(2), pp. 350–383. https://doi.org/10.2307/2666999
Goleman, D. (1995) *Emotional Intelligence: Why It Can Matter More than IQ*. New York: Bantam Books.
Goleman, D. (2017) 'Leadership that gets results', *Harvard Business Review*, 78(2), pp. 78–90.
Gov.uk (2023) *The NHS Constitution for England*. Available at https://www.gov.uk/government/publications/the-nhs-constitution-for-england (Accessed 28 February 2025).
Gov.uk (2025) *Handbook for The NHS Constitution for England*. Available at https://www.gov.uk/government/publications/supplements-to-the-nhs-constitution-for-england/the-handbook-to-the-nhs-constitution-for-england#principles-that-guide-the-nhs (Accessed 28 February 2025).
Health and Care Act 2022, Available at https://www.legislation.gov.uk/ukpga/2022/31/contents (Accessed 27 March 2025).
Health and Social Care Act 2008: Regulated Activities Regulations 2014. Available at https://www.legislation.gov.uk/ukdsi/2014/9780111117613/contents (Accessed 27 March 2025).
Hersey, P. and Blanchard, K.H. (1969) 'Life cycle theory of leadership', *Training and Development Journal*, 23(5), pp. 26–34.
Jelphs, K., Dickinson, H. and Miller, R. (2016) *Working in Teams*. 2nd edn. Bristol: Policy Press.
King's Fund (2025) *Improving NHS culture*. Available at https://www.kingsfund.org.uk/insight-and-analysis/projects/improving-nhs-culture (Accessed 31 March 2025).

Lewin, K. (1939) 'Field theory and experiment in social science: Selected theoretical papers', in Cartwright, D. (ed.) *Field Theory in Social Science*. New York: Harper and Row.

Mannion, R. and Davies, H. (2018) 'Understanding organisational culture for healthcare quality improvement', *BMJ*, 363, p. k4907. https://doi.org/10.1136/bmj.k4907

McKimm, J. and McLean, M. (2020) 'Rethinking health professions' education leadership: Developing 'eco-ethical' leaders for a more sustainable world and future', *Journal of Medical Education*, 54(5), pp. 516–523.

Myszkowska, A. and Łużniak-Piecha, M. (2022) 'Nurturing teamwork and team dynamics in a hybrid work model', *Central European Management Journal*, 30(4), pp. 506–530.

Nembhard, I.M. and Edmondson, A.C. (2006) 'Making it safe: The effects of leader inclusiveness and professional status on psychological safety and improvement efforts in health care teams', *Journal of Organizational Behaviour*, 27(7), pp. 941–966.

NHS Leadership Academy (2025) *Programmes to help you grow as a leader*. Available at https://www.leadershipacademy.nhs.uk/programmes/ (Accessed 26 February 2025).

O'Daniel, M. and Rosenstein, A.H. (2008) 'Professional communication and team collaboration', in Hughes, R. G. (ed.) *Patient Safety and Quality: An Evidence-Based Handbook for Nurses*. Rockville, MD: Agency for Healthcare Research and Quality, pp. 1–15.

Rajamani, S.K., and Iyer, R.S. (2023). Networks in healthcare: A systematic review. *BioMedInformatics*, 3(2), pp. 391–404. https://doi.org/10.3390/biomedinformatics3020026

Reeves, S., Pelone, F., Harrison, R., Goldman, J. and Zwarenstein, M. (2017) 'Interprofessional collaboration to improve professional practice and healthcare outcomes', *The Cochrane Database of Systematic Reviews*, 6(6), p. CD000072. https://doi.org/10.1002/14651858.CD000072.pub3

Schein, E.H. (2010) *Organizational Culture and Leadership*. 4th edn. Jossey-Bass, San Francisco, USA.

Stoller, J.K. (2021) 'Building teams in health care', *Chest*, 159(6), pp. 2392–2398. https://doi.org/10.1016/j.chest.2020.09.092

Swanwick, T. (2019) 'Leadership and management: what's the difference?', *BMJ Leader*, 3(4), pp. 99–100. https://doi.org/10.1136/leader-2019-000153

Tuckman, B.W. (1965) 'Developmental sequence in small groups', *Psychological Bulletin*, 63(6), pp. 384–399.

Wenger, E., McDermott, R. and Snyder, W.M. (2002) *Cultivating Communities of Practice: A Guide to Managing Knowledge*. Boston, MA: Harvard Business School Press.

West, M.A. (2012) *Effective Teamwork: Practical Lessons from Organisational Research*. 3rd edn. Oxford, UK: Blackwell/British Psychological Society.

West, M.A. and Lyubovnikova, J. (2012) 'Real teams or pseudo teams? The changing landscape needs a better map', *Industrial and Organisational Psychology*, 5(1), pp. 25–28. https://doi.org/10.1111/j.1754-9434.2011.01397.x

West, M.A. and Lyubovnikova, J. (2013) 'Illusions of team working in health care', *Journal of Health Organization and Management*, 27(2), pp. 134–142.

West, M.A., Lyubovnikova, J., Eckert, R. and Denis, J.L. (2014) 'Collective leadership for cultures of high quality health care', *Journal of Organizational Effectiveness: People and Performance*, 1(3), pp. 240–260.

Wu, X. and Zhu, Y. (2022) 'Ethical leadership and sustainable healthcare organizations: Balancing short-term needs and long-term responsibilities', *Journal of Healthcare Management*, 67(3), pp. 188–198.

Ystaas, L.M.K., Nikitara, M., Ghobrial, S., Latzourakis, E., Polychronis, G. and Constantinou, C.S. (2023) 'The impact of transformational leadership in the nursing work environment and patients' outcomes: A systematic review', *Nursing Reports*, 13(3), pp. 1271–1290. https://doi.org/10.3390/nursrep13030108

Yukl, G. (2013) *Leadership in Organizations*. 8th ed. Pearson Education, New Jersey, USA

21 10 essential requirements for doing a successful health and social care degree

Clive Sealey

The aim of this chapter is to:

- **Connect together the learning from the previous chapters**
- **Outline key requirements for successfully doing a health and social care degree**

The aim of this book is to help you in studying for your health and social care degree. It has attempted to do by clearly outlining key context, skills and knowledge that are essential to studying health and social care. Understanding these context, knowledge and skill is very important for anyone who has an interest in studying and working in health and social care.

The focus of this concluding chapter is to connect together the learning from the previous chapters to detail ten essential requirements to help you on your health and social care degree.

1 Studying health and social care requires understanding their 'cradle to grave' importance to our lives and the lives of others

As discussed in the Introduction, we have all had reason to use health and social care in the past, and are very likely to use it in the future. Reading this book, you have hopefully observed from the topics that health and social care has both a direct and indirect effect on us throughout our lives on a daily basis, from our cradle to our grave. Directly, this can be through receiving care at times when we need it, such as when we are sick, injured or due to our age. Indirectly, health and social care legislation and regulation protects us without us often realising it. We can say that health and social care is all around us, meaning that the study of health and social care is the study of the needs that we have through our lifetime. Individuals use and need health and social care primarily to improve the quality of their lives. This can refer to major improvements or minor improvements in their life. For example, consider that when people access GP services, go to A&E, use care homes and access mental health services, they do so because their quality of life is somewhat diminished to greater or lesser extents, and they require care to improve it. So we can say that when people access these and other health and social care services, they do so in the expectation that it improves the quality of their lives. This is different from studying many other degrees because of its focus on trying to solve real-life issues that can literally be a matter of life and death. This is a degree where changing your life and the lives of others occurs on a daily basis, and it is possible to literally see right in front of your eyes the difference that you are making. This importance of health and social care to our lives and the lives of others from cradle to grave cannot be underplayed or underestimated.

DOI: 10.4324/9781032619309-24

2 Studying health and social requires thinking and treating health °–°and social care as equally important

Health needs are often prioritised over social care needs, and more resources are often devoted to health care than social care. This can be understandable as sometimes health issues can immediately threaten the life of an individual, such as an injury or condition like a heart attack, while the immediacy of social care needs can be less apparent. However, the fact is that both health and social care needs can seriously impact on an individual's life. Just as having health needs like cancer can significantly impact a person's life, so having social care needs like loneliness, depression and isolation can also have a serious impact on a person's life. Linked to this is the fact that people can have both health and social care needs at the same time. For example, a person with a broken leg not only has health care needs to fix the leg, but also social care needs to ensure that they do not become lonely and isolated due not being able to physically walk. And individuals can also have conditions that are caused by both health and social care issues, such as myalgic encephalomyelitis/chronic fatigue syndrome. This shows that health and social care are not only intricately linked together, but also that they are equally as important as each other, and should not be seen as having anything other than having equal importance in relation to each other. Considering both the health and social care needs that an individual has is a key aspect of studying health and social care.

3 Studying health and social care requires acknowledging the existence of different perspectives

This book has shown that there is always an alternative way to provide health and social care, and health and social care does not simply happen, but occurs from the different perspectives that we have. This book has provided various definitions of different aspects of health and social care. The book starts with definitions of health and social care, and continues with definitions of legislation, regulation, safeguarding, children's rights, disability and ageing, amongst others. However, what should have become evident from these definitions is that there is always more than one way to define something. For example, consider the different definitions of medical, social and biomedical models of health in Chapter 9 and the different effects these definitions had on care. Or consider the different definitions of safeguarding outlined in Chapter 11, where we saw that we can define safeguarding narrowly focussed specifically on harm, or widely focussed on preventative, proactive and progressive actions. What this shows is that definitions guide how we understand an issue and ultimately what we do in practice. These different definitions reflect different perspectives, and understanding these different perspectives is crucial for health and social care practice. By considering the various definitions of health, practitioners can better support individuals in achieving their full potential and living fulfilling lives. Analysis of the importance of how we define things is essential to studying health and social care.

4 Studying health and social care requires distinguishing between fact and theory

When we talk about facts, we talk about things that are true all the time in all circumstances. Facts are important to use because they give us certainty and clarity in terms of knowing what is going to happen. When we talk about theory, we talk about things that we cannot say for certain is true all the time. Theories are important to us because they provide us with an explanation for things that we really do not understand. Health and social care is a mixture of fact and theory, and separating what is fact from what is theory is an important part of your degree. For instance, consider where a young person is needing care due to mental health issues. We can use what we know for certain about the young person's brain development to understand what is happening to the young person. These facts can help us to consider what is likely to be the most effective treatment for the young person. However, there is no certainty that this treatment will be effective, as we are using theory to consider this. In this way, if the treatment is not successful, we can consider other treatments that could be successful. So we can say that facts give us context, while theory gives us options, and we should be ready to change our mind in the light of events that does not support what we believe. If we understand that while theory and facts are closely linked but they are not the same, this opens our mind up to thinking and acting in ways that are most beneficial to the individual. Understanding the difference between fact and theory is an essential requirement of studying health and social care.

5 Studying health and social care requires learning that is wide and comprehensive

The study of health and social care covers a comprehensive range of topics, ranging from physical health, mental health, legislation, regulation, rights, anatomy and physiology, safeguarding, anti-discrimination and anti-oppressive practice, demographic changes, theories and perspectives. This range is wider than most courses, and it is very likely the case that no two health and social care degree courses are the same. For some, this may seem daunting and overwhelming, but it means that it is a degree that provides you with a comprehensive range of knowledge that is hard to match. Some of this knowledge is specific to health and social care, but a good majority of it is things that are relevant to your everyday life and you can use outside of the degree. For example, learning about anatomy and physiology is important to your degree, but is also something that you can use in everyday life. Similarly, learning about safeguarding is important to your degree, but is also something that is relevant to your everyday life and which you can apply in other situations. This shows that the uniquely comprehensive knowledge that you acquire from your health and social care degree is relevant to your everyday life.

6 Studying health and social care requires the willingness to challenge established ways of thinking and doing

As detailed above, studying health and social care means that you come across many different theories and perspectives. Additionally, there is no single way to provide health and social care; it can be provided in many different ways. This is because of the wide-ranging nature of health and social care, which means that there is no single health and social care professional or provider, but many professionals and providers of social care. For example, health and social care is provided by nurses, doctors, care workers and support workers in hospitals, GP surgeries, care homes and in the community. The majority of the theories, perspectives and care that you come across is relatively easy to understand and is likely to make sense to you. However, there are times when these do not make sense to you, or you do not agree with them. You should not see this as a problem, as it would be very weird if you agree with everything that you come across in the degree. This is fine as you are not expected to agree with everything that you see. Studying health and social care is not a training course, it is a degree, and a key requirement of degrees is to challenge your learning. Without such challenging, it is hard for things to improve. At the same time, you need to be prepared for your ways of thinking to also be challenged by others, and not see this as a threat to you. So be prepared to challenge your learning and your practice, and for your learning and practice to be challenged, as this is expected of you.

7 Studying health and social care requires applying critical thinking and critical reflection

Critical thinking and critical reflection refer to the way that we process information that we receive. It helps us to decide if something is relevant, suitable and reliable. In health and social care, we receive information from lots of different sources to help us to make decisions, and it is easy to become overwhelmed by this information and decide to make the quickest or easiest decision. For example, when an individual has a health or social care need, there are different ways that we could meet their need. However, it is important to be critical when we make such decisions. Critical in this context does not mean arguing, it means questioning and analysing before we make our judgement. So rather than making quick decisions, critical thinking is about taking time to think about what the best course of action is. Critical reflection is where having made our decision, we go away and think about the decision that we have made, in terms of whether it is the best decision we could have made. Applying critical thinking and critical reflection are not things that just immediately happen but need practice and time to think and consider our actions. The benefits of critical thinking and reflection are evident when they lead to the best outcomes for the individual.

8 Studying health and social care requires developing creative and inventive thinking

Solving problems is at the core of health and social care. It is about meeting needs that individuals have. However, one thing that soon becomes evident is that while individuals are similar, their needs are unlikely to be the same. While the needs that they present with may be similar, the causes may be different. For example, two children who are not developing well may have needs that are related to their family circumstance, their school circumstance or their social circle. It is unlikely that trying to meet these needs in the same way would be relevant here. Instead, this requires thinking of ways to meet these different needs that are creative and inventive. Creative thinking requires taking time to identify and consider a range of possible solutions to problems before coming to a decision. It means considering your ideas from different perspectives to see the possible consequences of each. It can mean making connections between old ideas to come up with new ideas. Thinking creatively not only improves the chances that your solution best meets the needs that an individual has, but also helps us challenge the assumptions that we have and find out new things that we did not even know about.

9 Studying health and social care requires making time to think to give yourself the best chance of succeeding

As detailed above, studying health and social care requires wide and comprehensive learning, a willingness to challenge established ways of thinking, critical thinking and reflection and creative thinking. These are all things that have to be worked at, developed, experienced, felt and sometimes suffered. They do not appear immediately but require time. Thinking time is a very important part of doing a degree. It is something that has to be built into your study. The absence of such thinking time brings pressure on you and clouds your judgement, and the degree becomes harder and less enjoyable. You are also more likely to make errors when time is limited. Thinking time allows you to consider a range of options and choose the best from these options, it allows you to construct logical and coherent arguments, and it allows for trial and error in your decisions. Making thinking time is an essential element of studying health and social care, and also for wider life itself.

10 Studying health and social care exemplifies optimism for the future

This book has been written during a period of crisis in health and social care, as characterised by cuts to the funding and the scope of health and social care. At the time of writing, there is an ongoing cost of living crisis that is continuing to affect health and social care. It is easy to be pessimistic in such a context. However, the positive effect that health and social care can make and the way health and social care has transformed our society from what it was in the past is often overlooked. We can say that health and social care has positively transformed our society from what it was in the past, and it is very likely that it continues to do so in the future, and this is not something that many fields of practice can say. Over the last 50 years or so, people have been living much longer than they did, are surviving diseases and conditions that would have killed them such as cancer, and many more people are participating in society in ways that they would not have been able, which have all occurred due to significant developments in health and social care. There are key social, demographic and technological changes occurring as we speak which are likely to continue to transform society in the future. For instance, these changes can lead to 'healthy ageing' rather than ageism. For health and social care, the key issue that these changes pose is the question of 'who cares?'. This is because the changes have not only disrupted traditional patterns of care, but introduced new care requirements. There is the potential for technology to answer this question to some extent through making care easier, quicker and cheaper, and therefore continue to enable health and social care to continue to positively transform the society that we live in. This provides optimism for the future.

Index

Note: Bold page numbers refer to boxes.

For Product Safety Concerns and Information please contact our EU
representative GPSR@taylorandfrancis.com
Taylor & Francis Verlag GmbH, Kaufingerstraße 24, 80331 München, Germany

www.ingramcontent.com/pod-product-compliance
Ingram Content Group UK Ltd.
Pitfield, Milton Keynes, MK11 3LW, UK
UKHW050230200926
475702UK00020B/2949

* 9 7 8 1 0 3 2 6 0 8 5 2 5 *